From Neuropsychology to Mental Structure

From Neuropsychology to Mental Structure

TIM SHALLICE
Medical Research Council Applied Psychology Unit
Cambridge
and
National Hospital
London

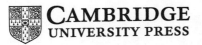

CAMBRIDGE
UNIVERSITY PRESS

Published by the Press Syndicate of the University of Cambridge
The Pitt Building, Trumpington Street, Cambridge CB2 1RP
40 West 20th Street, New York, NY 10011-4211, USA
10 Stamford Road, Oakleigh, Melbourne 3166, Australia

First published 1988
Reprinted 1990, 1991, 1993

Printed in the United States of America

Library of Congress Cataloging-in-Publication Data is available.

A catalogue record for this book is available from the British Library.

ISBN 0-521-30874-7 hardback
ISBN 0-521-31360-0 paperback

To my mother

Contents

vii

Preface

Interest in neuropsychology has increased greatly over the past 20 years. This has mainly occurred for direct clinical reasons, such as the increase in the ability of neuropsychological investigations to assess the crippling problems in thought, memory, and language that can occur from brain damage. There is, though, a second reason for the increase of interest in the subject. The human brain is still the organ we understand least well, and the process by which its highest function – cognition – operates remains mysterious. The dramatic effects of brain damage appear to provide valuable evidence about how the systems underlying cognition operate. The aim of this book is to assess this evidence. Is neuropsychological evidence of any real value in understanding normal cognition? If so, what form or forms should this evidence take, and what substantive conclusions can be drawn?

The relevance of neuropsychological findings remains controversial because neuropsychology – in a somewhat parallel fashion to psychology – has rejected much of its former doctrines in virtually every generation. The approach that is the subject matter of this book, cognitive neuropsychology, is hardly a generation old. In many respects, cognitive neuropsychology seems very healthy. Interest in it is increasing rapidly, and surprising findings are frequently being made. Yet its practitioners use conflicting methodologies, each of which balances on a set of barely examined assumptions.

In the 1970s, I wrote two articles (Shallice, 1979a, 1979b) that assessed, in a positive fashion, a methodological approach then unfashionable within neuropsychology – the single-case study. Since then, this approach has become very popular and is now being claimed as the only way to carry out neuropsychological research relevant to normal function. Some years ago, I decided that the position I had earlier adopted was in certain respects glib and that a more thorough assessment would be appropriate. That assessment has grown into this book.

The book is addressed both to neuropsychologists and to those in neighbouring fields who may wish to draw on neuropsychological research findings. It is structured in terms of an overall argument on the relevance of neuropsychological findings and the types of methods used. I argue for an approach between the more traditional neuropsychological procedures, with their emphasis on group studies and the anatomical localisation of deficits, and the more fashionable 'ultra-cognitive' methods, which ignore anatomical and other neuroscience considerations and are concerned only with the results of single-case studies. I have attempted to ground the argument in discussions of those topics where cognitive neuropsychology has been most successful. The somewhat idiosyncratic ordering of the topics arises from their place in the overall argument. No attempt has been made to provide complete coverage of the literature; the set of potentially relevant neuropsychological findings and theories of normal function to which they might relate is far too large. This has meant that certain important areas (e.g. agrammatism) are dealt with in less detail than they objectively deserve.

The selection of topics and their ordering in the overall argument has been strongly influenced by where I have worked. Although cognitive neuropsychology is now an approach that is used world-wide, many of its roots lie in research in Britain in the late 1960s and 1970s, and a number of the topics addressed are those that became current in that period. More specifically, in the late 1960s, as a cognitive psychologist at University College, London, I began to collaborate with Elizabeth Warrington at the National Hospital. In her department I had the very good fortune of working where the range of patients seen for clinical purposes and, more particularly, the variety of research problems encountered – both clinical and basic research – were to become as great as those in any neuropsychological centre in the world. Most of my empirical work has continued to be carried out there, and I remain convinced that the best environment for neuropsychological investigations is a clinical department where work on clinical and basic research problems can be mutually supportive. Mutually beneficial contacts between basic research workers and clinicians also reduce the ethical problems of studying a devastating illness for reasons other than the direct benefit of the patient. The particular approach I advocate here is strongly influenced by the methods used in the National Hospital.

The other strong influence on selection of topics has been the other part of my work environment – the Medical Research Council Applied Psychology Unit, Cambridge, where I have been based for the past 10 years. The type of cognitive psychology theorising with which cognitive neuropsychology methodology dovetails effectively is very well represented by the work of Alan Baddeley, John Morton, Tony Marcel, Karalyn Patterson, and my other colleagues. The extensive discussions that take place at the APU have kept focused the other half of the project – the understanding of normal function to which neuropsychological research relates.

A book of this length cannot be written without much help and support. During a period when the excellent research environment that British scientific institutions used to provide has become a part of our history rather than our current reality, I have been most fortunate to work for the Medical Research Council and their Applied Psychology Unit. Without the support of the MRC and the encouragement of Alan Baddeley, the director of the APU, this book could not have been written.

I am grateful to many people for their assistance. During the whole period of the development of the idea of the work, I was much helped by Deborah Hodgkin. Much of the first draft was written while I was on leave of absence as a visitor to Jacques Mehler's CNRS unit in Paris and as a visiting professor of the University of Padua. I very much appreciated the facilities provided and the warmth of the welcome at both institutions. Elizabeth Warrington kindly read most of the first draft; she helped me to eliminate many errors and rococo meanders. Marie-France Beauvois, Jacqueline Derouesné, David Howard, John Morton, Don Norman, Karalyn Patterson, Eleanor Saffran, and Alan Wing all read chapters; I much appreciated their cogent comments. The book was produced with an antiquated technology – the biro; my secretary, Sharon Gamble, somehow managed to translate the obscure scrawls produced into a coherent text with remarkable speed and accuracy. I thank her very much and would also like to thank Carmen Frankl and Alan Copeman, who prepared many of the figures.

The work would never have been completed without the support of Maria, my wife, whose encouragement of the hours I spent on it never failed to astonish me. Finally, I would like to thank Susan Milmoe and the staff at Cambridge University Press, who produced the manuscript with much skill and speed.

Part I

Introducing Cognitive Neuropsychology

1   From the Diagram-Makers to Cognitive Neuropsychology

1.1   Why Neuropsychology?

For 100 years, it has been well known that the study of the cognitive problems of patients suffering from neurological diseases can produce strikingly counterintuitive observations. From time to time, research workers studying normal function have been strongly influenced by such observations or by the ideas of the neurologists who made them. Bartlett (1932) and Hebb (1949) are two examples. However, in general, neuropsychology has had little impact on the study of normal function.[1]

With any knowledge of the history of clinical neuropsychology, it is easy to understand why this neglect occurred. The standard of description of the psychological impairments of patients was low, often being little more than the bald statement of the clinical opinion of the investigator. There was frequently a dramatic contrast between the vagueness of the psychological account of the disorder and the precision with which anatomical investigation of the lesion that had given rise to it was carried out at post-mortem. Also, the field, like psychology itself, could agree on little but the most obvious and basic theories. Typical are the disputes about the existence of the syndrome visual object agnosia, a specific difficulty in the perception of objects when both sensation and the intellect are intact. The syndrome was widely accepted as real in the golden age of the flowering of neuropsychology (1860–1905) (e.g. Lissauer, 1890). Yet its existence was still being denied nearly a century later (e.g. Bay, 1953; Bender & Feldman, 1972).

It is now clear that there are patients whose impairment is appropriately characterised as a visual object agnosia (for reviews, see Rubens, 1979; Ratcliff & Newcombe, 1982; Warrington, 1985; chapter 8). However, other syndromes described in earlier periods have fared less well. In chapters 2 and 4, it will be argued that two syndromes first described in the 1920s and much debated since – the Gerstmann syndrome and stimultanagnosia – are not functional entities. More critically, if clinical neurologists with an extensive knowledge of brain-damaged patients frequently considered major 'syndromes' described by earlier workers to be artefacts,

---

1. The term *neuropsychology* will be used to refer to the investigation of the disorders of perception, memory, language, thought, emotion, and action in neurological patients. The word *cognitive,* too, should be interpreted widely to include the higher levels of perception, memory, and the more central aspects of the control of action.

3

was it not entirely reasonable for research workers concerned primarily with normal function to ignore the field?

Within the past 15 years, the situation in neuropsychology and its neighbour, neurolinguistics, has changed dramatically. Quantitative descriptions of disorders are now standard. A spate of interesting findings has resulted in theories that seem to be compatible with those developed for the study of normal cognition. In turn, a considerable number of research workers interested primarily in normal function have responded. However, this response has been patchy; within cognitive psychology, some standard textbooks hardly mention neuropsychological findings.[2]

The reason for this neglect is perhaps that explicitly argued by Henderson (1981) and Crowder (1982a) – that neuropsychological investigations merely follow ones in the normal subject; they do not provide leads. A related possibility is that it arises from the type of empirical assessment produced by Fodor, Bever, and Garrett (1974), which reads a little oddly in the light of the later writings of at least one of the authors – Fodor (1983) – 'remarkably little has been learned about the psychology of language processes in normals from over a hundred years of aphasia study' (p. xiv). More probably, it is a result of the argument given by Postman (1975) in a major review article on memory. He dismissed neuropsychological findings, stating merely, 'The existing data do not impress us as unequivocal, more important extrapolations from pathological deficits to the structure of normal memory are of uncertain validity' (p. 308). This type of argument was put forward in an elegant fashion much earlier by Gregory (1961):

Suppose we ablated or stimulated various parts of a complex man-made device, say a television receiving set. And suppose we had no prior knowledge of the manner of function of the type of device or machine involved. Could we by these means discover its manner of working? . . . If a component is removed almost anything may happen: a radio set may emit piercing whistles or deep growls, a television set may produce curious patterns, a car engine may back-fire, or blow up or simply stop. . . . In a serial system the various identifiable elements of the output are not separately represented by discrete parts of the system. . . . The removal, or the activation, of a single stage in a series might have almost any effect on the output of a machine, and so presumably also for the brain. . . . The effects of removing or modifying, say, the line scan time-base of a television receiver would be incomprehensible if we did not know the engineering principles involved. Further, it seems unlikely that we should discover the necessary principles from scratch simply by pulling bits out of television sets, or stimulating bits with various voltages and wave forms. (p. 320–322)[3]

The theoretical problems in drawing inferences from neuropsychological findings will be assessed in detail in chapters 9, 10, and 11. Assume for the present, however, that they can be surmounted, at least in most cases. Neuropsychological

---

2. Anderson (1980) is an example.
3. Gregory (1961) was not arguing against the use of neuropsychological findings, but for their interpretation in terms of a model of the whole system. Marin, Saffran, and Schwartz (1976), in the early days of cognitive neuropsychology, record meeting essentially this argument in a cruder form: 'What can you possibly learn about the way a car works (or a vacuum cleaner, or a computer) by pounding it with a sledgehammer' (p. 868)! To which the authors pointed out that random decomposition results in theoretically useful results – for instance, in high-energy physics!

evidence has two very beguiling qualities that are best seen by contrast with 'normal' experimental evidence. Empirical phenomena in the corresponding study of normal processes – human experimental psychology – are very slippery things. Many factors affect any experimental procedure. Make a slight change in one aspect – rate of presentation, stimulus material, recall delay, amount of practice, and so on – and the effect disappears or reappears, although according to theory, it should not. Thus even if a phenomenon is narrowly robust, the experimental result provides only a most insecure platform for theoretical inferences. The consequence is that it is easy to take an inessential aspect of the experimental situation as the critical one and enter a theoretical blind alley. So progress remains slow, and the field remains as full as ever of its theoretical Jeremiahs.[4]

Given the task of understanding the organisation of the cognitive system, the first attraction of neuropsychological evidence is that the effects that occur can be both large and counterintuitive. The myriad factors that affect a subject's performance – degree of learning, amount of effort expended, individual differences, characteristics of the stimulus material, and so on – shrink in significance when compared with the magnitude and specificity of the observed deficits. One appears to be receiving a privileged view into the structure of the information-processing system.

The weakness of the empirical methods available in 'normal' human experimental psychology has a second consequence; we have little conception of the extent of the problems that need to be tackled. Empirical investigations in other sciences are often stimulated by the availability of novel techniques. In psychology, they are often triggered by the investigation of novel procedures, a phenomenon that Tulving and Madigan (1970) called the functional autonomy of methods.[5] Such procedures become fashionable when widely thought to provide answers to important theoretical questions. Ten years and a flood of papers later, the apparently simple original experimental finding is found to be very complex indeed, and its theoretical value is much less clear. So a pessimist could view the history of 'normal' human experimental psychology as a succession of mirages. The end result consists of islands

---

4. Consider Neisser (1981) referring to memory, but almost certainly he would intend his message to apply more generally: 'The results of a hundred years of the psychological study of memory are somewhat discouraging. We have established firm empirical generalizations, but most of them are so obvious that every ten-year-old knows them anyway. We have made discoveries, but they are only marginally about memory; in many cases we don't know what to do with them, and wear them out with endless experimental variations. We have an intellectually impressive group of theories, but history offers little confidence that they will provide any meaningful insight into natural behavior' (pp. 11–12). His response was to call for the study of memory outside the psychological laboratory, not limited to the artificial products of the investigator's narrow set of concepts. Neuropsychology certainly qualifies! It is ironic that in his summary dismissal of what investigators have learned about memory, Neisser should have failed to mention amnesia and its many dramatic and far from artificial aspects, which challenge clinicians whatever their theoretical predilections.
5. Examples include the Peterson procedure, the recency effect in free recall, the Sternberg procedure, the stimulus suffix effect, the word superiority effect, the use of pattern masking, and Wason's four-card problem.

of detailed empirical knowledge surrounded by a sea of ignorance, whose size we conceal from ourselves by vague theorising; in any case, its magnitude could hardly be known because we have few independent means of assessing it (see Newell, 1973).

Neuropsychology can help in this second respect, too. Advanced clinical practice contains the distilled 'craft' knowledge of over 100 years of observation of patients by neurologists and neuropsychologists; this understanding is well represented in books such as those by Hécaen and Albert (1978), Lesser (1978), Walsh (1978), De Renzi (1982), Heilman and Valenstein (1985), and Stuss and Benson (1986). This knowledge is rooted in the problems that neurological patients themselves experience. Experimental psychologists may not have investigated drawing or writing, say, because effective techniques for quantification have been difficult to develop for use with normal subjects. However, if a patient loses the skill as a result of disease, it is soon apparent to physicians. So relevant disorders, such as constructional apraxia or agraphia, are well known, and detailed clinical accounts of subvarieties exist (see Warrington, 1969; Marcie & Hécaen, 1979). As neurological disease affects every part of the brain – if with different incidence rates – the disorders that have been described will probably encompass damage to nearly all the cognitive mechanisms. 'Inverting' the set of disorders that exist might enable us to map the subcomponents of mind. Whether an inversion procedure is conceptually possible and at present practicable is a subject that will be directly addressed later. For two reasons, then, cognitive neuropsychology would be of value for the understanding of normal function if it were demonstrated to be effective.

1.2 Paradigm Shifts in Neuropsychology: The Diagram-Makers and their Critics

In the past, it was to some extent justified for those interested in normal cognition to neglect neuropsychological findings. To understand why the situation has changed, one needs to consider the history of neuropsychology. This has other benefits, too. Without a knowledge of the history of neuropsychology, its terminology is almost impossible to understand. Names like transcortical sensory aphasia, central aphasia, constructional apraxia, Gerstmann syndrome, and lexical agraphia all reflect different conceptual approaches.

There is, though, a more critical reason why the assessment of modern neuropsychology requires some understanding of its history. The evolution of thought about impaired cognitive functioning has a remarkably dialectical quality. Just like experimental psychology, but independently of it, neuropsychology became an embryonic science in the second half of the nineteenth century. Very schematically, its history may be divided into four stages, each dominated by particular schools: the rise of the so-called diagram-makers, with their elaborate models of the mental machinery (1860–1905); the reaction against them (1905–1940); the switch to group studies (1945–1970); and the development of cognitive neuropsychology (since the late 1960s). In present-day cognitive neuropsychology, the long-rejected central core of the diagram-makers' approach has been resurrected. Therefore, if cognitive neuropsychology is to be successful, it must obviously guard adequately against the fatal flaws that were present in the approach of 100 years ago! Yet there are signs that this elementary precaution is being neglected.[6]

Broca's claim in 1861 that the seat of language is in the inferior posterior portion of the left frontal lobe is often cited as the event that initiated neuropsychology as a science. In fact, related claims having less anatomical precision had been made a number of times in the preceding 40 years. According to the historian of science Young (1970), the date 1861 is remembered because Broca's demonstration of the localisation of a cognitive function occurred at a time when the scientific community was prepared to treat the idea seriously, events in other sciences having made it an acceptable possibility. Broca's claims certainly provoked a flowering of research. The next 40 years saw a mass of clinical observations and theoretical analyses.

There were two main aspects to the initial claim. The first was that language is a function that can be damaged separately from other cognitive processes. The second was that the function is localisable. The dissociation of language processes from cognitive ones was soon refined much further. In 1869, Bastian differentiated disorders of reading and writing from disorders of speech and to account for the differences used hypothetical anatomical diagrams with processing centres and transmission pathways. In 1874, Wernicke isolated a further form of language disorder, now known as Wernicke's aphasia, and produced a model of a sensory and a motor language centre joined by a transmission pathway. Damage to the motor language centre, he argued, would lead to the form of aphasia that Broca had described; that to the sensory language centre would produce the syndrome that he had discovered. He predicted the existence of a third form of aphasia, conduction aphasia, which should result from damage to the pathway. Ten years later, Lichtheim (1885), having deduced that conduction aphasics should have a specific deficit in repetition, described the first case in which such a difficulty was a central aspect. He then went much further and described four more aphasia syndromes! Two more syndrome labels date from his account: 'transcortical motor aphasia' and 'transcortical sensory aphasia'.

The diagram-makers not only isolated a number of distinct syndromes, but also produced a theoretical framework to explain them. The disorders were predicted from 'interruptions' to different functional components of what were basically processing diagrams. Lichtheim's (1885) theory is especially worth examining. On its appearance, it 'excited universal interest', according to a historian of the period, Moutier (1908). For instance, the influential German neurologist von Monakow,

---

6. The idea that modern cognitive neuropsychology should learn from the fate of the diagram-makers is derived from Morton (1984). My view of what should be learned is, however, somewhat different from his.

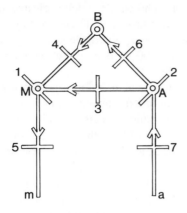

Figure 1.1. The simple version of Lichtheim's (1885) theory. *A* stands for the centre for 'auditory word-representations'; *M,* for the centre for 'motor word-representations'; *B* is where 'concepts are elaborated'; *a* and *m* are auditory input and speech motor output, respectively. The numbers 1 to 7, which correspond to 'interruption points', are discussed in the text.

who later broke with the diagram-makers, said that he was 'overwhelmed by the achievement' (quoted in Moutier). Even Head (1926), an arch-enemy of the school, admitted that it had had a profound influence on the clinical theories of the day, although more characteristically, he said that Lichtheim's paper 'reads like a parody of the tendencies of the time' (p. 65). In my view, the paper must be ranked today as one of the finest in the nineteenth century relevant to psychology.

I will consider only the simpler version of the theory in which reading and writing are ignored (Figure 1.1). Lichtheim actually put forward his suggested diagram of the subcomponents of the language system on mainly a priori grounds. His separation of a centre for 'auditory word-representations' from a centre for 'motor word-representations' appears to have been based on Wernicke's (1874) empirical findings. He then argued that children learn to speak by imitation so that a route from one of these centres to the other would be expected to exist. Concepts were then simply assumed to be separately located. From these a priori arguments, he inferred that each of seven 'interruption points', marked in Figure 1.1, should give rise to a different syndrome. Thus for Broca's aphasia, it is at position 1; Wernicke's aphasia, 2; conduction aphasia, 3; transcortical motor aphasia, 4; and transcortical sensory aphasia, 6. Examples were given or a reference cited for each of the claimed varieties of aphasia.

According to Moutier (1908), ten models of this type were produced between 1870 and the beginning of the twentieth century. To the information-processing psychologist of today, some of the diagrams look far more modern than the theories that were appearing in the psychology texts of the time. Consider, for instance, replacing the terms that Lichtheim used most frequently, 'centre for auditory images' and 'centre for motor images', by, say, 'auditory input logogen' and 'articulatory (or phonological) output logogen'.[7] The separation between the two systems is then analogous to that made by Morton (1979a) in later versions of the logogen model. Indeed, Morton (1984) has shown that in the language field, rival models of the period tend to have their modern equivalents. For instance, the models of Kussmaul (1877) and Bastian (1898) contrast with those of Wernicke (1874) and Lichtheim (1885) in having a single centre at the non-semantic level for perceiving and producing speech; an equivalent assumption is the essence of Allport and Funnell's (1981) model, produced 100 years later!

This sort of theoretical development, although most developed for language, was not restricted to it. For instance, with respect to the perception of objects, Lissauer (1890) differentiated between two types of agnosic disorder, in both of which intellect and visual sensation are intact. In apperceptive agnosia, the patient is unable to differentiate between two visually similar items, such as a walking stick and a rolled-up umbrella. In associative agnosia, the patient does not lack the ability to differentiate between visually similar objects, but loses their significance or meaning. Similar developments took place with respect to disorders of reading (Dejerine, 1892) and the organisation of skilled movement (Liepmann, 1900). However, it was over the models of aphasia that the controversy was most fierce and where the most critical defeats occurred.

Despite the modern appearance of the diagram-makers' models to our eyes, their ideas soon come under strong attack, two early critics being Freud (1891) and Bergson (1896). In the first 30 years of the twentieth century, the critics became dominant. The arguments of Marie (1906a) in France, of von Monakow (1910) and Gelb and Goldstein (1920) in Germany, and of Head (1926) in Britain led to general rejection of the approach as pre-scientific. Typical of the contemptuous attitude to their forebears in the field of aphasiology was Head's (1926): 'Incredulous of such scholastic interpretations they [i.e., neurologists in general] lost interest in a problem of so little practical importance. . . . The time was ripe for a ruthless destruction of false gods' (pp. 65–66). It is a historical irony that Wernicke and Lichtheim are now much better remembered than Head.

Hardly surprisingly, given the tone of such criticism, the matter was not just one of intellectual argument. In France, for instance, Dejerine – the principal representative of the diagram-makers' approach – and Marie – the principal critic – never spoke after Marie's challenge, except to enter into gladiatorial public debate. After Marie's victory, the followers of Dejerine were not appointed to the bureaucratically powerful positions within French neurology, even those who were widely

---

7. One of the most influential information-processing models of language has been Morton's (1969, 1979a) logogen model. The most critical assumption of the model is that a number of interface systems – logogen systems – lie between lower level perceptual (or motor) processes and those systems responsible for semantic and syntactic operations. In the earlier versions of the theory, there was only one such interface system; in the later versions, there are four: phonological input, phonological output, visual input, and visual output for listening, speaking, reading, and writing. Any given logogen system is composed of a set of morphemic units, each of which accumulates information about whether a particular word is present.

acknowledged as being extremely able. At one stage, the bitterness between the two schools even resulted in a formal challenge to a duel, although over an issue related to another area of neurology (see Lhermitte & Signoret, 1982).

The rejection of the diagram-makers was by no means total. Neurology was too decentralised and international a subject for a basically progressive school of thought to be bureaucratically eliminated. Neurologists like Henschen (1920), Kleist (1934), and Nielsen (1946) continued the diagram-makers' tradition, but until the extensive work of revival by Geschwind (1965), such thinkers were very much in the minority.

The diagram-makers' approach was vulnerable to attack on three main fronts. First, they argued that the functions they postulated could be precisely localised. The evidence on which this was based was very shaky. Thus Marie (1906a), in a famous paper, reanalysed the classic cases of Broca (1861) and argued that in both the critical patients, the lesions had extended far beyond the region that Broca had claimed, so-called Broca's area, in the inferior posterior part of the left frontal lobe. In complementary fashion, patients described as functionally of a Broca type had lesions outside Broca's area (see Moutier, 1908). For the more subtle syndromes described by Lichtheim (1885), the anatomical correspondences claimed for his centres and connections were almost entirely speculative.[8] The strict reductionist framework in which both the diagram-makers and their critics operated meant that once the anatomical part of their theorising was shaken, the credibility of the psychological side of their position was greatly weakened.

They were also being attacked on quite a different front. It was argued that the psychological concepts they had used were inadequate. For instance, the explanation given by the diagram-makers for Broca's aphasia is that it results from a 'loss of motor images'. In fact, one of the most salient features of the prototypic motor aphasic of the type described by Broca is the inability to construct whole sentences even when individual content words can be uttered. This aspect of Broca's aphasia is now known as 'agrammatism' and is frequently explained as an impairment in syntactic operations. Hughlings Jackson pointed out as early as the 1870s that such difficulties were not at all adequately captured by the concept of 'loss of motor images'. At a more general level, the overall theoretical approach of the diagram-makers must have seemed completely outdated by about 1920, when conceptual frameworks like behaviourism, Gestalt psychology, and mass action were in the ascendance. To adherents of these schools, the approach of the diagram-makers must have seemed medieval.

In accounts of the diagram-makers, it is to these two factors that their defeat is normally attributed (e.g. Luria, 1973). The insubstantial nature of the neuropsychological evidence they produced is probably an equally important factor. If their

8. For modern evidence that is, oddly, compatible with both sides of the argument, see, for example, Kertesz, Lesk, and McCabe (1977), Mohr et al. (1978), and Poeck, De Bleser, and Von Kayserlingk (1984a). Some of the brains that Broca analysed have recently been reanalysed yet again by Signoret, Castaigne, Lhermitte, Abelanet, and Lavorel (1984) using CT-scan procedures. Ironically, their conclusion was that Broca, not Marie, was right!

empirical accounts of cognitive deficits had been strong, they may well have been able to withstand the theoretical attacks on their position. In fact, their empirical accounts were normally weak. Take the doyen of the approach, Lichtheim. As pointed out earlier, his theoretical system was based on a priori notions of how children learn to speak. He then deduced that certain types of patient should exist, and either described a patient of his own or referred to one in the literature. The process was theory driven, not data driven. Sometimes, as in his empirical account of transcortical sensory aphasia, he produced a fairly impressive case, if one accepts his terse clinical summary on faith. On other occasions, the evidence is flimsy. Thus much of the evidence for his case of transcortical motor aphasia is based on the testimony of the patient's wife. The essential part of his own observations is, 'His vocabulary is copious, but he does not talk much, and speaks in a drawling manner. From time to time he misses a word or construction. . . . He repeats correctly whole sentences, if not too long' (Lichtheim, 1885, pp. 448–449). Anyone who doubted that repetition could be preserved in the absence of spontaneous speech, as required by an interruption at point 4 (see Figure 1.1.), would have little difficulty in disposing of Lichtheim's evidence. Therefore, to give much credence to many of these case descriptions, one has to have personal experience of a virtually identical patient. Yet this is not generally possible. The types of patients whom Lichtheim described are not common. Thus Freud (1891), one of the first major critics, would not accept conduction aphasia as a syndrome. He had never seen such a patient (see Green & Howes, 1977).[9]

By the early twentieth century, even the few neurologists generally favourable to the diagram-makers, such as Henschen (1920) – who made the most thorough survey of their work ever attempted – were forced to admit that the clinical data were frequently insufficient. Opponents, such as Head (1926), were dismissive. He held that even in his own time, 'the methods in general use were too crude to provide satisfactory records' (p. 140). What was required, he said, was 'systematic empirical observation of the crude manifestations of disease' (p. 66). When he undertook this, his overall conclusion was that the more carefully the patient is examined, the less certainly his disorder corresponds to any preconceived category. Indeed, if one tries to press every patient seen in the clinic into one of the diagram-makers' categories, this comment is justified.

Head's criticisms exposed another problem in Lichtheim's approach. One of Lichtheim's most important contributions was to make a methodological distinction between a 'pure case', in which, according to his own model, there was only a single deficit, and a 'mixed case', in which there were multiple deficits. 'Mixed' cases, he argued, were not of theoretical interest. Yet the effects of most lesions will correspond to more than one deficit on his model. Thus it follows that the types of patient whom clinicians see most of the time should be those who have a com-

9. Not all empirical descriptions of this period are so inadequate. Lissauer's (1890) description of associative agnosia is far more detailed. However, in the critical language field, detailed clinical descriptions were not generally available until after 1910 (see De Bleser, 1987).

bination of difficulties. This is in fact the case. So even though the rarity of 'pure cases' is quite compatible with Lichtheim's approach, it was natural that a rival theory developed; it postulated a central core aphasia with differing degrees of additional comprehension or expressive problems (e.g., in essence, Marie, 1960b; Head, 1926; Schuell & Jenkins, 1959).

To counter such an approach, one needs to be able to select 'pure cases' that are empirically convincing in their own right and to explain why they are more relevant than the mass of other 'mixed cases'. Not only were Lichtheim's empirical accounts of his own pure cases inadequate, but so was his discussion of cases that seemed potentially troublesome for his theory; his arguments that they could be treated as 'mixed' were brief and unconvincing. Worse still, there appeared to be a difficulty in applying the concept of a 'pure case'. Which patients are in this category depends on one's theory. If one were to reject Lichtheim's theory, could one not argue that a different set of cases was critical? Is not the whole approach circular?[10]

In fact, this argument is not valid. If two particular theories of functional organisation are in competition, then each theory can produce its own set of relevant pure cases. An assessment can be made of which of the two theories explains all these cases best. More critically, one needs to differentiate between different uses of neuropsychological evidence: those of theory testing and those of theory development. It is of theoretical value to describe the impairment of any patient – pure or mixed – if to explain it is difficult on the basis of an existing theory. For the development of a new theory, however, it is much more useful to work with pure patients, and this is what Lichtheim was doing. For either purpose, the set of patients who deserve detailed description depends on the development of theory in much the same way as does the set of experiments that are carried out in most areas of science. However, from an empiricist atheoretical perspective, such as that of Head, Lichtheim's procedure would seem totally unconvincing. It was much more natural to base theorising on the types of patient most frequently encountered.[11]

The view that there are no qualitative differences among the aphasias was probably always a minority one among clinicians – even those who rejected the diagram-makers' approach – and is now completely abandoned. Moreover, until the rise of information-processing models, none of the many other frameworks suggested seemed more theoretically plausible than the Wernicke–Lichtheim one or as useful clinically as a means of categorising the bewildering variety of aphasic patients into a tractable number of categories. With its adoption by Goodglass and Kaplan (1972) as the conceptual basis of the most popular standardised aphasia battery, it has become, in a historically curious fashion, an almost indispensable conceptual system for clinical practice. So the terminology of Wernicke (1874) and Lichtheim (1885) survives nearly a century after their theories were discarded.

10. Rarely is there a clearer example of the potentially theory-laden nature of scientific data so frequently claimed in modern philosophy of science – for example, Hanson (1958), Kuhn (1962), Feyerabend (1975).
11. The question of which patients should receive most empirical attention is as much a difficulty for modern cognitive neuropsychologists as it was for the diagram-makers. Lichtheim's criteria, in my view, remain valid. I will return to the problem in later chapters.

1.3 The Diagram-Makers' Successors

After the defeat of the diagram-makers, neuropsychology became much less interesting. The major methodological development was the rejection of the single-case approach. The impairments of a series of patients began to be assessed systematically. Inclusion in the series depended only on the patients satisfying some rather general criteria, such as being clinically capable of being tested, being willing, and having a relevant lesion or the appropriate broadly defined functional deficit, such as being aphasic. More critically, the tests, too, became more standardised and quantifiable. In aphasia, the work of Head (1926) and Weisenburg and McBride (1935) exemplified this approach. Ironically, their substantive theoretical conclusions are now almost totally forgotten. In another area, a yet more sophisticated methodology – the use of matched normal controls – was used in a very interesting investigation of frontal lobe function by Rylander (1939). Rylander provided a justification for the need to base theoretical inferences on the results of formal testing and not on clinical observations, which is simple but hard to improve on. The clinical examination, he argued, is 'something of an experiment. But it is a poorly organised experiment and difficult to control, the conditions under which it is performed are never fixed, and the results present a tangled skein of objective observations and subjective opinions' (p. 50).

The crucial legacy of this period was that clinical observations alone became an insufficient basis for theoretical speculation, although many papers that flout this simple rule are still produced and accepted by journals. Another manifestation of mainstream scientific influence was the trend towards the use of group studies. This became much stronger when psychologists began to work in the area in greater numbers, which occurred at roughly the time of the Second World War; before this period, the field had been dominated by neurologists. Group studies remained the dominant approach until the end of the 1960s. For the Halstead–Reitan school, in particular, group studies were addressed primarily to detecting whether a patient had sustained brain damage and, if so, where it was located; the psychometric procedures employed were based on a fixed battery of quantitative tests. The approach was typical of the empiricism that characterised experimental psychology methodology of the period, and few major advances in theory were made.

Of much greater theoretical interest were group studies addressed to specific types of deficit, such as those of the Milan and London groups on perception (e.g. De Renzi & Spinnler, 1966; De Renzi, Scotti, & Spinnler, 1969; Warrington & James, 1967) and of the Montreal group on memory and on frontal lobe functions (e.g. Milner, 1963, 1965, 1968). In this type of study, patients are assigned to particular groups on the basis of the gross anatomy of their lesion sites (e.g. right parietal lobe), and the groups are contrasted to determine whether they have the same pattern of deficits over a set of tests. De Renzi and his colleagues (1969) found that on certain perceptual tests, the right hemisphere patients were significantly more impaired, but on others, the left sided lesions had the greater effect. The distinction between the two types of test corresponded to that between apperceptive and associative agnosia, developed by Lissauer (1890) nearly 80 years before on the basis of a single-case study. The tests that the right hemisphere group found more difficult were those that, according to Lissauer, stress apperceptive processes, while the left hemisphere patients had more problems with the associative tests. These group studies, therefore, put Lissauer's functional distinction on a more solid empirical basis; they will be discussed further in chapter 8.

Studies of this general type were done in a number of other areas of perception (e.g. De Renzi & Spinnler, 1967) and also on constructional abilities (e.g. Piercy, Hécaen, & Ajuriaguerra, 1960). But if the future theoretical development of neuropsychology were to have relied on the results of empirical methods of this type, progress would inevitably have become slower and slower. As will be discussed in more detail in chapter 9, group studies of this type are very lengthy. Patients differ greatly in their premorbid level of performance and in the severity and nature of their illness. So a large number of patients generally have to be tested to obtain significant group differences. Thus studies like that of De Renzi, Scotti, and Spinnler (1969) involved between 100 and 200 patients, and yet some critical results were only at the .05 level.

It takes a long time to complete such investigations, even when the criterion for inclusion is that the lesion is limited to one hemisphere only. Just consider applying a similar approach to, for instance, two subcomponents of the reading process. All the relevant systems are probably located in the posterior part of the left hemisphere. Therefore, separate groups of patients with all patients in a group having a lesion in one part of the posterior left hemisphere but not in the other relevant part, would have to be found, even granting the assumption that the two subcomponents have different clearly defined localisations that are fairly constant over patients. In fact, many, if not most, patients with posterior left hemisphere lesions would tend to have damage to both sub-regions and would therefore have to be excluded from the series. The collection of appropriate patients by a single research group would probably require a decade or possibly longer. In addition, given the inaccuracy in localising the precise region that is actually functionally damaged, the procedure would be much more susceptible to error than that of comparing groups having lesions in different hemispheres. So the method seems almost inevitably to be limited to the establishment of gross functional dissociations.

In the mid-1960s, then, neuropsychology did not appear to outsiders to be a very exciting field. The laborious group-study methods then standard seemed likely to produce a decreasing return for theory on empirical time and effort. The rococo splendours of the field's youth were generally forgotten.

1.4   The Rise of Cognitive Neuropsychology

Outside the neuropsychology mainstream, there were some encouraging developments during this period. In 1965, Geschwind made a powerful and scholarly plea for resurrecting the early achievements of the field from their neglect. A few studies of individual patients or of small groups of functionally similar patients had considerable impact, as in the work on amnesia (e.g. Milner, 1966), aphasia (e.g. Goodglass, 1968), and more specific disorders (such as simultanagnosia, Kinsbourne & Warrington, 1962b). The more clinical studies of Luria (1966) were gaining wider recognition, and links with cognitive psychology and linguistics were beginning to develop (e.g., Marshall & Newcombe, 1966; Wickelgren, 1968).

Within 15 years, from these and a few similar strands was to develop an approach that would transform the field. Now known as cognitive neuropsychology, this approach had three major aspects – concerning its theories, methods, and programme. All brought the field more in line with its conduct a 100 years before! Together, they were critical to the progress made in the field.

The most important change was at the theoretical level. The rise of information-processing models within cognitive psychology in the 1960s and 1970s provided a springboard for explanations of abnormal function. There was no obvious way to extrapolate Hullian theory or Gestalt theory to account for the impaired performance of neurological patients. An information-processing model can, though, be easily 'lesioned' conceptually. So the processing systems or transmission routes assumed by cognitive neuropsychologists to be damaged can be subcomponents of models of normal function that either have been or can be postulated. Figure 1.2 illustrates the way that agraphia syndromes can be generated from a model of the normal spelling process suggested by Morton (1980a). (These particular syndromes will be discussed in chapter 6.)

The methodological change concerned the status of the case study. Instead of being treated as a somewhat disreputable legacy of the nineteenth century, the case study began to be considered the most powerful empirical procedure for making inferences to normal function. As we will see in chapter 2, this does not mean that a case study is conducted as it was in Lichtheim's time. Rylander's (1939) comments on the inadequacy of treating clinical reports as scientific data still apply. The critical point is that the results of single-case studies have become as legitimate a type of evidence with which to support or criticise a theory as the results of group studies. Moreover, it is held in cognitive neuropsychology that the individual case study is much more likely to produce strong evidence for discriminating among theories of normal function.

The programme stressed the relevance of neuropsychological evidence for the understanding of normal function. A good example is the statement of Marin, Saffran, and Schwartz (1976):

We are arguing that the behavior of the patient with organic brain disease largely reflects capacities which existed in the premorbid state. We should therefore be able to make some inferences about the organization of normal language function from *patterns of functional preservation and impairment:* if process X is intact where process Y is severely compromised or absent, and especially if the converse is found in other patients, there is reason to believe that X and Y reflect different underlying mechanisms in the normal state. At the very least, the resulting matrix of intact and impaired functions should yield a taxonomy of functional subsystems. It may not tell us *how* these subsystems interact – but it should identify and describe *what* distinct capacities are available (e.g., it might, to take a hypothetical instance, describe a semantic process that is distinct from a syntactic process). The method is, of course, limited by the functional topology of the brain. Because functions may overlap in

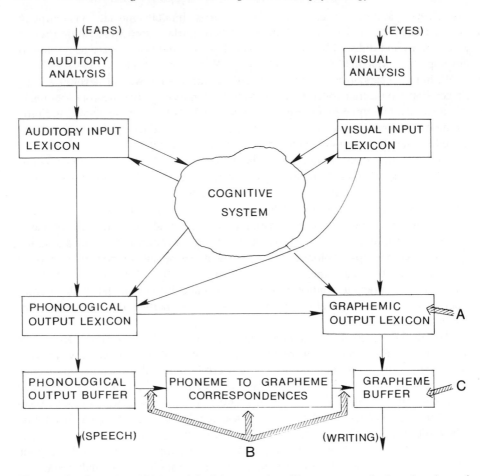

Figure 1.2. Morton's (1980a) model of the normal spelling process and where locations of impairment would be on the model to account for three modern agraphia syndromes: lexical agraphia *(A);* phonological agraphia *(B,* three alternatives); and graphemic buffer agraphia *(C).*

their anatomical substrates, we cannot state with assurance that every functional system which *could* be observed *will* be observed. But *positive* evidence that functions are organized independently should be significant for a theory of the language process. (p. 869–870)

The detailed contents of the programme were not original to cognitive neuropsychologists. Many neurologists and physiological psychologists had long held a similar position on the effects of lesions. Methodologists had developed related inference procedures in considerably more detail (e.g., Teuber, 1955; Weiskrantz, 1968; Kinsbourne, 1971). What was new was the stress on individual cases and, more particularly, the confidence that an information-processing approach provides that a link-up is possible with the study of normal higher cognitive processes.

Basing explanations of impaired performance on models of normal function means that, unlike its nineteenth-century precursor, the cognitive neuropsychology approach allows, or rather encourages, cross-talk between explanations of normal and impaired performance. It is obvious that one should try to use the best possible models of normal function when trying to explain impaired function. However, cross-talk implies more than that. It means that the understanding of normal function can be enhanced by learning about impaired function, too. The purpose of this book is to assess this claim. Can cognitive neuropsychology do more than provide support for theories derived from already existing studies on normal subjects?

I intend to assess this claim in two ways. For the argument to have any power, it must be based on solid empirical evidence, not on some version of what Gall believed and Broca found. In chapters 3 to 8, I therefore consider a number of areas in which cognitive neuropsychology has been fairly well developed. I examine what theoretical conclusions about normal function can be derived from the empirical findings, whether they square with those obtained by more standard experimental methods using normal subjects, and, if so, how independent the two approaches really were. The neuropsychological effort will be judged successful if the two approaches independently arrive at conclusions that are similar and not intuitively obvious. In my discussion of these areas, I take a particular approach within cognitive neuropsychology; this will be described in chapter 2. As the individual topics are discussed, it should become clear that theoretical inferences from impairment to normal function are based on a considerable number of assumptions; these are assessed in chapters 9 to 11.

In the final part of the book, I assess the question of whether cognitive neuropsychology provides valuable findings for understanding normal function in a rather different fashion. I make the strong assumption that the methods outlined in the first half of the book do work. Then I take some difficult and important aspects of cognition where study of normal subjects has not yet led to widely accepted conclusions and ask whether cognitive neuropsychology provides any direction in these areas. These topics are knowledge, the allocation of cognitive resources, planning, episodic memory, and consciousness. The second half of the book is therefore much more speculative than the first.

2   The Cognitive Neuropsychology Approach

2.1 On Modularity

If Lashley's (1929) idea of mass action were valid, then neuropsychology would be of little relevance for understanding normal function. Any form of neurological damage would deplete by a greater or lesser degree the available amount of some general resource, say the mythical g. Knowing which tasks a patient could or could not perform would enable us to partition tasks on a difficulty scale. It would tell us little, if anything, about how the system operated.

If one considers the design principles that might underlie cognitive systems, a rough contrast can be drawn between systems based on equipotentiality (e.g., those that follow principles such as mass action) and more modular ones. At a metatheoretical level, some form of the 'modularity' thesis is probably the most widely accepted position in the philosophy of psychology today (e.g. Chomsky, 1980; Morton, 1981; Marr, 1982; Fodor, 1983). Over the past 30 years, the arguments for the position have become increasingly compelling and diverse; they are of a number of different types: computational, linguistic, physiological, and psychological.

The most basic argument is the computational one, which we owe to Simon (1969) and Marr (1976). In Marr's words,

Any large computation should be split up and implemented as a collection of small sub-parts that are as nearly independent of one another as the overall task allows. If a process is not designed in this way, a small change in one place will have consequences in many other places. This means that the process as a whole becomes extremely difficult to debug or to improve, whether by a human designer or in the course of natural evolution, because a small change to improve one part has to be accompanied by many simultaneous compensating changes elsewhere. (p. 485)

Empirical support for these conclusions can be obtained at a number of levels. The most abstract concerns domains of competence, such as the ability to walk, to catch objects, to see depth, or to know whether English sentences are grammatical. Take the last of these; modern post-transformational theory of syntax holds with considerable internal evidence that the grammatical status of a very wide range of sentences can be determined using only a restricted set of rules (for a tractable account see Radford, 1981). It seems plausible, too, that the rules are specific to the language domain; very different ones would, for instance, describe the input–output relations of the subsystems responsible for binocular vision. Moreover, within the language domain, the rules seem to be specific to syntax and relatively independent of conceptual and pragmatic considerations. The simplest way to explain this relative independence of our competence in a particular domain is to assume that it is the product of a subsystem that is itself relatively independent of other subsystems. This is Chomsky's (1980) conclusion about the existence of what can loosely be called a module for grammatical competence.[1]

On a much more concrete level, an argument compatible with Marr's position comes from neurophysiology. It is based on the observation that there are a number of different areas in the posterior third of monkey cortex that are highly specific in the types of stimulus attributes – colour, movement, position, depth, and so on – to which they respond (see, e.g. Van Essen, 1979; Cowey, 1985). Why should regions of visual cortex have such highly specific responses? Cowey (1982) argues that the vast majority of neurons in the cortex are local circuit interneurons and that they are involved, often in inhibitory fashion, in the fine-tuning of the response of single neurons to such features as orientation, disparity, direction, velocity, wavelength, and size. Each neuron coding a feature needs to be interconnected with others involved in analysing the same attribute. To attempt to carry out these different operations on all features in one area would create great demands on the process that specifies the correct local connections in development. Regional specialisation on the contrary, means that columns of cells can simply be connected with all or most of their immediate neighbours that have related functions. The average length of the interneurons can also be kept shorter.

The argument that anatomically distinct subsystems exist to carry out separate micro-functions can be extended further to explain not only why different regions of cortex respond differentially, but also why they have the detailed neurophysiological and neuroanatomical properties they do. A particularly elegant example of this is Zeki's (1980) work on the properties of colour-sensitive cells in area V4 of the visual cortex. Functional modularity has thus been a very productive assumption for visual neuroscience.

There are also many relevant arguments on the psychological level (see, e.g., Sternberg, 1969; Posner, 1978; Fodor, 1983). For instance, McLeod, McLaughlin, and Nimmo-Smith (1985) have shown that the catching response can be triggered by the visual stimulus of an expanding image on the retina – corresponding to an approaching ball – with, on average, an accuracy of better than 5 msec! McLeod and his colleagues argue that such precision would not be possible if the response were produced by a system influenced by many factors; instead, they argue, some specific module directly responsive to the rate of increase in size of the image must be involved.[2]

1. Of course, the question of how autonomous syntactic operations are is a live issue within both linguistics and psychology. The linguistic arguments do, however, seem to be fairly powerful. For objections from within linguistics, see Lakoff (1980), but note also the fairly devastating reply of Chomsky (1980).
2. The most famous psychological procedure that produces evidence for the specificity of subsystems is Sternberg's (1969) 'additive factors' method: separability of processing is inferred from the additive effects of two different factors on reaction time.

These four arguments for modularity – from computer science, linguistics, neurophysiology, and cognitive psychology – differ in level of abstraction and in how closely they relate to empirical evidence. In addition, three of them are based on specific examples; they do not demonstrate that modularity is a *general* property of the systems underlying human cognition. However, they make it a reasonable assumption to use as a first pass in the interpretation of neuropsychological findings.[3]

This discussion presupposes that we know what the word *module* means. Intuitively, it is easy enough to grasp. Most machines are made up of subcomponents whose interactions with other parts of the machine are different in complexity and kind from their own internal workings. Moreover, modularity is a basic principle that we often use to understand natural systems.[4] Recently, though, an intuitive idea of modularity has been considered to be insufficient. One attempt to characterise it more adequately has received much attention – Fodor's (1983) theory, in which the term is given an explicit and detailed interpretation. A module, for Fodor, is a subsystem with a particular set of properties: it is domain-specific, innately specified, not assembled from more basic elements, hard-wired, 'computationally autonomous', and 'informationally encapsulated' and has a characteristic pattern of development. By 'computationally autonomous', Fodor means that a module does not share attention, memory, or other general-purpose processes with other modules. By 'informationally encapsulated', he means that a module has access to only a very restricted amount of information contained in the system as a whole. Presented so baldly, Fodor's view of the module no doubt seems like a forbidding jungle of abstractions. In fact, his account is most elegant. But for neuropsychological purposes, the criteria he suggests may well be too specific and the systems to which they are supposed to apply, too limited.[5]

Marr's (1982) view of modularity is less explicit and more useful for neuropsychological purposes. He uses the concept in a processing sense, in terms of the *amount* of interaction between two systems (p. 356). On this view, systems differ

3. The more complex possibility suggested by Fodor (1983), that modularity applies to only certain parts of the cognitive system, will be discussed in chapters 12 and 14.
4. Rosenthal (1984) has, indeed, argued that we may use modularity just because it is the only procedure we have for understanding anything about the world rather than because it is a property of the natural world per se. In fact, field theories show that it is not the only procedure we have. Nor does his position account for why the concept of modularity has been successfully employed for understanding the natural world. However, there is a degree of intuitiveness in the arguments of Chomsky (1980) and Marr (1982) that gives Rosenthal's position a certain subversive persistence. To put it briefly: Is the set of non-modular systems characterisable other than by exclusion – that is, negatively? If not, how could one know that there were not non-modular systems that had the properties that Chomsky and Marr explain by assuming modularity?
5. On Fodor's (1983) approach, the reading system, for instance, could not be modular, since it has a number of properties that clash with his definition; for instance, the system could hardly be innately organised. Moreover, it seems impossible, for example, that impairments to the adult nervous system – which is the subject of this book – could give evidence about whether or not a system has been assembled. Finally, in our present state of knowledge, is it possible to determine whether or not a system has been assembled? I doubt it. For critiques of Fodor's position, see Marshall (1984a), Putnam (1984), Schwartz and Schwartz (1984), and Shallice (1984).

in their degree of modularity, and a relatively modular system may require or be able to call upon some general resource, such as Kahneman's (1973) concept of 'effort'.

I will use the terms *module* and *modular* in this latter sense. However, it will be shown in Chapter 11 that neuropsychological evidence does not speak definitively to the question of modularity even under this weaker interpretation; moreover, Marr's approach also needs to be operationalised, which it has not been. I will therefore tend to use the vaguer phrases 'functional subsystem' and 'isolable subsystem', derived from Posner (1978). Tulving (1983) has expressed rather nicely what this type of concept implies. For two subsystems to be functionally different, he argues, means

that one system can operate independently of the other although not necessarily as efficiently as it could with the support of the other intact system. The operations of one system could be enhanced without a similar effect on the operations of the other; similarly the operations of one system could be suppressed without a comparable effect on the activity of the other. The functional difference also implies that in important, or at least in non-negligible ways, the systems operate differently, that is, that their function is governed at least partially by different principles. (p. 66)

For an overall system composed of subsystems of this type, I will for convenience use the term *modular*.

2.2 What Can Be Learned about Normal Function from Impaired Behaviour?

The basic question that this book addresses can be approached in two distinct ways. The first is to make an assumption about the overall structure of the system – say, that it is broadly modular in Marr's (1982) sense. One then asks what neuropsychological findings tell us about its detailed functional architecture. What are the basic cognitive-processing elements, the modules? How are they interconnected? The result is a sort of surveying operation, a very complex and difficult one, but with the fundamental concepts about how the system is constructed already accepted.

The second approach is more abstract. If one drops the initial assumption, it can then be asked whether neuropsychological findings tell us anything about the types of basic elements out of which cognition might be constructed. Can, for instance, neuropsychological findings indicate that the basic elements are modular in Marr's sense or that they are isolable subsystems or what? In other words, can neuropsychological evidence be used to buttress the four arguments on modularity with which this chapter began?

The rest of this chapter and chapters 3 to 8 will be concerned with evidence relevant to the first of these issues. Most of chapters 9 and 10 will be concerned with an overall assessment of neuropsychological evidence from this perspective. In chapter 11, the second, more abstract issue will be tackled: What type of system could in principle, if 'lesioned', mimic neuropsychological findings? The last five chapters assume the answers developed there.

Assume, then, that cognition is carried out by isolable subsystems.[6] Marr (1982) makes the critical point that there are a number of different levels on which one can understand how a modular system operates. For individual component:

At one extreme, the top level, is the abstract computational theory of the device, in which the performance of the device is characterized as a mapping from one kind of information to another, the abstract properties of this mapping are defined precisely, and its appropriateness and adequacy for the task at hand are demonstrated. In the center is the choice of representation for the input and output and the algorithm to be used to transform one into the other. And at the other extreme are the details of how the algorithm and representation are realized physically – the detailed computer architecture, so to speak. These three levels are coupled, but only loosely. The choice of an algorithm is influenced for example, by what it has to do and by the hardware in which it must run. But there is a wide choice available at each level, and the explication of each level involves issues that are rather independent of the other two. (pp. 24–25)

The two lower levels apply to the operation of particular isolable subsystems. The highest level, though, has two aspects. We need to know both what is the overall organisation of the major computational subcomponents – the isolable subsystems – and what each of them does, what technically it computes. It may seem that the answers to these two questions are rather tightly connected, but that need not be so. For instance, as far as the history of the understanding of the anatomy of the body was concerned, it was possible to provisionally identify organs without any knowledge of what they did. It will be argued in this book that a related process can operate for the mind. The mapping of the functional architecture may be possible with only a loose specification of what each subsystem actually does.

If one accepts an approach of this general type, the wider theoretical relevance of neuropsychological research will depend on what can be learned about the operation of such a multi-level system from its global behaviour when parts of it are damaged. Marr (1982) extends his discussion of levels of explanation by arguing that to understand the normal functioning of such a system, one has to proceed from the highest level down; to attempt a mechanistic explanation on the level of hardware or hypothetical hardware in the absence of functional or algorithmic specifications is, he claims, likely to prove arid. In particular cases, this may prove to be too sweeping a position because the particular hardware available (e.g. slow parallel circuitry) may make some types of (mathematical) functions much easier to compute than others. However, Marr's argument does seem apposite if one considers attempting to determine how a hypothetical subsystem might work from observing the way in which macroscopic behaviour can be impaired by a lesion. To attempt to assess how the subsystem operates at the mechanistic level from that type of evidence would be like trying to deduce how computer hardware works by exam-

6. I will assume that output can flow from one such subsystem to a second in other than all-or-none fashion. They can therefore be part of a so-called 'cascade' system (McClelland & Rumelhart, 1981) (see chapter 11). I will also presuppose that modularity applies down to only a certain level of detail (e.g. Allport 1985).

ining the malfunction of a program caused by a fault in the machine when one has no knowledge of the program's structure. This would almost certainly be a hopeless task, and inferences to the algorithmic level would be almost as difficult.

If one turns instead to the task of determining the overall organisation of the modular structure – and, particularly, what functionally isolable subsystems exist and, in very general terms, what each does – the picture is altogether more promising. Were a single subsystem to be severely damaged, then the ability of the organism to perform a particular micro-function would be grossly impaired. This would not necessarily manifest itself in behaviour in a sharply defined way given appropriate tests. Thus damage to a subsystem like the one that Kahneman (1973) has suggested is responsible for 'effort' would necessarily lead to impaired performance on many tasks. However, in many cases, specific consequences would be expected. Consider, for instance, damage to a hypothetical subsystem concerned with only the recognition of faces or another responsible for just the syntactic structure of a sentence being produced. Specific damage to a transmission route between subsystems is also likely to have fairly selective consequences. The critical point is that if in these cases one looks at the whole range of tasks that the organism can perform, the set of tasks on which performance is impaired is likely to be relatively insensitive to the specific nature of the impairment within a subsystem (or transmission route), provided that the impairment is fairly severe. The set of tasks on which impaired performance occurs will be relatively unchanged when there is a change in the nature of the impairment *within* the subsystem.

One consequence of this rather simple argument is that recent manifestos arguing that it is essential – not merely desirable – for neuropsychological theory to be based on artificial-intelligence models, as in 'Neurolinguistics must be computational' (Arbib & Caplan, 1979; see also Allport, 1985), are misguided. The most favourable level for effective mediations between neuropsychology and the theory of normal processing seems likely to be not that of the detailed operation of computational models, but that of the more global functional architecture.

In practice, the situation is frequently not as straightforward as in the case of the face-recognition subsystem hypothesised earlier. If a subsystem lies within a complex modular network, then the consequences of damage may not be very simple, even if the effects are gross. The organisation of the interconnections among subsystems would be critical. The level of theorising necessary would, however, be one of those within human information-processing psychology. Within that field, the task faced by research workers of trying to determine at the same time the correct functional organisation, the correct algorithm, and the correct means by which it is computed is clearly not practicable with the weak experimental procedures available. A split developed between those research workers who were, in practice, the first modular theorists, who attempted to capture the rough essentials of the functional organisation of the cognitive system – represented, say, by the work of Broadbent (1958), Morton (1969), and Posner (1978) – and those who desired precision or theoretical rigour and used approaches more influenced by mathematical psychology and computational theory.[7] Within the looser information-processing framework, neuropsychological findings have the potential to produce evidence relevant to particular models in a rather analogous fashion to certain chronometric procedures, such as those used by Sternberg (1969) and Posner (1978). In both cases, the evidence relates to the global organisation of subsystems rather than to the details of their operation. Thus there is an existing level of theorising about cognition to which neuropsychological findings should relate.

The research programme to be assessed in the first half of this book starts, then, with a basic assumption. The cognitive difficulties experienced by neurological patients are to be understood to a first approximation in terms of the functioning of the normal information-processing system, with certain isolable subsystems or transmission routes operating in an impaired fashion. The effects in patients of theoretical interest are assumed to be sufficiently gross that, subject to the considerations discussed in the last few paragraphs, one does not require a detailed theory of the functioning of the relevant subsystems. From studying the disorders of these patients, it is assumed, one can obtain useful information about the global modular structure.

This approach is conceptually simple. Its effective application can, however, be byzantine in its complexity. The pattern of impairments to the modular system cannot provide a complete account of a patient's behaviour. It is the product of many factors other than the systems that are damaged. Patients do not arrive at the neuropsychological clinic with anything like the uniformity of age, intelligence, background, views about being tested, and so on that one expects of the students who typically serve as subjects in normal experimental psychology. On the physical level, there is the possibility of neurological reorganisation taking place during the recovery process; if the lesion is restricted to one hemisphere, complementary but qualitatively different systems in the other hemisphere might conceivably replace in some way those that have been damaged. At another level, one needs to take into account the strategies that patients develop to compensate for the difficulties they experience. Moreover, for patients, the test situation is not the fairly neutral hour passed by the typical subject in a 'normal' psychological experiment, but is intimately linked with one of the major events of their life – their illness. It is undoubtedly the case that in the theoretical disputes concerning the interpretation of certain disorders, some of these points were initially neglected and later turned out to be relevant. I will, however, assume that, in general, these are second-order issues as far as theoretical inferences to normal function are concerned. The assumption will be assessed in detail in chapter 10.

---

7. The former type of approach has been much criticised for its looseness in failing to specify how subcomponents work. However, the response has been that more detailed assumptions are inappropriate at this stage of theorising (see, e.g., Broadbent, 1958; Baddeley, 1976), and, indeed, this choice is the one that fits better Marr's (1982) levels-of-explanation principle.

2.3 Neuropsychological Facts

Any effective science needs a means of generating interesting facts. Philosophers used to argue that meter readings or similar 'microscopic' acts of measurement are the bedrock of the scientific process. However, the information against which rival theories are assessed is, in fact, a much more complex beast and is specific to a particular science at a particular time.[8] Thus a fairly embryonic fact of present-day experimental psychology – a finding just published – normally concerns an effect of particular independent variables on a dependent variable averaged across a group of subjects and requires the use of control groups, factorial designs, ANOVAs, and so on. What corresponds to this in neuropsychology?

The obvious answer, and one adopted by psychologists when they first began to work systematically with neurological patients, is that neuropsychological findings are about the performance of groups of patients when the criteria for group membership are objectively defined. However, as discussed in chapter 1, unless each group is selected in some way that is very tightly defined functionally, the patients in a group are likely to have damage to different subsystems. Therefore, summing performance over a group can produce a reported average that is qualitatively different from that of any individual patient – a so-called averaging artefact – or, more prosaically, can lead to the disappearance of theoretically interesting effects due to inter-subject variability.

A good illustration of this type of problem comes from the lengthy debates about facts that took place in amnesia research in the 1970s. Amnesia is one of the most dramatic phenomena that occurs in clinical neuropsychology as well as one of the most widely known. In a severe case, the patient may appear to have little recollection of events that happened in the past, even as recently as a minute or two before, and this clinical impression is amply supported by quantitative results on a wide range of tests. As an illustration, Figure 2.1 shows the performance of 11 amnesic patients of Warrington and Weiskrantz (1978) and 200 controls on a verbal forced-choice recognition memory test of Warrington (1984). It can be seen that there is virtually no overlap between the two groups.

The 1970s debate about facts concerned the specificity of the disorder. Clinically, it had long been claimed that amnesia can be a highly specific disability, that intelligence and 'knowledge', for instance, can be spared (see Talland, 1965). However, modern quantitative investigations of amnesia employed two methodologies that produced differing conclusions on this issue.

One approach was used by Milner and her colleagues in Montreal (e.g. Scoville & Milner, 1957; Milner, Corkin, & Teuber, 1968) and later by Warrington and her collaborators in London (e.g. Baddeley & Warrington, 1970; Warrington & Weis-

---

8. Latour and Woolgar (1979) give an interesting account of the social process involved in a reasonably advanced science – neuroendocrinology – in the development of a fact from its initially being claimed to its general acceptance.

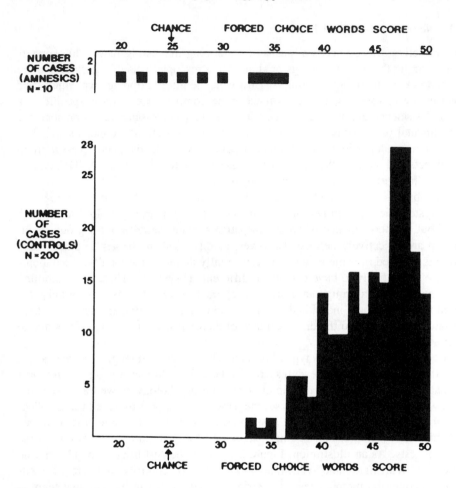

Figure 2.1. Performance of 200 control subjects (below) and 10 amnesics (above) on the Warrington 50-item forced-choice recognition memory test. From Warrington and Weiskrantz (unpublished).

krantz, 1970). Patients were chosen for study according to the selectivity and severity of their amnesic difficulties. In Lichtheim's (1885) terms, the aim was to obtain severe, but *pure,* cases. The absolute number of patients tested was considered much less important, and the aetiology of the lesion – the disease process that had given rise to it – was treated as of less importance still.

The alternative approach, adopted by Butters, Cermak, and their colleagues in Boston (e.g. Cermak & Butters, 1972), was more in accord with standard modern experimental psychology practice. Patients were selected according to their aetiology, and the groups tended to be of greater size than those studied by, say, Warrington and Weiskrantz. The studies normally involved patients with a Korsakoff

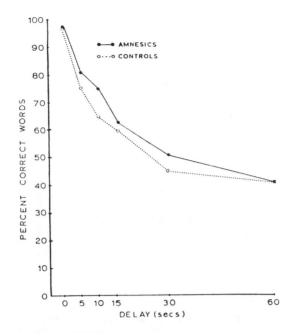

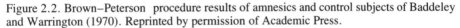

Figure 2.2. Brown–Peterson procedure results of amnesics and control subjects of Baddeley and Warrington (1970). Reprinted by permission of Academic Press.

syndrome stemming from chronic alcoholism, since this is a relatively frequent aetiology for amnesic difficulties. With Korsakoff patients, they tried to ensure that their groups had a mean IQ of roughly 100.

In practice, the two procedures led to different results on a number of issues. Two were whether amnesia involved short-term memory as well as long-term memory – and, in particular, whether the use of the so-called Brown–Peterson procedure[9] did or did not give normal results in amnesic patients (e.g. Baddeley & Warrington, 1970, vs. Cermak & Butters, 1972) (Figures 2.2 and 2.3) – and whether semantic encoding could be normal in amnesia (see, e.g., Meudell, Mayes, & Neary, 1980, vs. Butters & Cermak, 1976).

The procedure of using a reasonably sized group of Korsakoff patients led to the findings that an association existed between an amnesic disorder and other deficits. Amnesics, for instance, were found to have difficulty with some short-term memory tasks and with semantic coding. From these findings, a theory of amnesia was developed that was fashionable in the 1970s – the encoding deficit theory (Butters & Cermak, 1975). Amnesics were thought to encode stimuli in a superficial fashion, and, following levels-of-processing theory (Craik & Lockhart, 1972), this was held to produce weaker memory traces.

9. In the Brown-Peterson procedure, the subject has to retain information over short intervals of time (e.g. 15 sec), which are occupied by a highly demanding filler task.

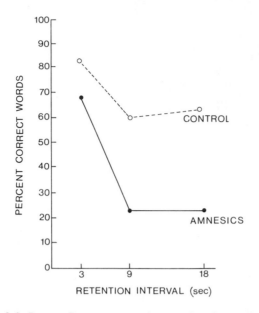

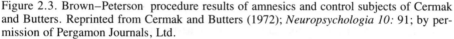

Figure 2.3. Brown–Peterson procedure results of amnesics and control subjects of Cermak and Butters. Reprinted from Cermak and Butters (1972); *Neuropsychologia 10:* 91; by permission of Pergamon Journals, Ltd.

This explanation of amnesia has now been abandoned for a variety of reasons (e.g. Mayes, Meudell, & Neary, 1978, 1980; Meudell et al., 1980). However, the critical methodological point is that the facts as represented by Figures 2.2 and 2.3, significance tests and so on, differed between the two sets of investigations. Taking the Brown-Peterson procedure as an example, various hypotheses were developed about which result was the valid one. For instance, it was argued that the filler task used by Baddeley and Warrington (1970), who claimed that amnesics could be normal on this task, was insufficiently demanding and that the amnesics could in effect rehearse while undertaking it (Butters & Cermak, 1974). This argument collapsed as a general explanation of intact amnesic performance on the test on discovery of an amnesic who, when tested by the procedures used by the Boston group, produced results similar to those obtained by Baddeley and Warrington (see Cermak, 1976). The patient studied by Cermak had, in fact, had an encephalitic illness, so it might appear that aetiology was the critical variable. However, individual Korsakoff patients can also produce entirely normal Brown-Peterson curves even if they are performing a demanding filler task – for example, adding a random series of numbers at the same level as controls (see Warrington, 1982a).

The most plausible explanation for the discrepancy in the pattern of results on these sets of tests is that it reflects a difference in the population of patients selected for study by the two types of methodology (for more extensive discussion, see Baddeley, 1982a). Although Korsakoff's psychosis can arise with only a very restricted area of sub-cortical neurological damage (e.g. Brierley, 1977; Mair, War-rington, & Weiskrantz, 1979), it also frequently occurs in the setting of widespread pathological changes (see Victor, Adams, & Collins, 1971). Indeed, 80% of Kor-sakoff amnesics are said to have frontal lobe damage (Butters, quoted in Mosco-vitch, 1982), and Korsakoff patients can fail on tasks associated with frontal lobe pathology (e.g. Oscar-Berman, 1973). Thus it is now commonly argued that some of the characteristics of Korsakoff amnesia claimed by the Boston group arise from associated frontal lobe impairments (e.g. Moscovitch, 1982; Mayes, Meudell, & Pickering, 1985).

One can conclude that any group of patients that is selected primarily because they have a Korsakoff aetiology will probably contain many patients with damage to a number of systems. Nor is the use of a group with mean IQ 100 (see Butters & Cermak, 1974) an adequate safeguard that all cortical systems are intact, other than those where damage leads to amnesia. The patients may have been of higher mean IQ premorbidly. Therefore, in this type of group study, it is virtually impossible to rule out the possibility that any association observed between two different deficits arises not because the same functional subsystem is responsible for both relevant processes, but because more than one functional subsystem has been damaged in some of the patients in the group.

Two types of conclusion have been drawn from consideration of these sort of problems. One relates to the relative reliability of *associations* and *dissociations* between symptoms as bases for functional inferences, a matter to be discussed shortly. The other is that group studies are not a reliable source of neuropsychological facts in so far as inferences to normal function are concerned. In chapter 9, I will question this assessment. This brief account of one aspect of amnesia research, together with the arguments from chapter 1, does, however, suggest a slightly more complex con-clusion: associations between deficits based on the results of group studies are a dan-gerous basis for an inference to normal function, and, as discussed in chapter 1, dis-sociations between deficits based on group studies are difficult to obtain. As studies employing the single-case methodology – described in later chapters – appeared more productive in other areas of neuropsychology (e.g. acquired dyslexia and dys-graphia), it began to be argued by many, but not all, cognitive neuropsychologists that the most significant data pertaining to normal function are to be obtained in single-case studies or in studies of very small groups of functionally equivalent patients. It has even been argued that *only* the results of what individual patients do are scientific facts (e.g. Caramazza, 1986). Yet an earlier school of neuropsychol-ogists who employed the single-case approach – the diagram-makers – had fallen completely out of favour. How was cognitive neuropsychology to avoid its fate?

2.4 The Single-Case Approach

Can a theoretically productive science really be based on 'facts' that are observa-tions of the behaviour of individual patients or small groups of patients who are supposedly functionally equivalent? It might seem premature to attempt to answer this question before giving examples of the approach. Yet the provisional answer will determine the way specific disorders are discussed in later chapters.

For a start, how does cognitive neuropsychology avoid the three major criticisms that led to the downfall of the diagram-makers: over localisation, over conceptual tools, and over empirical descriptions of patients?

Cognitive neuropsychologists have tended to duck the issue of localisation. It is argued that once the functional architecture has been sorted out, and only then, should we start worrying about its neurological implementation. This assumption neatly insulates psychological theorising from refutation involving anatomical evidence. However, it is probably pragmatically justified because the mapping relation among the levels may well be more complex than the localisation of functions in macroscopic centres assumed in classical neurology.[10] The response on the second point has been more satisfactory. With respect to the theoretical tools available, information-processing models provide a much more suitable conceptual base than was available to the diagram-makers.

As far as the third point is concerned, it is now accepted that a study of an individual subject is of no value unless it employs quantitative and reasonably controlled procedures during a period when the patient's clinical condition is qualitatively and preferably quantitatively static. It should also be a general rule that studies of individual patients contain the results of standard clinical 'baseline' tests, such as the Wechsler Adult Intelligence Scale (WAIS) (Wechsler, 1958), the Boston Aphasia Battery (Goodglass & Kaplan, 1972), some memory battery (e.g. Warrington, 1984), or their equivalents. In practice, otherwise well-conducted studies neglect this simple rule. Yet without the results of such baseline tests, it is very difficult for others to obtain a global impression of the patient's condition. This is vital both for comparing the results of different patients and for assessing whether the results of a series of potentially interesting but narrow experimental investigations have some major clinical flaw; the results of apparent theoretical interest may simply reflect an impairment in another domain that would have been picked up by more adequate clinical testing. Thus reading can be confounded by a speech difficulty, an apparent picture-naming difficulty may arise from a perceptual problem, and so on. For these reasons, single-case studies lacking quantitative data or adequate baseline tests will, in general, be ignored in this book.

Few cognitive neuropsychologists would challenge these elementary principles. Yet do the findings obtained on any single patient constitute a scientific fact? The natural temptation is to dismiss this question as one of arcane metaphysics over which sensible scientists do not concern themselves. The temptation should, however, be resisted. Cognitive neuropsychologists have answered this question in different ways, and as a consequence, they have tackled case studies using very different approaches. The epistemological choice has practical implications.

To illustrate these divergences, consider the studies reported in *Deep Dyslexia* (Coltheart, Patterson, & Marshall, 1980), which other neuropsychologists have viewed

---

10. See chapter 9 for further discussions of this issue.

as the first major book entirely within the cognitive approach.[11] It was thought to illustrate both the narrowness and the uniformity of the approach. Indeed, Brown (1981), in a long and generally favourable review, described it as being more like the work of one researcher than that of many individuals. Yet the book contains at least three very different approaches on how the selection of relevant patients and generalisations about results should proceed.

2.5 Facts Are Only What Individual Patients Do

The first approach to be considered, that of Morton and Patterson (1980), seems at first glance to be extreme: 'We do not believe there *is* such a thing as a deep dyslexic identifiable by some "qualifying examination". We are primarily looking at individual patients and it is only required that our accounts be self-consistent for each individual' (p. 97). Moreover, they were not discussing just deep dyslexic patients. Their position was that facts in neuropsychology are what individual patients do, and only that. They held syndrome labels like deep dyslexia to be useful only because they shorten and facilitate communication among those who share research interests.

As far as the logic of the scientific process is concerned, this approach seems attractive. Yet although science is a rational process, its rationality functions in a social realm, not in logic along. From the perspective of a realistic practice of science, the approach contains flaws. If each patient is treated as unique, then replication of an observation on another patient becomes impossible. Yet there is no reason to assume that neuropsychologists are more competent and careful than investigators in other fields where non-replicable results have been obtained. Indeed, the situation is made worse because the subject of a case study could be a patient who has developed an idiosyncratic coping strategy or could even be a hysteric or malingerer.

Caramazza (1986) has developed a related position in a more explicit and formal manner. His argument rests on the fact that if patterns of performance differ between two patients, there is no way of knowing whether this is a failure of replication or just arises from their having different functional lesion sites. He considers that one need not be worried by the lack of ability to replicate findings, arguing that what counts is the overall pattern of data:

The evidential weight of any single result is determined by the total body of evidence available to us at any point in the course of the scientific enterprise – in general, the larger the available body of relevant evidence the smaller the weight assigned to any single result. (p. 61)

Is this Bayesian process really the way the scientific process works? Did, say, the theoretical importance of Galileo's observations of the mountains on the moon

---

11. The syndrome deep dyslexia will be discussed in chapter 5. It has a number of characteristics, principally that patients make different types of errors in reading words – semantic, visual, and 'derivational' – and find certain types of words, such as function words and abstract words, particularly difficult to read.

or of the moons of Jupiter arise, just to use another of Caramazza's arguments, because it was 'congruent, under some explanatory account, with the vast majority of established evidence in the field' (p. 61)? Results that are anomalous because they do not fit established views are, of course, crucial in science. Yet it is not their mere number that counts. Unreplicated anomalies have much less weight than replicated ones.[12]

Whatever is the 'correct' position in the philosophy of science concerning replication, there are, in practice, more prosaic problems. If neuropsychology abandons the possibility of empirical generalisations not totally dependent on the theory they are being held to support, then the field is liable to drown in a sea of data. Individual theoreticians can work only with a data-base of limited size. Indeed, a tendency already exists for theorists to explain the disorders of their own patients and to ignore those of others. With the increasing popularity of the approach, a set of rival theories that implicitly use different data-bases could arise, as occurred at the time of the diagram-makers.

Another factor makes this danger greater. With the unique-case approach, one has, in principle, a set of theories being compared with what could become a very large set of cases for which pretheoretical generalisations are not allowed. Where, however, do these theories come from? At present, cognitive psychology does not provide such riches. We have only fairly crude and tentative hypotheses. According to this approach, then, the only rational grounds both for selecting patients for study and for not allowing results to become forgotten in the back numbers of journals are the relevance that individual patients seem to have for particular theories that may well turn out to be inadequate. Given the natural tendency for frequently seen impairments to receive more attention, rare and theoretically interesting cases may be swamped – a process that contributed to the decline of the diagram-makers. In addition, syndrome labels would act not merely as a theory-free means of facilitating communication – even if that is what they theoretically should be – but also as a practical guide to the selection of relevant patients. Since syndrome labels would be considered 'unscientific', what in practice would pass for a syndrome would remain chaotic. The unique-case version of the single-case approach, then, may be satisfactory as regards the logic of science, but as a guide to a realistic practice, it seems insufficient.[13]

2.6 Symptom Complexes

Other authors in the *Deep Dyslexia* collection were less purist than Morton and Patterson (1980). They attempted to generalise empirically over patients and to use

---

12. Other aspects of Caramazza's (1986) position are discussed in chapters 9 and 10. The difficulty of reproducing Galileo's observations testify to how critical replication was historically in this case (see, e.g., Feyerabend, 1975, chapters 9 and 10).

13. Deep dyslexia – in its present usage – is an example of a syndrome label frequently used in an atheoretical and unprincipled fashion (see section 5.3).

procedures for selecting patients for study that were not totally dependent on existing theories.

One such strategy – the symptom-complex approach – which can be traced back
at least to Wernicke (1874), was adopted by Coltheart (1980a) in his review of the
deep dyslexia 'syndrome' and by Marshall and Newcombe (1980). It contrasts sharply
with that used by Morton and Patterson. In his analysis, Coltheart begins with the
most intuitively striking of the symptoms of the postulated 'syndrome' deep dyslexia, the production of so-called semantic errors (e.g. *air* → *fly*) by a patient in
reading aloud. He then asks,

Are there other symptoms which such a patient will invariably display? If deep dyslexia is
defined by the occurrence of semantic errors, and is in addition a symptom-complex, then it
must be possible to identify a collection of symptoms which are consistently associated with
the occurrence of semantic errors. The symptom-complex may turn out to have a different
logical structure: for example, it may turn out to be necessary to define deep dyslexia in
terms of two necessary symptoms, whose joint occurrence is always associated with the
remaining symptoms of the symptom-complex. Another possibility is that the symptom-
complex has no such logical structure, that it consists of N symptoms and that these are all
of equal status as far as the definition of deep dyslexia is concerned. A detailed examination
of the symptoms displayed by deep dyslexic patients will permit adjudication between these
various possibilities. (p. 23)

This approach sounds logical. In Coltheart's elegant review of deep dyslexia, it
seems satisfactory; he argues that a patient who makes semantic errors will have 11
other characteristic difficulties.[14] What theoretical inferences should follow from
the different logical structures that Coltheart discusses? The version of the symptom-complex position that seems least liable to result in misleading conclusions is
to make inferences to normal function only when there is a completely consistent
relation among symptoms across patients. Caramazza (1984) has termed this type
of symptom complex a 'psychologically strong' syndrome. This approach, though,
has the opposite problem to that of the Morton and Patterson one. Instead of an
excess of facts, no safe facts exist at all. Any fact might disappear tomorrow when
an unfortunate new patient is observed with only some of the symptoms that occurred regularly together. Cognitive neuropsychology would have an unstable empirical base that would be liable to be eaten away as fast as it was laid down. There
is even no guarantee that two types of damage to the same functional subsystem
would lead to exactly the same pattern of symptoms. So a cluster could be discarded
when both it and the particular discrepant set of findings in fact resulted from damage to the same single functional subsystem. Moreover, one possibly aberrant un-
replicable finding would, if the logic is properly applied, lead to the abandonment
of the syndrome complex as a satisfactory functional entity.

The alternative would be to use a probabilistic type of logic. Symptoms that often
occur together would be the cluster to be used as a springboard for theoretical

14. Coltheart (1980a) does in fact accept that his account is complicated by the existence of one aberrant
   patient, AR. However, such specific empirical complexities of the deep dyslexia syndrome are not
   directly relevant here. The issue is discussed in chapter 5.

inferences. Caramazza (1984) has termed such a cluster a 'psychologically weak' syndrome. It would correspond to the way that the term *syndrome* is used in clinical practice (see, e.g., Kinsbourne, 1971). The danger of using such a cluster as a basis for inferences to normal function is well known from the history of clinical neuropsychology. A good illustration is the 'Gerstmann syndrome'. Patients with left parietal lesions can at times have a striking cluster of deficits: acalculia, a difficulty in performing arithmetic calculations; right–left disorientation; pure agraphia; and finger agnosia, a difficulty in locating the relative position of the fingers by touch alone (for a review, see Benton, 1977). This syndrome was widely accepted as a clinical entity from the 1920s to the 1960s. Theories about why these impairments should occur together ranged from a disturbance of the 'body schema' (Gerstmann, 1930) to impairments of 'directional sense' (Lange, 1930) or 'configurational thinking' (Conrad, 1932). However, following the extensive quantitative group studies of Benton (1961), Heimburger, Demyer, and Reitan (1964), and Poeck and Orgass (1966), it became accepted that the 'syndrome' was not a unitary functional entity. Each of the components occurred as frequently with non-Gerstmann characteristics as with one another. They are now considered to cluster – in so far as they do – merely as a result of their common left parietal anatomical basis.

Another syndrome that probably has no unitary functional basis is simultanagnosia, a disorder of reading and scene perception once considered to be a disorder of the apprehension of visual wholes conceived of as the final step in perception (Wolpert, 1924) (see chapter 4). More familiar examples are Broca's aphasia and conduction aphasia, as originally described. Each is now widely accepted to be what Lichtheim (1885) termed a 'mixed syndrome'; it does not have a unitary functional basis (see Mohr, 1976; Berndt & Caramazza, 1980; Schwartz, 1984; Badecker & Caramazza, 1985; chapters 3 and 7). Both probably arise as commonly observed entities due to the geography of the vascular system (Poeck, 1983). Historically, then, clusters of impairments found in common across patients have proved a treacherous foundation on which to build a bridge to normal function.

2.7   The Importance of Dissociations

The potential dangers of the symptom-complex approach are sufficiently well known that a number of cognitive neuropsychologists with a clinical background adopted a different one. It is represented in *Deep Dyslexia* by the approach taken by Warrington and me, but a number of others at about that time held related positions (see, e.g., Marin, Saffran, & Schwartz, 1976; Beauvois & Derouesné, 1979). Not all who utilise this approach would subscribe to quite the same position. However, all distinguish one type of neuropsychological finding as having a special status – *dissociations*. The dissociation is an old concept in neuropsychology, a methodological account having been given by Teuber (1955). In chapter 10, I will differentiate three sub-types. But for the present purposes, a dissociation occurs when a patient performs extremely poorly on one task – preferably way outside the normal range – and at a normal level or at least at a very much better level on another task.

The importance of dissociations stems from an inferential asymmetry between associations and dissociations, if observed impairments faithfully reflect damage to an underlying modular system. If one patient shows an association between two types of deficit and a second shows a dissociation, with one of the abilities being preserved, then a simple explanation of the overall pattern exists. The observed dissociation can be presumed to arise from a lesion that has affected only one side of a functional line of cleavage in the modular system; the association is presumed to result from a lesion that has crossed this line. On this account, if the association is actually observed later, it does not affect any interpretation that may have been made of the dissociation, but if the dissociation is observed after the association, it undermines any interpretation made of the association symptom complex as a unitary functional entity.

On the dissociation approach, the characteristics of an impairment may be divided into two parts. The primary aspects of the disorder are those describable in terms of what will be called a *set of dissociations*. In a theoretically useful case, a large number of functions should be intact and only a limited number, impaired; the disorder should be highly selective.[15] As will be seen in chapter 10, a single dissociation – unlike an association between deficits – may be sufficient to present serious difficulties for a theory of normal function. However, positive support for a theory is normally best based on a set of dissociations, which can potentially correspond to specific damage to a single subsystem. The secondary aspects of the disorder are those describable in terms of an association between deficits, together with the more detailed qualitative and quantitative aspects of the behaviour. These aspects of the behaviour of a patient are viewed as having a much more tentative status than the set of dissociations as regards inference to normal function. Moreover, although the total set of characteristics of a patient may in principle not be replicable, since lesions inevitably differ somewhat, the primary set of dissociations can be observed again.[16] And if a later patient is described in whom certain of the associated impairments – the secondary aspects – dissociate, then the previously observed syndrome is said to be a *multi-component,* or *mixed,* one that has *fractionated.*[17] The later patient is more likely to be what Lichtheim called a 'pure case', having a single-component syndrome. It will be shown in chapter 10 that fractionation of a syndrome does not necessarily imply that the more selective of the two disorders is the more pure. In general, however, the application of a fractionation procedure for the determination of which cases are theoretically more relevant will help to refine the data-base. Unlike the strong form of the symptom-complex ap-

---

15. Theoretically, the complementary situation – a selective preservation of a function – is also valuable, but it rarely occurs.
16. Dissociations can be so intuitively surprising that, in my view, a replication is of considerable importance in justifying that such a dissociation should be treated seriously.
17. The term *functional syndrome* refers to a set of symptoms held to arise from damage to a single processing subsystem (in the pure syndrome case) or to two or more subsystems (in the mixed case). It should be noted that in labels such as 'Gerstmann syndrome', the term *syndrome* has the definition common in clinical practice – a group of symptoms that frequently co-occur.

proach, the data base produced by a dissociation–fractionation procedure is not in perpetual danger of losing its functional relevance.

A very different type of complication for functional inferences in neuropsychology has long been known: an observed difference in a patient's performance level on two tasks, A and B, does not mean that the two tasks require a different set of processing systems. Task A may simply be easier than task B. Therefore, when considering the theoretical implications of an apparent dissociation, one needs to consider whether the tasks involved could differ only in the amount of cognitive resources they require. One remedy – first suggested by Teuber (1955) – is to obtain a *double dissociation,* in which a second patient is found who shows the complementary dissociation, the previously spared task being the one now impaired. As Kinsbourne (1971) pointed out, one does not know that both patients have different *specific* deficits; but given modularity assumptions, one does know that at least two subsystems are required to explain the overall pattern of performance. At least one of the dissociations cannot arise from what will be called a 'resource artefact'.[18]

This is only the simplest of the problems that can occur in making theoretical inferences within the dissociation–fractionation framework. A more detailed discussion of these issues will be delayed until chapters 10 and 11, by which time illustrative material will be available so that the problems can be discussed in concrete contexts. The broad conclusion is that if powerful information about the organisation of the cognitive system is to be obtained from single-case studies, then the dissociation–fractionation approach is the most likely one to provide it.

It will be argued that what this approach provides is a methodological heuristic for obtaining theoretically useful information, not an automatic induction procedure. However, at the level of formally relating observation to theory, the evidence that the method provides is entirely compatible with the unique-case approach. The dissociation–fractionation approach, then, can guide the selecting of patients, facilitate the obtaining of pragmatic reliability in results, and assist theorising in ill-charted areas. Each patient showing a particular pattern of dissociations can, when it is thought appropriate, be considered separately, and the individual results compared with alternative theories. Indeed, the more complex the theoretical domain, the more necessary may be discussion of the results of a number of individual patients within the context of existing models. It should not be forgotten, though, that in the understanding of modular systems, neuropsychological data may well prove to be more important for sketching the broad outlines of the organisation of subsystems than for testing the details of specific theories at the algorithmic or mechanistic levels.

In the chapters that follow, functional syndromes are generally introduced in terms of a set of dissociations. Patients with the appropriate set of dissociations who have

18. The word *resource* is used in the sense of Norman and Bobrow (1975). The assumptions and the artefact will be discussed in chapter 10.

been adequately investigated are usually considered together. It would be too lengthy to consider separately the characteristics of each patient exhibiting the basic syndrome. However, when the secondary aspects of a syndrome are being considered, the most appropriate procedure is to treat each patient as an individual test of theory. In practice, overlapping, but not identical, investigations have been done on different patients. At times, then, I will draw on evidence from different patients who have the same basic syndrome. I will, however, state for which patients the results have been obtained, and readers should bear in mind that arguments that involve cross-patient inferences are less rigorous than those that depend on only what a single patient does.

In this chapter, the reader has been presented with a rather abstract set of arguments generally unsupported by concrete examples. We are badly in need of some evidence! To illustrate the points made, I will take a fairly simple domain – one in which a single syndrome can be considered in relative independence from other ones – as a case study of the method. I will examine the short-term memory syndrome in detail, considering both how the syndrome is established and how the theoretical deductions drawn from studying it square with theoretical inferences about the same cognitive domain made by other means.

Part II

**Converging Operations: Specific Syndromes
and Evidence from Normal Subjects**

3   The Short-Term Memory Syndrome

3.1   The Syndrome

To isolate a new functional syndrome that does not have its characteristics mapped out by previous studies is a difficult and delicate process. The investigator has to be sensitive to the presence of a novel dissociation, itself a far from straightforward matter. Then a set of simpler and duller explanations in terms of syndromes that are already known have to be assessed. Only if they can be adequately rejected has a putative functional syndrome been isolated and only then can one begin to consider its theoretical implications. In this chapter, I am going to illustrate the process by considering a single syndrome – the short-term memory syndrome – from both a clinical and a theoretical perspective.

It is in clinical practice that new syndromes are detected. An unexpected result on a particular test is noticed and explored. In the present case, the unexpected result occurred on the Wechsler IQ battery. Many clinicians begin their assessment of a patient by using Wechsler subtests, not primarily to obtain an estimate of IQ but to see if any particular pattern of scores occurs across the different subtests (e.g. McFie, 1975; Lezak, 1976). In the late 1960s, Elizabeth Warrington was using this procedure to assess a patient, KF, who had sustained a severe head injury. He had a very low score on the Digit Span subtest, with performance on other subtests being relatively normal (Table 3.1) Obviously, no theoretical inferences can be made unless the deficit is reliable. With a patient like KF, however, repeated assessments even years later can give closely similar results. Moreover, the problem was not restricted to digits. KF performed as badly in repeating strings of words, and his performance with strings of letters was even worse.

When first observed, such a repetition deficit is most striking. Over a series of trials, on each of which just two digits were presented to KF, he could reliably give back only the first. Thus on a trial during which, say, '4' and '7' are spoken to the patient a second apart, he might well respond, '4 . . . I've forgotten the other.' As he could almost always repeat one digit reliably, Warrington thought that the deficit might well be arising from a problem of memory rather than of perception or production. As KF had a normal long-term memory, she thought it possible that the impairment was specifically related to short-term memory.[1]

---

1. Working as a mathematical psychologist and with an interest in memory and a Hebbian bent, I told Warrington that in my view, this was theoretically impossible. Waugh and Norman's (1965) impres-

Table 3.1. *WAIS subtest weighted scores (corrected for age) of the first two STM patients described*

	KF[a]	JB[b]
Arithmetic	5	8
Similarities	9	11
Digit Span	2	3
Vocabulary	7	9
Picture Completion	13	9
Block Design	11	7
Picture Arrangement	10	12

Note: Weighted scores have a mean of 10 and a standard deviation of 3.
[a] Warrington and Shallice (1969)
[b] Warrington, Logue, and Pratt (1971)

Since this difficulty was isolated in KF (Warrington & Shallice, 1969; Shallice & Warrington, 1970), a number of other patients with an essentially similar set of dissociations have been studied in detail: JB and WH (Warrington, Logue, & Pratt, 1971; Shallice & Butterworth, 1977); IL (Saffran & Marin, 1975); MC (Caramazza, Basili, Koller, & Berndt, 1981); PV (Basso, Spinnler, Vallar, & Zanobia, 1982; Vallar & Baddeley, 1984a); EA (Friedrich, Glenn, & Marin, 1984); and TI (Saffran, 1985a) (Table 3.2).[2] Not all these patients were initially diagnosed using the WAIS. For MC, PV, and EA, aphasia batteries were used; PV also performed at a high level on Raven's Matrices, a non-verbal IQ test. However, the basic diagnostic principle was generally the same – a gross impairment on span-type tasks by contrast with other language and intelligence tasks, the comparison being based on quantitative results of standardised tests.[2]

The patients were similar only in the psychological nature of their impairment. The neurological origins of their difficulties were different: one (KF) had had a head injury; five had had strokes; and one (JB) had had a meningioma, previously removed at operation. Although their lesions had different causes, they were in

---

sive paper had just appeared, and it seemed to settle the relationship between short- and long-term memory, with the short-term store (or primary memory) the vehicle for the laying down of traces in long-term storage. Fortunately, I was rash enough to attempt to justify my theoretical conviction by collaboration on the investigation of the patient's impairment. It rapidly became apparent that the Hebbian position I held could not easily account for the dissociation. I became a convert to the empirical interest of neuropsychological data.

2. When later in the chapter, a phenomenon is described in one of the patients with no specific reference given, the source is one of these papers. For most syndromes discussed in later chapters, a similar set of reference papers will be given.

Table 3.2. *Level of impairment of STM patients*

	Numbers	Letters	Words	Additional major impairments
KF	2.3	1.8	2.3	Halting speech, deep dyslexia, spelling problems
JB	4.0	3.0	3.0	—
WH	2.9	2.5	2.4	Expressive speech problems
IL	3.6	2.0	2.5	—
MC	1.8	—	1.9	Naming and comprehension difficulties
PV	4.0	1.8	2.8	—
EA	2.0 (approx.)	2.0 (approx.)	<2	Spelling problems
TI	3.5	—	1.9	Halting speech, spelling problems

Note: Span is defined as string length where 50% of strings are correct.
From reference papers on the syndrome (see p. 42)

roughly the same part of the cortex.[3] The anatomical aspects of the disorder will not be considered further. The syndrome is, however, a case in which a rough localisation principle seems to operate.

3.2 Simple Alternative Explanations

An isolated deficit on span tasks does not necessarily imply that the patient has a specific memory impairment. The establishment of a dissociation is an empirical starting point, not a theoretical conclusion. The second stage in the establishment of a new syndrome must be to consider alternative explanations of the disorder and in this case, the possibility of an impairment to one of the non-memory processes required to perform the task. In general, which other processes are considered is guided by clinical knowledge of the kinds of impairments that can occur. Span tasks, however, are fairly simple. Only two other processes seem relevant: the perception of the words involved and the ability to produce them. As a minor complication, one needs to consider how these processes operate not just when single words are presented, but when words are presented at the rate used in the span task itself. It is possible, for instance, that the speech perception system might become refractory if stressed or might be able to operate only very slowly.

The relation between short-term memory and speech perception is a complex one about which there are varying opinions, as we will see later. Clinically, the patients comprehend speech fairly well, provided that simple syntactic constructions are used; thus a primary speech perception difficulty seems unlikely. The possibility

---

3. The left inferior parietal (particularly posterior) and the superior left temporal lobes (see, in particular, Warrington, Logue, & Pratt, 1971). For converging evidence on localisation using a quite different technique, see Ojemann (1978).

that the patients cannot repeat because they cannot perceive the words can be tested in a straightforward fashion using the same type of input that occurs in span tests. In our initial investigations, we simply presented the patients with strings of 30 words, 10 of which were in a given category. The words occurred at a rate of one per second, and the patients were asked to tap when they heard any word in that category. KF, JB, and WH detected 93%, 100%, and 100% of the targets.[4]

The complementary possibility is that the patients might be able to remember adequately in the span situation, but not be able to produce the words sufficiently easily. They might lose the trace during an effort to articulate the words. In fact, replacing the speaking of digit names by pointing to digits on cards did not alter span materially in any of the patients with whom it was tested: KF, JB, IL, PV, EA, and TI. The initial selective deficit of span performance has therefore been refined further. It cannot be simply and artefactually explained away as the consequence of an impairment of speech perception or speech production.

3.3   A Simple Theoretical Account of the Dissociation

The existence of a selective deficit is most easily explained by assuming that a particular subsystem (or subsystems) is damaged. To determine the function of the subsystem, it is necessary to refine the tasks used. A characteristic of the cognitive neuropsychology approach is to consider disorders in conjunction with the study of normal function, which in this case is short-term memory.

For a few years in the late 1960s, when the initial investigations were taking place, a fair degree of theoretical agreement existed on short-term memory. Models in which a number of different memory stores are postulated were becoming standard. Since then, the agreement has dissolved. Multi-store theories began to seem outdated in the 1970s (e.g. Craik & Lockhart, 1972), and the demise of 'short-term memory' was announced in the 1980s (Crowder, 1982b). The death, however, turned out to be of only the 'modal model', in which information was held to be transferred directly from a short-term store (STS) to a long-term store (LTS) (e.g. Waugh & Norman, 1965; Murdock, 1967). Moreover, the major competitor of the multi-store position – levels-of-processing theory – had itself begun to look sickly by the late 1970s (e.g. Baddeley, 1978).

In my view, the multi-store model remains adequate, although in a form different from the modal model of the 1960s. In particular, it still seems most plausible that a number of short-term stores exist, each with a specific cognitive function (e.g. Morton, 1970; Baddeley & Hitch, 1974); the idea of direct transfer from short- to long-term storage does, however, need to be discarded (see, e.g., Shallice & Warrington, 1970; Tulving & Madigan, 1970). I will return to these assumptions later.

---

4. It might be argued that this test is not adequate because top-down information might assist a patient with some form of perpetual difficulty in the identification of words in a specific category when words in general could not be identified. Digits and letters are, however, members of very restricted categories, so that this explanation could not be applied to the grossly impaired digit span and letter span findings. I will return to the issue of whether the perceptual process is intact.

For an initial interpretation of the syndrome, I will assume, with certain provisos, that the debates of the 1970s on short-term memory can be considered an elegant detour and that a multi-store framework is the most useful one.

Within such a framework, it seems most likely that auditory–verbal span performance involves primarily a single short-term store. If more than one store were involved, complex interactions among the variables that affect span would seem likely in normal subjects. For instance, if one store were affected by the phonological confusability of the stimuli and the other were not (e.g. a phonological and a central short-term store), the degree to which the two were used would probably vary with rate of presentation, and an interaction would be found. To explain the general absence of interactions found in their extensive study of the effect of a number of variables on span, Sperling and Speelman (1970) concluded that the main contribution did come from a single store.[5] I will call the storage system that seems to be primarily involved the auditory–verbal STS; it could, though, be called the phonological input buffer, as we will see.

What form would an impairment to this system take? One consequence would be rapid forgetting when effective retention depended on this system. An obvious experimental paradigm to test this is the Brown-Peterson procedure, in which the presentation of the information to be retained is followed by a brief but demanding filler task.[6] Both KF and PV were tested with only a single auditorily presented item, which gives perfect repetition in immediate recall. Both patients showed a striking loss of information about the single item after only a few seconds of Peterson-type distracting activity (see Warrington & Shallice, 1972; Basso et al., 1982) (Figure 3.1). This decline is considerably more than occurs when a single item is presented to normal subjects (Murdock, 1961).[7]

5. Further support for this position can be obtained from studies by Baddeley (1968) and Lyon (1977). Watkins and Watkins (1977) have produced strong evidence that performance is controlled by two systems, not one system, in a serial-recall paradigm apparently quite similar to span; lists of eight words had to be recalled in order. They therefore argued that the early part of the list is recalled from secondary memory (LTS) and the later part, from primary memory (STS). They related their findings to results from more typical eight-item span situations – for instance, those in which the stimuli are digits (e.g. Routh, 1976). In fact, the results are not comparable. Watkins and Watkins used four-syllable words for which mean span is only 4.6 words (e.g. Craik, 1968a). Thus their lists were well above span length. As a result, their middle three serial positions produced very poor performance, with error rates of roughly 90%, as compared with, say, 30% for digit stimuli (Routh, 1976). Given the great quantitative difference in the pattern of performance, there are no grounds for assuming a qualitative similarity across the two situations in the underlying mechanisms.
6. It is sometimes assumed that the rapid decline in performance in Brown-Peterson tasks may not be reflecting the loss of information in STS because of the 'proactive interference' effects that occur over the first few trials, which are attributable to LTS (e.g. Crowder, 1982b). However, if recall can be from either LTS or STS, then for forgetting to occur, it must not be possible to retrieve information from either store. Thus an LTS locus for the deterioration in performance over the first few trials is quite compatible with the Brown-Peterson decline within a trial reflecting loss of information in short-term storage.
7. A variety of Peterson-type tasks have been used with these patients. If recall at zero delay is not already at a very poor level, they show a rapid decline in performance with auditory presentation. They do not show these effects with visual presentation (see section 3.6).

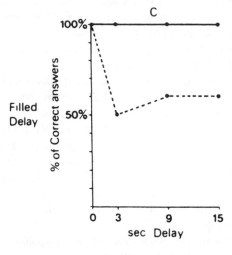

Figure 3.1. Brown-Peterson performance of short-term memory patient PV for 1 consonant in both auditory and visual modalities. The solid line is for visual input; the dotted line, for auditory. Reprinted from Basso, Spinnler, Vallar, and Zanobia (1982); *Neuropsychologia 20:* 268; by permission of Pergamon.

In addition to rapid forgetting, one would expect that the factors that affect the performance of normal subjects at the limits of their span should affect the patients when presented with much shorter list lengths. It is known that span is much influenced by phonological similarity, especially with respect to the order in which items are retrieved, and it is often argued that auditory–verbal STS is phonological in nature, with a strong temporal-ordering component (Conrad, 1964; Wickelgren, 1965; Baddeley, 1966; Healy, 1975; Lee & Estes, 1977).[8] STM patients are affected adversely by the use of phonologically similar material. With auditory presentation, an effect of phonological similarity was obtained with both KF (Warrington & Shallice, 1972) and PV. Thus with list lengths of two and three letters, PV was correct on 40% fewer of the lists in the phonologically similar condition than in the dissimilar condition. Using much longer lists, of six items, control subjects showed a virtually identical pattern; they were correct on 39% fewer of the similar than the dissimilar lists (Vallar & Baddeley, 1984a).

A second characteristic of normal performance when subjects reach the limit of their span is that order errors tend to be very frequent (Ryan, 1969). A similar effect occurred in the patients, but for much shorter lists. Thus on four-item lists, the

8. It is sometimes held that short-term stores also contain semantic information. Neuropsychological evidence that span does not depend on semantic processing will be provided in chapter 12. To preview the argument, 'semantic memory' patients showed no difference in span between known and unknown words (Warrington, 1975).

Table 3.3. *Performance of STM patients on tests of LTM*

	KF[a]	JB[b]	WH[b]	PV[c]	Control
Wechsler paired-associate learning (success score)	14	18	11	19	14.8
Ten-word learning (no. trials)	7	10	9	4	9
Warrington recognition memory (words correct)	—	45	—	—	45

[a] Warrington and Shallice (1969)
[b] Warrington, Logue, and Pratt (1971)
[c] Basso, Spinnler, Vallar, and Zanobia (1982)

percentage of order errors made by KF, JB, and WH was 40%, 17%, and 75%, respectively (combining over digits and letters) (see Shallice & Warrington, 1977a).[9]

3.4 The Dissociation Between Auditory–Verbal STS and LTS Performance

Another dissociation was what surprised us most when we first worked with these patients. They performed quite normally on a wide variety of tasks that tap long-term episodic memory, such as paired-associate learning, recalling a short story, learning 10 words given repeated presentation, and the 50-item forced-choice verbal recognition test discussed in chapter 2 (Table 3.3). If their long-term memory is spared, then on two-component memory tasks, in which measures of STS and LTS can be separately isolated, the deficit should be restricted to STS only.

It was often held that free recall of unrelated words is the standard test that allows this distinction to be made. Within a multi-store framework, the classic position was that the much better recall of the last few items compared with the earlier items that normal subjects show – the so-called recency effect – comes from these words still being represented in STS at the time of recall (e.g. Waugh & Norman, 1965; Glanzer & Cunitz, 1966).[10] The patients who have been tested on free recall are

9. The high rate of order errors is especially striking, given that it is often held that item information grows linearly with number of items, but order information grows factorially (Crossman, 1961; see also Crowder, 1979).
10. In the 1970s, it began to be argued that the recency effect in free recall does not reflect primarily retrieval from the short-term store also used in span (e.g. Baddeley & Hitch, 1977). In my view, although complications undoubtedly exist, there is considerable evidence that supports the classical view. Thus a number of experiments produce evidence that the information retrieved in the free-recall recency effect is primarily phonological, as is auditory–verbal STS (e.g. Craik, 1968b; Shallice, 1975; Glanzer, 1976; Broadbent, Vines, & Broadbent, 1978; Martin & Jones, 1979). At present, therefore, the simple classical assumption still seems more likely to be correct, although a considerable number of the anomalies still remain to be resolved.

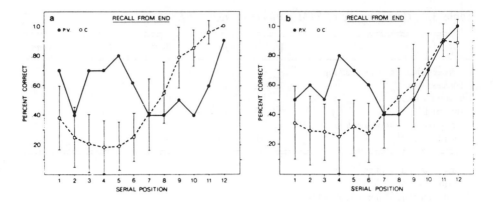

Figure 3.2. Free-recall performance of PV and control subjects for both (a) auditorily and (b) visually presented words. PV's recency effect with auditory is limited to the last item. The normal recency effect of PV with *visual* presentation relates to the preservation of visual STS in the STM patients, which is discussed in section 3.6. Subjects were instructed to try to remember the final words presented first. This produces a more reliable recency effect. Reprinted from Vallar and Papagno (1986) by permission of Academic Press.

KF, JB, WH, and PV. They showed a recency effect in immediate auditory free recall limited to at most one item (Figure 3.2). Comparison of immediate and delayed recall using a capacity estimation procedure devised by Baddeley (1970) shows them to have a normal long-term memory component.

It is useful to compare the performance of amnesic patients – discussed in chapter 2 – who have another type of memory problem, with that of the STM patients. It has long been known clinically that severely amnesic patients can repeat back even quite long sentences (e.g. Talland, 1965; Zangwill, 1966, case 1). Drachman and Arbit (1966) demonstrated in a more formal fashion that even though amnesics were far inferior to normal subjects, if required to learn supra-span lists, they did not differ from the controls on span. Figure 3.3 gives the performance of the amnesic patients studied by Baddeley and Warrington (1970) on free recall.

The performance of the STM patients and the amnesics form the two sides of a 'double dissociation' on the recency and non-recency parts of the curve. This is the first example that has been given of this methodological procedure, discussed in chapter 2. It is clear that the difference in performance between the two groups of patients cannot be explained by words in one or the other type of serial position being easier to retrieve. It is difficult not to conclude that two separable mechanisms are involved.

A simple conclusion is therefore compatible with both the 'negative' and the 'positive' arguments. Specific impairments of span appear to arise from damage to a phonologically based short-term store. Deficits in the other processes required for span performance cannot account for the result. In addition, the impairment has the

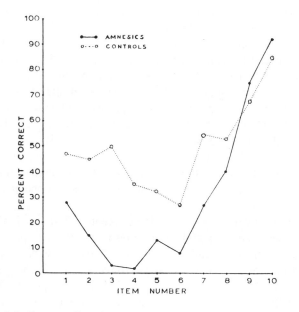

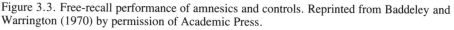

Figure 3.3. Free-recall performance of amnesics and controls. Reprinted from Baddeley and Warrington (1970) by permission of Academic Press.

characteristics that one would expect in the light of what is known of the operation of normal short-term memory.

3.5 More Complex Alternative Interpretations

This simple view did not go unchallenged. Whenever a potential new syndrome is isolated in neuropsychology, clinicians consider whether the impairment could be explained more simply in terms of conditions that have already been described. A critic of any interpretation of a neuropsychological patient is, however, in a difficult position. In other areas of science, if a critic feels that some factor in the explanation of an experiment has been overlooked, the experiment can be repeated with an appropriate variation included in order to test the importance of that factor. This is not, in general, a possible option for the neuropsychological critic, since the patient almost certainly has been tested in another place or at another time. The best empirical move that the critic can make is to find a patient who appears functionally similar to the one who is the subject of the dispute and to show that the criticism holds in regard to this second patient. This, however, leaves the critic open to the counter that the patients are not functionally equivalent in the appropriate respect.

The debate that developed within neuropsychology over the short-term memory syndrome illustrates this point well. It is not surprising that the interpretation of the impaired repetition performance of these patients in terms of a short-term memory problem was controversial. As discussed in chapter 1, the greatest feat of nine-teenth-century neuropsychology was the elaboration of the theory of specific apha-sias and the description of appropriate patients by Broca (1861), Wernicke (1874), and Lichtheim (1885). Central to their achievement was the identification of the syndrome of conduction aphasia, predicted by Wernicke and first described by Lichtheim. (On Figure 1.1, it corresponds to a disconnection at interruption point 3.) In the Wernicke–Lichtheim account, conduction aphasia had two main proper-ties. Spontaneous speech was held to be fluent but to contain 'literal paraphasias' (i.e. non-word utterances phonologically similar to the intended words). Much more important, the speech function that was held to be most impaired was repetition. Specific difficulties with span tasks therefore fit as neatly into the diagram-makers' category of conduction aphasia as into the information-processing conceptual ap-proach developed a century later.

This is not a matter of historical interest only! The conceptual framework of most later aphasiologists included a disorder with similarities to conduction aphasia, al-though it was frequently given a different name. By the 1970s, conduction aphasia was generally accepted in clinical practice as a syndrome (e.g. Goodglass & Ka-plan, 1972; Benson et al., 1973; Green & Howes, 1977), but interpretations still varied. It has been identified as a loss of inner speech, as in Goldstein's (1948) 'central aphasia'; as an impairment of the selection and in particular, of the ordering of phonemes in speech production (Dubois, Hécaen, Angelergues, Maufras De Chatelier, & Marcie, 1964); and even as a mild speech perception disorder (Kleist, 1916; see Stengel & Lodge Patch, 1955; Hécaen & Albert, 1978). The interpreta-tions differed, but they provided a rich set of frameworks within which to interpret what I have so far called STM patients.

Three types of alternative explanation were suggested from within a conduction aphasia conceptual framework.[11] Kinsbourne (1972) developed an explanation in the spirit of the classical Wernicke–Lichtheim theory. Tzortzis and Albert (1974), by contrast, argued from the Dubois et al. (1964) approach for a difficulty in the sequential programming of speech production. Finally, Strub and Gardner (1974) developed a position somewhat related to a combination of the positions of Gold-stein (1948) and Kleist (1916) – a central aphasic disorder involving the processing, synthesis, and ordering of phonemes.

Kinsbourne's (1972) modern version of the disconnection theory was based on his detailed study of two patients, JT and JO. Like the patients already discussed, JT and JO had very severe repetition difficulties. The span performance of JT was comparable with that of KF, his span being 1.75 digits. JO, though, was rather different. He could not repeat even one digit reliably or quickly, scoring only 73% with one digit and 45% with two. The starting point for Kinsbourne's alternative interpretation was an aspect of the performance of these two patients that much impressed him. They could perform well on judging whether two strings of four

---

11. Much later, a fourth alternative explanation was put forward by Allport (1984); it comes, however, from a very different theoretical tradition and will be discussed at the end of the chapter.

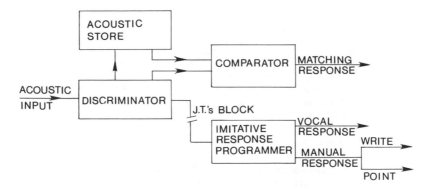

Figure 3.4. Kinsbourne's (1972) model of the locus of impairment in his conduction aphasic patients. I assume that information in the acoustic store can flow to the discriminator.

digits presented immediately one after the other were the same or different. One patient was 95% correct and the other, 80%. Both were perfect at the matching of two-digit strings. Kinsbourne therefore argued that his patients – and, by analogy, ours – did not have any critical impairment of short-term storage. Instead, he claimed that the problem consisted of the pathologically limited capacity of the communication channel by which information is passed from speech comprehension systems – including the acoustic store – to a response-programming system (Figure 3.4).

When one compares Kinsbourne's patients with patients like KF and JB, the importance of baseline tests is made clear. A striking characteristic is the lower overall level of their verbal IQ test scores, particularly that of JT, when compared with the STM patients (compare Table 3.4 with Table 3.1). Given how well they performed on some subtests, this is unlikely to be due to the patients' having had a low IQ prior to their illnesses.[12] The most plausible explanation is that the degree of speech production difficulties and/or general language difficulties is considerably greater than that of the patients with whom they are being compared. This can be clearly seen in the span performance of patient JO. Unlike for the earlier patients, there was a considerable improvement in his span when he was allowed to point to numbers instead of speaking them aloud (1.2 → 3.5). Thus JO's span difficulties do not speak to the interpretation of the patients discussed earlier in the chapter.

This leaves only the results of JT as potentially theoretically relevant. More

12. It is often an important clinical problem to assess the level of performance that might have been expected from patients before their illness (i.e. premorbidly). Occupation and education are rough guides. The WAIS subtest least affected by generalised brain damage is the Vocabulary subtest; it is often relatively preserved in dementing diseases (e.g. McFie, 1975; Nelson & McKenna, 1975). The best clinical measure available is the reading level of irregular words (in the absence of an acquired dyslexia disorder) (Nelson & O'Connell, 1978). This is even less affected than the Vocabulary subtest in dementing illnesses (see Nelson & McKenna, 1975; Nelson & O'Connell, 1978), probably because it requires only a low amount of cognitive 'resources' (see chapter 10).

Table 3.4. *WAIS subtest weighted scores of Kinsbourne's (1972) patients*

	JT	JO
Arithmetic	0	8
Similarities	0	3
Digit Span	0	1
Vocabulary	0	–
Picture Completion	11	9
Block Design	16	9
Picture Arrangement	13	11

detailed analysis of his performance indicates that there may well be a major STS component in JT's impairment. Thus presented with one item for recall, he was correct on 40/40 trials. Presented with two, but having to recall only the first, he obtained only 32/40, which is similar to his level of performance, 30/40, when having to recall both. This seems difficult for Kinsbourne's hypothesis to explain. The loading of the supposedly impaired transmission route is the same when only a single item and when the first of two items have to be recalled; in both cases, only one item has to be passed down it. The result can be simply explained on the basis of short-term memory theory in terms of the presentation of the second item reducing the trace strength of the first (e.g. Waugh & Norman, 1965).

What, however, is most critical is not the explanation of JT's disorder, but whether Kinsbourne's hypothesis will explain the impairment of the supposed STM patients.[13] A test that is clearly critical is a recognition-probe one, in which the subject has to decide whether a probe stimulus is or is not a member of the preceding string of stimuli. In that situation, as for matching, the transmission route has to provide information sufficient to program only a 'yes' or 'no' response – less than that necessary for single-digit recall. Three STM patients have been tested on this task, and all produced grossly abnormal levels of performance. KF made 35% errors on five-digit strings; JB, 37% errors on six-digit strings; and MC, 26% errors on four-word strings. The transmission-route theory cannot account for these results. In addition, the frequency of order errors and, more particularly, the rapid decline in retention over time in a Brown-Peterson task present grave problems for any inter-

---

13. For further analysis of JT's performance, see Shallice and Warrington (1977a). This article also discusses the anomalous matching result, on which his performance was not very different from one previously obtained with KF. In fact, matching appears to be a very easy test. The only occasion that the performance of such patients has been compared with that of controls was by Tzortzis and Albert (1974) for their conduction aphasic patients, to be discussed shortly. For two of their patients (C2, C3), matching performance was similar to that of JT and KF, but considerably worse than that of two *aphasic* controls. Thus no evidence exists that patients of this type have normal performance on this test.

pretation of the STM patients in terms of Kinsbourne's disconnection hypothesis. Thus it is not a tenable explanation for the STM patients.

The recognition probe and the Brown-Peterson results present equal problems for a very different explanation of specific span deficits, which was put forward by Tzortzis and Albert (1974). They argued that the deficit can arise from an impairment in the memory for the order of sequences, being led to their hypothesis because of the frequency of order errors in reduced span performance. Yet not all span errors are order errors, and frequent errors of that type are just what the short-term memory theory would predict, as discussed earlier. Order is, in any case, an irrelevant factor in probe-recognition tasks, in single-item Brown-Peterson recall, and in free recall, on all of which the STM patients are impaired. This alternative also seems implausible.

Strub and Gardner (1974) presented two further arguments against the STM hypothesis. Both were derived from the performance of a patient, LS, whose deficit had many characteristics in common with those of the STM patients. Presented with a pair of words to recall, he was successful on 53% of trials if there was a 2-sec gap between them, but on only 20% of trials if there was only a 0.5-sec gap. As span is relatively independent of rate of presentation in normal subjects (e.g. Sperling & Speelman, 1970), this result seems unexpected on the STM hypothesis. In fact, KF had shown an even more striking effect of this type – an improvement from 7% to 73% when going from the 0.5-sec to the 2-sec condition in two-item recall. However, when letters were used instead of words, he showed a much smaller improvement – from 17% to 40%. Why should this be? We had argued that it was because words, being meaningful, benefit more from long-term storage than do letters. Glanzer and Cunitz (1966) had clearly shown that although a slower rate of presentation does not affect the ability to retrieve information from short-term storage, it increases the amount retrieved from long-term storage. So the effect of rate of presentation on span is easily explained if one assumes that the patients make a disproportionate use of LTS in the span situation. Moreover, as Saffran and Marin (1975) pointed out, an abnormal reliance on long-term retrieval in the span situation would lead to problems in nonsense-syllable recall, which has been found with IL and EA and was used by Strub and Gardner as a second criticism of the STM theory. The criticisms of the STM theory made by Strub and Gardner therefore do not seem strong.

In this section, readers may have felt themselves in a thicket of detailed arguments based as much on the history of how debate on the syndrome developed as on what they need to know about it now. This very complexity, though, is important to illustrate. It is an almost inevitable consequence of considering competing interpretations of a syndrome. If two or more patients are being discussed, one always needs to consider whether their impairments are functionally equivalent. Clinical information, such as that obtained with baseline tests, and clinical knowledge of syndromes become as relevant as the detailed experimental results obtained.

One needs to hack a path through the thicket for another reason too. To draw theoretical conclusions about normal function from neuropsychology, one needs fairly secure effects. We have seen that in the past, neuropsychologists were continually in dispute about the existence of relatively basic disorders. Unless the internal neuropsychological arguments can be seen to be countered, one can hardly expect those interested in normal function to pay much attention to clinical claims.

3.6   General Theoretical Inferences

If it is accepted that specific span deficits do arise from damage to a particular short-term memory system, does the syndrome provide any reliable information about how that system operates in the normal subject? Indeed, it can tell us more than might be expected. Again, the key is the use of dissociations. Any function that dissociates from the span deficit must require little of the particular short-term memory resource that the span utilises. In this context, six different functions, at least, are of interest: long-term memory, general cognitive abilities, visual short-term memory, non-verbal auditory short-term memory, speech production, and speech perception. However, to present the evidence on only the different dissociations that exist would show that the approach has the potential to produce interesting theoretical conclusions, but it would provide no check on the reliability of the methodology. I will therefore also briefly discuss arguments from the normal literature that point to similar theoretical conclusions; in general, they were produced independently and later in time.

When short-term memory patients were first being investigated, their preserved long-term memory performance seemed the most surprising aspect of the syndrome. In models of the period – now conflated as the 'modal model' – it was assumed that the length of time that information remained in STS was critical for transfer to LTS (e.g. Waugh & Norman, 1965; Atkinson & Shiffrin, 1968). If the amount of information that could be stored in short-term memory was greatly reduced, then information would generally remain in STS for a much shorter time and so weaker long-term traces would be laid down. The LTM performance of the STM patients was difficult to reconcile with any simple version of the modal model. The obvious neuropsychological inference was that input to the LTS did not require STS (e.g. Shallice & Warrington, 1970). Elegant experiments on normal subjects performed soon afterwards also showed that the transfer assumption was invalid (e.g. Craik & Watkins, 1973). Thus normal and neuropsychological evidence was in agreement that the serial-store notion was incorrect.[14] The theory developed from the neuropsychological evidence incorporated the now-classical relation between the phonological and semantic type of processing and the different durations that the traces created last (e.g. Baddeley, 1966; Geiselman, Woodward, & Beatty, 1982) (Figure 3.5).[15]

14. Tulving and Patterson (1968) had earlier questioned the assumption on the basis of findings on normal subjects.
15. The normal experimental evidence was, however, generally interpreted in terms of levels-of-processing theory (Craik & Lockhart, 1972). Their objection to multi-store models was not based on just the transfer problem. For discussion of other critical points, such as the evidence for short-term storage of semantic information (Shulman, 1970) and problems of capacity, see Shallice (1975, 1979a). For more general criticisms of levels-of-processing theory, see Baddeley (1978).

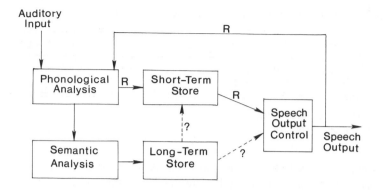

Figure 3.5. Shallice and Warrington's (1970) theory of the relation between the STS and the LTS involved in auditory–verbal recall. *R* refers to the rehearsal loop.

If a view fairly close to the 1960s position still seems appropriate from the neuropsychological perspective for the existence of a short-term store separate from a long-term one, is the same true about whether the short-term store is unitary? It is not. A fairly consistent characteristic of the STM patients is that their ability to retain verbal information presented visually over short intervals is much superior to their auditory–verbal STS capacities (Table 3.5; see Figure 3.1). Moreover, for visual presentation, the pattern of performance was very different from that of normal subjects. For PV, there was no effect of the phonological similarity between the letters in a list and the number recalled and no effect of preventing rehearsal by using so-called articulatory suppression (Vallar & Baddeley, 1982); the errors that KF made showed visual, not phonological, similarity effects (Warrington & Shallice, 1972). The pattern is simply explained if the patients have a visual STS that is larger in capacity than their impaired auditory STS. They would therefore make no attempt to transfer information to the auditory store by sub-vocalising, as normal subjects have long been known to do (e.g. Conrad, 1964; Sperling, 1967).

Within cognitive psychology, the idea that a separate visual short-term store exists is far from novel (e.g. Margrain, 1967; Sperling, 1967). There is now good evidence that even for verbal material, a sizeable short-term store can be used that is distinct from the standard phonological one (e.g. Broadbent, Vines, & Broadbent, 1978; Salamé & Baddeley, 1982). However, these authors point out that it is not clear whether it stores the products of visual processing or the results of some more central analysis.[16] Indeed, the direct evidence from STM patients that the store they use is purely visual is somewhat slender, being the visual errors made by KF. However, if the information in the intact store is not in visual (or orthographic) form, it is difficult to see why the STM patients cannot use it to retain auditorily presented material. In general, though, there is again a pleasing convergence of evidence from 'normal' and neuropsychological investigations.

16. The elegant experiments of Phillips and Christie (1977) show clearly that visual *non-verbal* short-term storage is separate from, say, auditory–verbal short-term storage.

Table 3.5. *Auditory and visual digit span for STM patients*

	KF	JB	WH	IL	MC	PV	EA	TI[a]
Auditory	2.3	4.0	2.9	3.6	1.8	4.0	<2	3.5
Visual	3.0	>4	>4	>5	>3	4.5	2.4	3.5

[a] TI is assumed to have a double deficit.
From reference papers on the syndrome (see p. 42)

Returning to the system that normal subjects use in span tasks, can the STM patients provide evidence about its function and contents? A common view is that it is a large, longer lasting echoic store or sensory register (e.g. Broadbent, 1971, 1984; Broadbent et al., 1978). If this were the case, then a deficit of auditory STS should show up for non-verbal as well as for verbal auditory material. We investigated the ability of KF and JB to remember sets of three familiar sounds presented at a one per 3-sec rate (Shallice & Warrington, 1974). To prevent controls gaining an advantage by saying the names of the sounds to themselves, the experiment was run under articulatory-suppression conditions – that is, subjects counted rapidly to themselves. The big difference between the patients and the controls that exists when three letters are presented in the same sort of situation no longer exists when familiar sounds are used (see Figure 3.6). Also, normal subjects perform significantly worse with sounds than with letters, so the phenomenon is not simply a ceiling effect. We concluded that the damaged store was used only by speech input.

This is one of the few cases where evidence appears not to be consistent from one STS patient to another. Tzortzis and Albert (1974) found a deficit in their conduction aphasics in the reproduction of sequences of taps. However, articulatory suppression was not used in their experiments, so no allowance was made for the assistance that normal subjects obtain from verbal mediation and rehearsal. Indirect support that this is an important factor comes from a test developed by Friedrich et al. (1984) on EA. Using random sequences of one or the other of two tones occurring at a two per 1-sec rate – too fast for effective sub-vocalising – EA scored within the normal range at reproducing sequences of six tones by tapping them out.

Converging evidence that the primary store for span is speech-specific comes from a variety of experiments on normal subjects. The most direct analogue is the comparison between short-term memory for words and for familiar sounds. In a serial-probe task, the subject has to give the item in the stimulus list that occurs immediately after the probe. Subjects perform much worse when the stimuli are familiar sounds than when they are words; this effect occurs in situations where free recall gives equivalent results for the two types of material (Philipchalk & Rowe, 1971; Rowe, 1974). Rowe therefore suggested that short-term memory for familiar sounds does not use the order-based short-term store that verbal material uses.

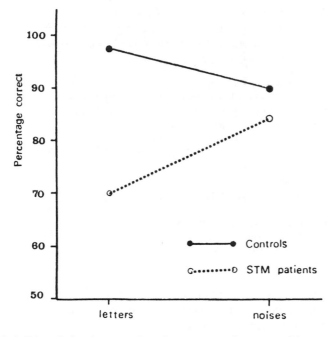

Figure 3.6. Dissociation between three-item span performance of letters and familiar non-verbal sounds between two STM patients and controls. Reprinted from Shallice and Warrington (1974); *Neuropsychologia 12:* 554; by permission of Pergamon.

3.7 The STS Deficit: Speech Production or Comprehension?

Both the comprehension and the production of speech require that information be retained at a phonological level over short periods of time. Many models presuppose that a representation related to 'surface structure' continues until clause and sentence comprehension is completed. In a complementary fashion, it is often assumed that the smooth flow of spontaneous speech requires that prior to articulation, the utterance be preserved in a compiled form in a buffer. It is therefore plausible that one or more specific short-term stores have evolved to perform these functions and that they can be selectively damaged. Indeed, many have suggested that the stores underlying span may have one or both of these language-related functions. Does neuropsychological evidence help select between these alternatives?

If the store primarily involved in span were the phonological holding mechanism required for speech production – say, Morton's (1970) 'output buffer' – then the STM patients should show considerable difficulties in spontaneous speech. One would expect them to exhibit a trade-off between making many phoneme-ordering errors and having much shorter phrase length with many pauses. In fact, this pattern corresponds quite closely to the classical clinical descriptions of conduction aphasia (e.g. Benson et al., 1973). 'Fluent with literal paraphasias' is the standard account,

Table 3.6. *Spontaneous speech of STM patients*

KF[a]	Halting; word-finding difficulties; circumlocutions; paraphasias rare
JB[b]	Fluent; virtually normal
WH[c]	Dysphasic
IL[d]	Minimal expressive difficulty
MC[e]	Fluent; 'moderate word-finding difficulties and paragrammatism'
PV[f]	Fluent; 'a few phonemic paraphasias and word-finding difficulties'
EA[g]	Fluent, with 'occasional phonemic paraphasic errors'
TI[h]	Fluent but hesitant; 'occasional literal paraphasias'

[a]Warrington and Shallice (1969)
[b]Shallice and Butterworth (1977)
[c]Warrington, Logue, and Pratt (1971)
[d]Saffran and Marin (1975)
[e]Caramazza, Basili, Koller, and Berndt (1981)
[f]Basso, Spinnler, Vallar and Zanobia (1982)
[g]Friedrich, Glenn, and Marin (1984)
[h]Saffran (1985a)

but excessive pausing and self-corrections also often occur. In conduction aphasia, the literal paraphasic errors typically consist of the reordering, omission, or addition of correctly pronounced phonemes (Dubois et al., 1964; Lecours & Rouillon, 1976).

Certain authors have indeed argued that the storage system impaired in patients with STM deficits is concerned with speech production (e.g. Tzortzis & Albert, 1974). However, the spontaneous speech of the STM patients described earlier is not consistently of the type clinically associated with conduction aphasia (Table 3.6). Indeed, three of the patients – JB, IL, and PV – had clinically normal or near-normal speech. Thus JB, who worked as a secretary, sounded quite normal to the clinician's ear. This was confirmed by a statistical analysis of her speech (Shallice & Butterworth, 1977). She was asked to describe her most recent holiday. Normal subjects are rather consistent in the proportion of speech time that consists of pauses, and they constituted 35% of JB's speech, by comparison with a mean of 37% for the controls. Her pauses were of mean length of 171 msec, by comparison with the normal mean of 163 msec. Her error rate was also completely normal, except for a slight increase in function-word errors (0.6 per minute, by comparison with 0.1 per minute for the controls). More critically, there were no literal paraphasias in this sample of her speech.

The normal quality of her speech – in particular, the absence of literal paraphasic errors and the normal rate of word production and pausing – suggests that any stores involved in speech production are intact. Therefore, from the dissociation principle, it would be inferred that the store involved in span is not a subcomponent of the speech production system. It could be argued instead that span merely requires much more of this resource than does spontaneous speech. This would, however, presuppose that a greater amount of the resource had developed or evolved than is required, which seems implausible.

Table 3.7. *Percentage of words recalled in Levy's (1971) study*

Presentation	Subject's activity	
	Repetition	Suppression
Auditory *and* visual	41	39
Visual alone	37	20

Note: Words were presented either in both modalities simultaneously or in only the visual modality. During presentation of each eight-letter list, subjects either repeated the presented words or continued saying 'Hi-ya' – the articulatory suppression condition.

If the store involved in span is not part of the speech output system, then patients who are typical of the classical symptom complex of conduction aphasia presumably have a 'mixed' syndrome involving two components. Their impairment would affect not only the auditory–verbal STS, but also part of the speech production system, possibly an output buffer or what Butterworth (1980) has called the phonological assembly system.[17] Indeed, a cluster analysis of the performance on language tests of a large group of aphasics suggests that not all patients classified as conduction aphasic have the same disorder (see Kertesz & Phipps, 1977).

This means that it should be possible to isolate at least two different deficits of repetition. Interesting in this respect is a report of Damasio and Damasio (1980) on a number of patients diagnosed as conduction aphasic according to the Boston Aphasia Battery diagnostic classification (Goodglass & Kaplan, 1972). All were said to have fluent, meaningful aphasic speech, in which phonemic paraphasias predominated, and a profound inability to reproduce verbal material correctly, although details were not given. Three of these patients, however, had digit spans of seven, and two had spans of six. Thus there is a strong suggestion that a dissociation complementary to that of STM patients exists, since phonemic paraphasias can occur in speech production in a patient who has an intact span.

The classical symptom complex of conduction aphasia appears to *fractionate* into at least two more basic functional syndromes. One – an impairment of STS – involves a specific inability to repeat a series of short, high-frequency items, or span. The other disorder – to the phonological assembly system – is an inability to *reproduce,* either in spontaneous speech or by imitation a long low-frequency word, even though span for short, highly familiar items is intact (see Shallice & Warrington, 1977a; Allport, 1984). The characteristics of both syndromes point to the primary auditory–verbal short-term store *not* being involved in speech production. Evidence from the normal literature is now leading to the same conclusion.

In the 1960s, the debate about whether the code involved in the phonological-

---

17. It may also involve the transmission routes between the input and the output systems, as will be seen in chapter 7.

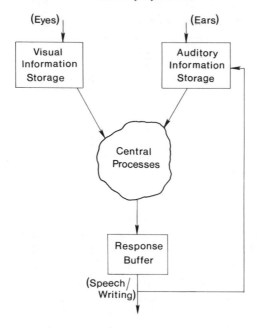

Figure 3.7. Sperling's (1967) theory of the retention of visually presented material in short-term memory. Suppression would preempt the use of the response buffer.

similarity effect was auditory or articulatory was not resolved. However, in 1971, Levy showed that articulatory suppression – in this case, continually saying 'Hi-ya' – produces a severe decrement in span if presentation is just visual. It also reduces the effect of phonological similarity (see also Murray, 1968). However, these effects do not occur if auditory input is used (Table 3.7). One simple interpretation is that subjects use inner speech based on sub-vocalisation to transfer visually analysed information to the auditory–verbal store. This is the old explanation of Sperling (1967) (Figure 3.7) for the effect of phonological similarity on visual span for letters with his 'Auditory Information Storage' made more specific. Levy (1971), however, suggested that the visual information is transferred only to an articulatory store and is interfered with there by suppression but that there is a separate auditorily based input store.

A series of experiments by Salamé and Baddeley (1982) makes the second position implausible. The phenomenon in which they were interested is one originally explored by Colle and Welsh (1976): speech to which the subject does not need to attend produces powerful interference on the short-term recall of *visually* presented information. Salamé and Baddeley showed in a number of ways that the effect cannot be caused by mere distraction. It is clearly easier to explain on the basis of Sperling's position than of Levy's.[18]

18. A possible explanation on the basis of Levy's (1971) position would be that auditorily presented words could preempt the articulatory system, by analogy with the effects of delayed auditory feedback, and so produce interference in the articulatory system. However, Salamé and Baddeley (1982)

The reader may well be wondering if there is any cognitive function that does not dissociate from a specific span deficit. If that were the case, the auditory–verbal short-term store would seem to have no function! In neuropsychology, it is logically impossible to obtain conclusive evidence that a dissociation does not occur. And six or so patients is a somewhat small sample from which to draw generalisations. The absence of a dissociation – or, to be more positive, the existence of an association between symptoms – is therefore always provisional.

There is one prime candidate for an association with a span deficit – a subtle impairment within the speech comprehension process. For a century, it had been assumed that conduction aphasic patients had intact comprehension. They could understand questions and instructions and take part in conversations seemingly with complete understanding.[19] The most salient aspect of the sentence comprehension of STM patients is, indeed, its normality. JB, for instance, is able to work as a secretary, a job that makes heavy demands on language comprehension. In line with the assumption that the damaged store is phonological, it was found when IL, JB, and MC were tested that they can retain the gist but not the surface structure of many sentences. Thus Saffran and Marin's (1975) pioneering study on IL included examples such as *The residence was located in a peaceful neighbourhood* being repeated as *The residence was situated in a quiet district*.

Sentences with a heavy information load, however, can defeat the comprehension abilities of the patients. Thus the Token Test of De Renzi and Vignolo (1962) requires subjects to perform an action like 'put the red circle between the yellow square and the green square.' It was performed at below-normal levels by all STM patients with whom it was used – namely, KF, JB, WH, MC, PV, and EA. When one turns to syntax, the situation is more complex. If the string is shorter than sentence span, then, as one would expect, a 'pure' STM patient shows no problem. Thus on the syntactic-comprehension test of Parisi and Pizzamiglio (1970), which assesses comprehension of word order, function words, and affixes, PV scored at a normal level (98% correct) (Vallar & Baddeley, 1984b). PV had a sentence span of about 6 words, and the mean length of the test sentences was 5.1 words.

When the test sentences exceed sentence span, however, syntactic processing

---

found that short words produced an effect identical to that of long ones, although they would preempt the articulatory system for only half the time. The classic Sperling (1967) position therefore seemed both the simplest and the most plausible explanation. In an interesting paper, Ellis (1979a) argued for an output-buffer locus for span. He showed that a number of properties of the errors that occur in the immediate recall of syllable strings are analogous to those found in speech errors. However, he failed to discuss why errors arising from the use of a phonological *input* store would not be expected to have similar characteristics.

19. Group studies of patients diagnosed as conduction aphasics have found them to have a subtle comprehension difficulty somewhat similar to that found in Broca's aphasia (Caramazza & Zurif, 1976; Heilman & Scholes, 1976; chapter 7). If the meaning can be inferred from the major lexical items in a sentence alone (e.g. *The apple the boy is eating is juicy*), then the comprehension of conduction aphasics is good. However, Caramazza and Zurif found that performance was at chance when syntactic processing is essential (e.g. *The boy that the girl is chasing is tall*). It is not, however, clear whether the problem can be characterised as an associated deficit.

Table 3.8. *Effect of semantic reversibility and the presence or absence of an introductory clause on repetition of passive sentences in IL*

| | Response sentences | | | |
Meaning	Passive Correct	Active Correct	Reversed	Incomplete —
Original sentence				
1 Clause: not reversible	9	0	0	1
1 Clause: reversible	6	0	2	2
2 Clauses: not reversible	3	7	0	0
2 Clauses: reversible	3	0	6	1

Adapted from Saffran and Marin (1975)

can give difficulty. Thus reversible sentences have been found to be more difficult to understand using a picture–sentence matching test than are non-reversible sentences by IL and MC, both of whom have shorter spans than PV. Table 3.8 shows the effect of an introductory clause and the semantic reversibility of a sentence on whether gist is preserved in sentence repetition. There is clearly an overall sentence-complexity factor.

A somewhat related effect was obtained by Vallar and Baddeley (1984b) in PV. Long sentences, per se, offered no problem to PV. Thus the silliness of long sentences such as *It is true that physicians comprise a profession that is manufactured in factories from time to time* could be detected as well by her as by normal subjects (93% correct). However, the situation was different if she was presented with sentences that are long and syntactically quite complex and in which semantically reversible nouns are switched. An example would be *One cannot reasonably claim that sailors are often lived on by ships of various kinds.* PV could not determine whether the result was meaningless or not (61% correct, by comparison with 83% in the controls).

As an added complication, Saffran (1985a), working with TI, discovered a dissociation between performance with picture–sentence matching or semantic-anomaly detection, on the one hand, and grammaticality judgements, on the other. Thus on detecting the *semantic* anomaly in sentences like *It was the bird that the worm swallowed,* TI was only 66% correct, by comparison with 90% for patients with right hemisphere lesions. However, he scored 85% correct on detecting the ungrammatical nature of sentences like *He let an old friend of his from out of town to drive the new car.* Here, the critical words (e.g. *let* and *to*) are separated by nine words. Moreover, lexical information about *let* must be being retained; if it were replaced by, say, *allowed,* which would preserve the sense, the sentence would no longer be ungrammatical. TI's performance was within the range of scores produced by right hemisphere control patients.

How are these patterns of findings to be explained? One possibility, espoused by

Butterworth, Campbell, and Howard (1986), is that the phonological STS is 'not necessary for sentence comprehension' (p. 204).[20] The difficulties that STM patients have could just be additional deficits. This seems unlikely because problems do not occur unless sentence span is exceeded.

There are a number of ways in which a short-term store could aid speech comprehension. The results make implausible the simplest position, that sentence comprehension depends on a working memory in which phonological representations are initially lodged and later replaced by propositions (e.g. Clark & Clark, 1977). PV's good performance on long padded sentences and TI's on grammaticality judgements are difficult to reconcile with this position.

A second possibility is that phonological representations are stored separately from the results of later syntactic and semantic analysis and are required for specific types of syntactic operations. Thus the Associated Transition Network framework of Wanner and Maratsos (1978) contains two different processes, for which temporary storage of relatively unprocessed information is required to obtain the correct syntactic interpretation. One is when the initial sequential attempt to parse the sentence fails. The system then backs up and reassigns syntactic functions. So in the example *The old train the young, train* is initially parsed as a noun; but when subsequent words make this interpretation untenable, it is reassigned as a verb. The second process, involving a temporary representation called HOLD, is used in the interpretation of relative clauses. A copy of the head noun phrase is placed on HOLD until the place in the clause (x) when its syntactic function for the clause can be assigned. For instance, in *The problem that the girl talked to the teacher about* (x) *is . . . ,* the noun phrase *the problem* is maintained in HOLD until after eight or more words have been interpreted.

The idea that the major function of the phonological store is to maintain information at the lexical level until such time as its syntactic role can be assigned is, however, made somewhat implausible by Saffran's (1985a) findings on grammaticality judgements. There the difficulty appeared to arise in the use of the compiled versions, not in the syntactic operations themselves. There is, however, a third possibility, that the store has a back-up function but not principally for syntactic operations; rather, it has a general-purpose back-up role in comprehension. For instance, the on-line compiling of an utterance into representations of its meaning is probably limited in the amount of new information – say, the number of propo-

---

20. They adopted this position as a result of an investigation of a student, RE, who had a developmental STM impairment, a digit span of only four, and yet no demonstrable comprehension deficits. In general, developmental disorders will not be considered in this book; there are plausible grounds for assuming that a developmental impairment will lead to other systems developing differently and to the subject utilising unusual strategies. However, in any case, the relative mildness of the disorder makes functional inferences dangerous. RE could at times repeat sentences of more than 15 words correctly (27%, as compared with 61% for *student* controls). This is far better than any STM patient considered so far and ample for most possible comprehension operations. For a more complex position which is roughly intermediate between that adopted by Butterworth, Campbell, and Howard (1986) and the position adopted in this chapter, see Caplan, Vanier, and Baker (1986).

sitions – that can be retained. If too much novel detail is being compressed into the utterance, a second pass would be needed; it, in turn, would require a back-up store. Additionally, it could have the function of aiding any form of higher level processing when, say, parts of the utterance are masked by noise or when attention was originally focused on some other activity – situations that frequently occur. If the store had this general role, it would tend to develop certain syntactic functions, such as facilitating any back-up requirement. These would not, however, be primary.

On this third view, the difference between grammaticality judgements and, say, sentence–picture matching could be that the sentence–picture matching requires a number of operations. In particular, a precisely compiled representation of the sentence must be retained over the time that the group of pictures is scanned. If there is any hiccup in these later processes, the normal subject can start again from the stored phonological representation. The STM patient cannot. Grammaticality judgements, by contrast, can be based on immediate on-line responses. This view is in accord with Vallar and Baddeley's (1984b) analysis of PV and the Token Test findings on a number of the patients.

How does the idea that a phonological input store has a speech comprehension function relate to findings on normal subjects? In normal subjects, retention of the literal representation of speech is known to be strongly subject to interference from subsequent speech, even when gist can be recalled (Sachs, 1967; Johnson-Laird & Stevenson, 1970). However, the amount hanging suspended in literal form is fairly substantial (Jarvella, 1971, 1979; Glanzer, Dorfman, & Kaplan, 1981). Glanzer et al. (1981), for instance, using sentences of 7.5 words, showed that the last sentences in passages were perfectly recalled, as were over half of the penultimate ones. There was, however, very little literal recall of the sentence before that. If the auditory–verbal STS is not useful for comprehension, it is difficult to see why literal recall of that duration should be possible in a speech-specific store.

Certain characteristics of auditory–verbal STM as known from memory research clearly fit with the idea that it is a relatively low-level back-up store for speech comprehension. These include the effects on span of phonological confusability (Baddeley, 1968) and word length (Baddeley, Thomson, & Buchanan, 1975) and the strong representation of order information (e.g. Healy, 1975). There does, though, appear to be a problem. It is often claimed that the short-term store holds only two to three items (e.g. Glanzer, 1972), which is a useless amount for comprehension purposes. In fact, such estimates come from the use of the recency effect in free recall, which is a particularly unsuitable means for measuring the capacity of a speech-related store.[21] Overall, a speech comprehension function for the phono-

21. The strategy being used by a typical subject towards the end of a free-recall list is oriented towards the meaning of the words and is not designed to utilise auditory–verbal STS effectively; it is not a form of maintenance rehearsal (see Shallice, 1975). Even span is likely to provide an underestimate of STS capacity usable in speech comprehension. Partially degraded phonological information may be sufficient to complete the semantic and syntactic construction of a sentence, but it is too weak to support retrieval of an isolated word in span. Moreover, the stimulus in span is an unnatural staccato series of words uttered in a monotone, lacking many of the retrieval cues potentially available in continuous speech. If the short-term store has a speech comprehension function, then it should be possible to use other cues to aid retrieval in addition to the one preserved in span – order. In fact,

logical buffer fits with the normal memory literature and with the neuropsychological evidence. The precise role that the auditory–verbal STS plays in speech comprehension, however, remains an open question.

3.8   An Anomaly

Neuropsychology would not be psychology if there were not a few complications
for this tidy picture. A basic challenge to the position taken in this chapter has been
made by Allport (1984). Allport accepts that the primary auditory–verbal STS is
part of the speech perception system but argues that it should not be considered to
be a subsystem separate from the processes involved in the ongoing phonological
categorisation of the speech input – a view related to levels-of-processing theory
(see also Crowder, 1982b). It should be underlined that Allport's position is very
different from the one dismissed earlier in the chapter. Allport is not arguing that
JB has a poor span *because* she fails to perceive the words.[22] His view is more
subtle. He is claiming that no modular distinction should be drawn between the
systems involved in phonological processing in word perception and the type of
short-term storage that maintains a transitory phonological trace. For him, the STM
deficit is a more sensitive sign of damage to the system than are most direct tests of
phonological processing in perception.

His evidence was derived primarily from a study of JB, who, he argued, has a
general phonological-processing problem. Most of the evidence he cites does not
favour this view over that of a deficit specific to STM. For instance, he found that
JB was unable to perform same–different matching with nonsense syllables satisfactorily when the different pairs differed by only one distinctive feature; she made
26% errors. This he views as a phonological-processing problem. However, Saffran
and Marin (1975) had already pointed out that a deficit in retaining nonsense syllables is to be expected with a severely impaired auditory–verbal STS.[23]

some of these types of cues have already been shown to affect STM capacity. Thus Glanzer (1976)
found that speaking word lists with intonation increased capacity, although admittedly he was using
recency as a measure. Frankish (1985) has shown that adding pauses, even of very short duration,
in order to produce grouping, facilitates retrieval. The increased pauses that Frankish used to induce
grouping mirror very well the increases in word duration used as syntactic boundary markers in
continuous speech. If a possible speech comprehension function is taken seriously, the apparent
problem of capacity dissolves.

22. Many of the experiments discussed later in the chapter support the earlier conclusions, including
this one. For instance, the preservation of gist, but not of surface structure, is an elegant demonstration that the memory difficulties of these patients are not just a consequence of a failure to perceive.

23. A second point that Allport raises – the occasional inability of JB to reproduce single infrequent
abstract words (she scored 44/50 in my unpublished data) – is also not relevant. In order to reproduce a word, a patient with an impaired STM will tend to rely either on semantic mediation or on
the direct input–output lexical connection. A word-reproduction error requires that the use of both
routes should not be effective on that trial and that the patient cannot use STM. The error then
becomes equivalent to an error in reproducing a nonsense syllable, so the point relates to the one
discussed in the text. Friedrich, Glenn, and Marin (1984) have made a general argument similar to
that of Allport, so, again, the difficulty their patient, EA, had on these tasks could arise from her
short-term memory difficulty.

The one finding of Allport's that was not clearly confounded by the tests having an obvious STM loading concerned JB's performance on lexical decision – deciding whether a stimulus is or is not a word. He used auditorily presented low-frequency words and 'distractors' that differed from a word by only one distinctive feature on only one consonant. JB missed 20% of distractors, compared with 8% by normal controls, and she made 7% false positive errors on the words, whereas the controls made hardly any. It is, however, possible that to detect a mispronunciation in a word reliably requires that one should at times internally replay the word, and a short-term storage deficit would lead to trouble in this process. The finding does suggest, though, that JB has a mild phonological-processing problem. Auditory lexical decision is a difficult task for patients, and JB's deficit is at most mild. It would seem likely that many patients with much larger spans than JB would have this level of deficit, but this remains to be shown.

Evidence from other patients is conflicting (Vallar & Baddeley, 1984a). EA showed a less sharp categorical boundary in a so-called voice-onset time analysis than do normal subjects; her phonetic categories for stop consonants were held to be more 'fuzzy'. However, much more critically, PV was perfect (60/60) on same–different matching of consonant–vowel pairs that differed by one or two distinctive features. Allport might argue that consonant–vowel pairs impose less general strain on the phonological processing than does a syllable. However, the dissociation seen in PV seems strong evidence against his position.[24] It remains quite conceivable, if not very likely, that Allport is correct that short-term storage processes are so inextricably mixed up with on-line-processing ones that no clear split can be made between the two.[25] The essential point remains that the neuropsychological evidence points to the existence of an auditory–verbal short-term store as an integral part of the speech perception system.

3.9   Conclusion

In this chapter, I have looked at a single syndrome in considerable detail. One reason has been to give the reader a flavour of the many levels on which arguments in cognitive neuropsychology must necessarily operate. However, one additional general point can be made. The conclusion reached about short-term memory from the neuropsychological evidence may not seem particularly surprising from the perspective of the recent literature in cognitive psychology. Both sets of evidence give short-term storage a much less central place in cognition than was customary in about 1970. However, over the past 15 years, human experimental psychology has contained many widely different views about short-term memory. For instance, one

24. A result similar to that found in PV has been obtained by Berndt (personal communication). From a theoretical perspective, one would expect that the function of short-term storage would help determine its properties. Auditory–verbal short-term storage has very different characteristics from, say, visual STS. It does not seem likely to be merely an epiphenomenal after-effect of the mechanisms that categorise words phonologically.

25. Structures intermediate between modular and non-modular ones are discussed in chapter 11.

fashionable position was that it is related to consciousness (see Atkinson & Shiffrin, 1971). Over this period, the neuropsychological positions did not merely follow those in orthodox human experimental psychology. Indeed, a number of the theoretical conclusions discussed were probably developed within cognitive neuropsychology before they became standard in human experimental psychology (see Baddeley, 1982b).

There may be a general reason for this. If the theoretical conclusions reached in this chapter are valid, human experimental psychology has attempted to study phenomena that are essentially in one domain – sentence comprehension – using empirical and theoretical techniques derived from another domain – memory. This mismatch between subject matter and techniques has resulted in a mass of anomalous findings and a variety of theoretical detours that are only now being resolved. As the neuropsychological approach works with effects that are so much grosser than those in experimental psychology, it was much easier to avoid many of the detours. More important, the present independent convergence of inferences from cognitive neuropsychology and human experimental psychology in the area supports the view that the cognitive neuropsychology approach works.

4   The Peripheral Dyslexias

4.1   Why the Acquired Dyslexias?

In this chapter and the next, I consider whether the cognitive neuropsychology research programme is working at a level more complex than a single functional syndrome. Can the approach provide information about the organisation of a group of subsystems, and not just about the functioning of a single one? If each potential subsystem could be shown to be damaged by a pure syndrome specific to it, the power and plausibility of the approach would be greatly increased.

What domain should one choose to explore in detail in order to assess whether the breakdown of related functions in different patients is caused by damage to different components of a modular organisation? It might seem natural to take a domain like language or object perception, in which any such modular organisation would have been honed by evolution. Instead, I am going to consider the breakdown of reading, a skill that is specific not only to one species, but also to what is, from an evolutionary perspective, a tiny time period. A prerequisite for taking such a domain as a prototype is that contrary to one of Fodor's (1983) assumptions, the human modular structure must be affected by the experience of the organism, with respect to not only the operation of individual subsystems, but also the organisation of the functional architecture itself.

There are a number of reasons for choosing the reading system and the syndromes that occur when it is damaged – the acquired dyslexias. The first is that this is the group of syndromes that has been investigated most intensively by single-case methods because some of their characteristics have proved challengingly counterintuitive. The second is that it is technically much easier to observe and document a disorder of and perform adequate experiments on reading than to do so in a comparable domain that appears biologically more basic, such as speech perception. An extensive literature on the behaviour of normal subjects can also be drawn on. Finally, modern theories of the reading process tend to view it as modular (e.g. Morton, 1969, 1979a; Allport, 1977) or at least as containing functionally isolable subcomponents (e.g. McClelland & Rumelhart, 1981).[1] If this approach to the reading process is an appropriate one and the underlying assumptions of cognitive

1. 'Cascade' theories related to McClelland and Rumelhart's (1981) theory will be considered in chapter 11.

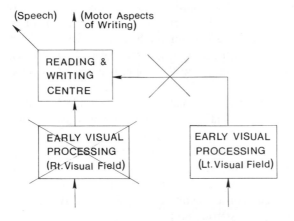

Figure 4.1. Information-processing representation of Dejerine's (1892) theory of alexia without agraphia. The crosses represent the two lesion sites held to be required to give rise to the syndrome.

neuropsychology are valid, then it should be possible to isolate a number of types of acquired dyslexia, each corresponding to the particular subcomponent of the reading process that is impaired.[2]

It is only in recent years that there has been strong neuropsychological interest in the acquired dyslexias. Until 1973, the area was generally considered rather secondary. It had had only one really notable event in its history. At the end of the nineteenth century, the French neurologist Dejerine (1892) had distinguished two main dyslexic syndromes: alexia with agraphia, an impairment of reading, together with one of spelling or writing; and alexia without agraphia. He assumed that a centre existed for the visual images of letters, which he placed in the angular gyrus region of the left parietal lobe and assumed to be necessary for both reading and writing. The first type of patient was held to have an impairment to the centre itself. For the second, the centre was thought to be intact, but lesions isolated it from the visual areas, right visual-field input being lost through the existence of a hemianopia – a total loss of visual sensation in one half-field – and left visual-field input through a disconnection of the right occipital lobe and the left angular gyrus (Figure 4.1).

The next 70 years produced a few additions and refinements, but nothing substantial changed – neither the syndromes that Dejerine had described, nor the anatomical theory by which he had explained them (see, e.g., Benson & Geschwind,

2. Throughout these chapters, I will be concerned with alphabetic languages, principally English, French, and Italian. With the exception that certain syndromes are less easy to detect in an orthographically regular language, such as Italian, no essential differences have yet been observed among the syndromes occurring in the different alphabetic languages, and it will be assumed that they do not exist. The one major class of acquired dyslexia studies that is thereby excluded consists of those performed with the more complex writing systems of Japanese. Interested readers should consult Sasanuma (1980, 1985) for detailed and sophisticated analyses.

1969; Hécaen & Kremin, 1976).[3] The anatomy became refined. The prototypic pair of lesion sites for alexia without agraphia became the posterior section of the corpus callosum – the splenium – and the left occipital lobe (see Hécaen & Albert, 1978). The primary theoretical issue discussed was how this basically anatomical theory could explain occasional patients in whom the lesion site was apparently anomalous.[4]

The establishment of the psychological nature of the disorders lagged far behind the anatomical analysis in sophistication, the authors of most papers on the syndromes having contented themselves with a cursory clinical account. Moreover, from a theoretical perspective, the relation between reading and spelling processes remains a matter of considerable theoretical dispute, as will be discussed in chapter 7. Dejerine's assumption of the existence of a centre common to the two skills is no longer generally accepted. For a functional analysis of the reading process, it therefore makes an inappropriate starting point.

Change began to occur in the 1960s, but it was not until 1973 that a major development took place. Marshall and Newcombe, in a very influential paper, developed a previously neglected method and introduced two new syndromes and a new theoretical framework.

In the long period when the acquired dyslexia field was relatively quiescent, a few workers had been interested in the nature of the reading errors that patients make (e.g. Low, 1931; Schuell, 1950; Kinsbourne & Warrington, 1962a). In general, though, interest in an acquired dyslexic patient concerned the symptoms that are associated with the reading difficulty (e.g. agraphia) and not its detailed characteristics. Marshall and Newcombe's paper produced a dramatic change. They demonstrated that dyslexic patients can have error patterns that are individually consistent and yet very different from one another. The first of the two main reading disorders that Marshall and Newcombe (1973) suggested they called *surface dyslexia,* in which most errors were held to be 'partial failures of grapheme–phoneme[5] conversion' (p. 183): *insect → 'insist'* (hard to soft *c*), and *incense → 'increase'* (soft to hard *c*). The second disorder they called *deep dyslexia,* in which the predominant class of error was a semantic substitution: *speak → 'talk', sick → 'ill',* and *berry → 'grapes'.*[6]

3. An exception was the study of reading difficulties arising from unilateral neglect (see chapter 12).
4. Patients with alexia without agraphia do not necessarily have either lesions of the splenium or a hemianopia, so ingenious anatomical speculations are required to maintain the theory as a general account (see, e.g., Greenblatt, 1973; Ajax, Schenkenberg, & Kosteljanetz, 1977; Vincent, Sadowsky, Saunders, & Reeves, 1977).
5. Following Coltheart (1978), the term *grapheme* will be used to refer to any letter or letter group corresponding to a phoneme.
6. Marshall and Newcombe (1973) also suggested the existence of visual dyslexia. However, one of the patients they described, AT, appears to have had bilateral lesions and potentially general visual problems (see also Marshall & Newcombe, 1977). The other, JL, had a right hemisphere lesion, and the errors he produced are typical of neglect dyslexia, which can arise from such lesions (Kinsbourne & Warrington, 1962a); this syndrome is discussed in chapter 13. Visual dyslexia was not an influential concept. Deep dyslexia was, in fact, described empirically by Marshall and Newcombe in 1966. Their detailed theoretical account is, however, in their 1973 paper.

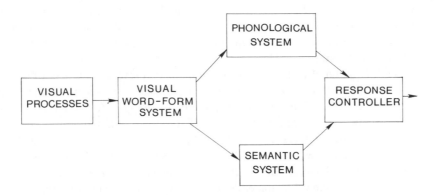

Figure 4.2. Marshall's and Newcombe (1973) 'two-route' model of the reading process. (The model and nomenclature have been changed a little to bring them into line with those used more generally in chapters 4 and 5; in particular, their visual addresses have been changed to visual word-forms, discussed in section 4.4.)

In addition to showing that there can be great differences in the errors that individual acquired dyslexic patients make, Marshall and Newcombe put forward an interesting and plausible theory to explain the different types of error pattern. They used a model of the reading process in which the semantic system can be accessed either directly from visual and orthographic processes or indirectly through phonological mediation (Figure 4.2). Surface dyslexia, they argued, involves damage to the first route and deep dyslexia, damage to the second.

It is now becoming increasingly standard to adopt a 'multiple-route' model in which one route provides direct access to the semantic system from orthographic processes while in one or more others, phonological mediation is required. However, at the time that Marshall and Newcombe (1973) put forward their model, the most fashionable approach was to assume that reading for meaning necessarily involved an intermediary phonological stage (e.g. Rubinstein, Lewis, & Rubinstein, 1971). By the mid-1970s, it was becoming clear in cognitive psychology, too, that a semantic reading procedure existed (e.g. Kleiman, 1975; Green & Shallice, 1976). As with the short-term memory syndrome, discussed in chapter 3, the popularity of multiple-route models of normal reading followed their use in neuropsychology.

Many of the arguments advanced by Marshall and Newcombe have been criticised since 1973. It is probable that neither of their key syndromes is a unitary functional entity. It is also universally agreed that their model is too simple, although there is no agreement about how it should be elaborated. It will be argued that the correspondences between the syndromes and the theoretical deficits they suggested are essentially valid, but for different types of patients from the ones they discussed! Yet the syndromes they proposed and the correspondences they suggested have left an enduring mark on cognitive neuropsychology. Their paper opened up the possibility of fruitful interaction between neuropsychology and cognitive psychology in the field of reading. After 1973, new disorders were described at a rapid rate – one in 1977, two in 1979, one in 1980, and one in 1981. Moreover, the two main syndromes originally suggested by Marshall and Newcombe have been subject to detailed debates and developments. There are even books on each of these two disorders!

The description of research in acquired dyslexia presents a number of problems. Since the single-case approach has been most widely applied in this area, much material is available. But the most frequent methodology adopted has been to characterise particular patterns of dyslexic difficulties as symptom complexes; this is how both surface dyslexia (Marshall, 1976; Coltheart, Masterson, Byng, Prior, & Riddoch, 1983) and deep dyslexia (Coltheart, 1980a) have been most widely viewed. As discussed in chapter 2, this methodology has serious difficulties.

A second problem is that major defining features of the symptom complexes have been the predominant error type made by patients. In fact, the type of errors produced by a patient is a fascinating but slippery datum that should be used with caution. It is fallacious to assume that the existence of different predominant error types across patients necessarily implies that different underlying subsystems have been damaged or that apparently qualitatively similar errors arise from the same cause.[7]

Fortunately, another type of observation can be made that is much closer to the dissociation approach discussed in chapter 2 and to procedures standard in human experimental psychology. I will call it the 'critical-variable' approach. The probability that a dyslexic patient will read a word is often influenced by the rating of the word on one or more dimensions. For instance, it is common for certain dyslexics to be much more likely to read a word if it is highly imageable (e.g. *potato*) than if it has a low imageability rating (e.g. *duration*) (see, e.g., Richardson, 1975; Shallice & Warrington, 1975). The interpretation of such a finding by itself is beset by the standard problem of correlational data. One end of the dimension may just be easier. However, it is possible for results of this type to be combined in a fashion analogous to a double association. If another patient is also impaired by a roughly equivalent amount in the performance of the task but is not influenced by this critical variable, then the most direct modular interpretation is that the two patients have damage to different subsystems.[8] The inference from patterns of performance to the existence of distinct functional systems is stronger if another word dimension influences reading in the second patient but not in the first. In a review paper, Patterson (1981) elegantly illustrated the way that real functional distinctions had been established among a number of different forms of acquired dyslexia using this approach. In general, though, investigations of dyslexia symptom complexes have stressed error types more than critical variables. My presentation will be more concerned with the effects of critical variables.

A third problem for discussing the acquired dyslexias is that certain dyslexic

---

7. Examples will be given later in this and in the next chapter.
8. The issues that arise in assessing the validity of such an inference are similar to those that arise with orthodox double dissociations (chapter 10).

syndromes are closely related to non-dyslexic disorders and do not speak directly to the issue of multiple reading routes. They include neglect dyslexia (Kinsbourne & Warrington, 1962a), attentional dyslexia (Shallice & Warrington, 1977b) and semantic access dyslexia (Warrington & Shallice, 1979). They will be discussed in chapters 12 and 13, along with the disorders to which they relate.

To simplify the discussion of those acquired dyslexic difficulties that are related to the theoretical issue of multiple reading routes, I will use the distinction between the peripheral and the central dyslexias. Before a word can be understood or pronounced, it must normally be categorised as an orthographic entity. I will refer to this process as the attainment of the visual word-form. Any dyslexic disorder that results in the visual word-form not being satisfactorily achieved is classified as a peripheral dyslexia. If the impairment is at a later stage, the dyslexia is classified as a central dyslexia.[9]

This chapter is concerned primarily with the peripheral dyslexias and the next, with the central dyslexias. One complication concerns the symptom complex surface dyslexia. It was originally conceived of as a disorder of transmitting information to the semantic system – that is, a form of central dyslexia. However, many patients so characterised may be peripheral dyslexics. I will, therefore, begin the discussion of surface dyslexia in this chapter.

4.2. Letter-by-Letter Reading

There are three syndromes in which the attainment of the visual word-form is impaired. Two – neglect dyslexia and attentional dyslexia – are, however, better considered with other disorders of visual attention. The most basic and best known form of peripheral dyslexia is alexia without agraphia, the syndrome first isolated in the classic study of Dejerine (1892); it has a variety of other names: 'pure alexia', 'agnosic alexia', 'spelling dyslexia', and 'word-form dyslexia'. This disorder is undoubtedly a syndrome in the clinical sense, many cases having been described (for reviews, see Benson & Geschwind, 1969; Hécaen & Kremin, 1976; Kremin, 1982).

Studies of series of such patients show that, characteristically, the reading of letters is better than that of words (Alajouanine, Lhermitte, & Ribaucourt-Ducarne, 1960); indeed, according to Pere (1978 quoted in Kremin, 1982), in 19 of the 100 cases he reviewed, letters were read perfectly. Clinically, the patients appear to read by building up the word from its constituent letters in a very laboured sequential process. The letters are said one by one, normally silently but sometimes aloud. Thus a patient presented with the word *book* might actually say, 'B-O-O-K . . . book.' Whether reading is successful depends mainly on how accurate the patient is in reading each letter explicitly, given that he or she can spell.

The laboured analytic process that the patient adopts when reading results in long

---

9. This classification was introduced by Shallice and Warrington (1980). The word-form differs from the visual logogen of Morton (1979a), as it is held to apply also to the processing of orthographically regular non-words (see later in chapter).

Table 4.1. *Reading characteristics of letter-by-letter reading patients ordered roughly in terms of severity*

	Average time to read word (in secs)		Letter reading errors (%)
	Three- to four-letter words	Seven- to eight-letter words	
RAV	1.8	3.0	0
BY	1.5	3.8	8
ML	3.5	10.0	0–8
JDC	6.7	—	5
TP	7.6	15.5	4
MW	12.8	24.3	10
KC	10.5	26.0	17
CH	16.9	47.5	50

From reference papers on the syndrome (see p. 74)

words taking much more time to read than short ones, and many patients also make more errors on them. Gardner and Zurif (1975), in a brief study that confounded part of speech and word length, showed that two patients of this type read two- to three-letter non-nouns much more rapidly than four- to eight-letter nouns (1 sec vs. 9 sec; 8 sec vs. 19 sec, respectively). By contrast, three patients described as having alexia with agraphia with minimal anomia were significantly faster on the nouns.

Four studies have provided a more detailed analysis of patients whose selective reading deficit had the main characteristic of a gross effect of word length on reading speed, which in general was very slow. These four reference studies are Staller, Buchanan, Singer, Lappin, and Webb (1978) (patient BY), Warrington and Shallice (1980) (patients JDC and RAV), Patterson and Kay (1982) (patients MW, CH, TP, and KC), and Shallice and Saffran (1986) (patient ML).[10] The basic results, shown in Table 4.1, support the clinical view of the syndrome and the patients' own reports that reading involves building up the word consciously from its component letters. All the patients showed a large effect of word length, being much slower at reading longer words than shorter ones; in many cases (e.g. BY), the time taken is close to being a fixed multiple of the word length. Moreover, reading speed and accuracy seem to depend on the accuracy of identifying individual letters.[11]

10. A study by Friedman (1982) describes a patient who showed a strong effect of word length on errors and was described as a case of alexia without agraphia, although in fact he appeared to suffer from an agraphia syndrome, lexical agraphia (Beauvois & Derouesné, 1981), to be discussed in chapter 6. However, because no latency data were presented, the patient's deficit is difficult to analyse, and it will not be considered further. Latency measures were obtained for only one word length with JDC. However, she read very slowly, taking, on average, more than 6 sec to read four-letter words, made numerous errors – more on longer words – and showed other characteristics of the syndrome, so she will be included.

11. The minor anomaly of BY, making 8% letter-identification errors, can probably be explained by his having identified letters very rapidly in the relevant test (0.85 sec/letter).

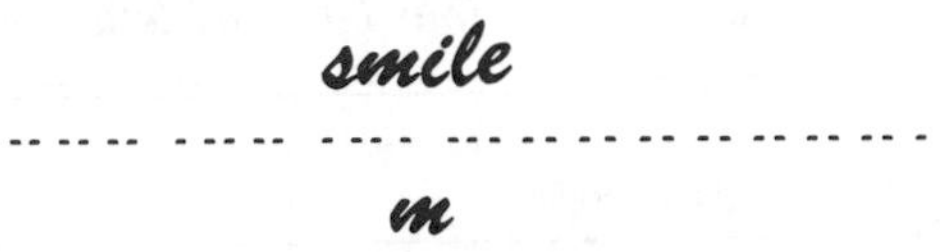

smile

-- -- -- - -- -- --- - -- -- -- -- -- -- -- -- --- -

m

Figure 4.3. Script that produces difficulty for letter-by-letter reading patients. Note the ambiguity of single letters presented in isolation. Reprinted from Warrington and Shallice (1980); *Brain 103:*105; by permission of Oxford University Press.

Two other aspects of their behaviour support the notion that the patients normally have to use an explicit letter-by-letter process to read a word. The presence of script rather than print makes the use of a letter-by-letter strategy much more difficult. The use of a very simple Letraset script (Figure 4.3) increased RAV's reading time by nearly 50%, and related effects were observed with JDC and ML. Similarly, presenting the stimuli briefly for a second or so has been shown to markedly impair the reading of all the patients for whom it has been tested (Table 4.2).

In the past, there was much debate over whether letter-by-letter reading results from an impairment specific to orthographic processing or whether it is a consequence of some more general disorder of visual perception. This issue is of wider significance, since if the deficit is limited to written stimuli, then systems or at least transmission routes specific to the reading process exist. All the patients listed in Table 4.1, except BY, who had a more limited field defect, are like most of those previously clinically described as having a hemianopia and therefore a restricted visual field. Could it be that the letter-by-letter reading of the patient is simply a consequence of the restriction in the visual field? Theoretically, a single visual field is sufficient for most words to be read rapidly, as is obvious from the visual-field studies on normal subjects. Also many patients with a hemianopia can read satisfactorily. However, the possibility of the hemianopia giving rise to the impairment can be simply refuted with these patients. RAV was given the task of reporting two numbers at opposite ends of an eight-letter word exposed for 150 msec (e.g. 7*thinking*4). He scored 10/10 correct. TP scored 10/10 on a seven-letter version of the same task. There seems little problem with the effective field of view of these patients.

4.3 Simultanagnosia

There is a more interesting way of explaining the disorder as the consequence of an impairment not specific to reading. As in the discussion of the interrelation of the short-term memory syndrome and conduction aphasia, the symptoms have to be considered in the context of a syndrome described in an earlier period of neuropsychology's development.[12] This syndrome, which has the benefit of the evocative name simultanagnosia, was first described by Wolpert (1924). Wolpert's patient was severely impaired in interpreting complex pictures and was a letter-by-letter

12. The other classic account – Dejerine's own (!) – will be discussed later.

Table 4.2. *Tachistoscopic performance of four letter-by-letter readers*

	Tachistoscopic			Unlimited exposure
	Exposure duration	Word length (in letters)	Correct percent	Correct percent
RAV[b]	500 msec	4–7	82	98
ML	2 sec	4–8	17	95
JDC	500 msec	6	0	?
TP[a]	1 sec	3–9	46	84

[a] In TP's case, the tachistoscopic score comes from a lexical decision experiment corrected for guessing. In all other cases, the results are from reading aloud.
[b] The relatively good performance of RAV can be explained through his relatively intact visual span; see section 4.3.
From reference papers on the syndrome (see p. 74)

reader. He explained this pattern of difficulties as stemming from a disorder of the 'highest level of perception', which he characterised in the manner appropriate for his time through the Gestalt notion of the 'formation of the whole out of its parts'. Wolpert's concept was widely accepted (see, e.g. Hécaen & Angelergues, 1963). However, in an acute critique, Weigl (1964) showed that the empirical evidence on which Wolpert and others had based the syndrome was very thin. He also pointed out that conceptually, the hypothesis

turns out to be extremely controversial as soon as one confronts that problem of what actually is, in each case, to be understood by the expressions 'whole' or 'part'. In the field of optical recognition, for example, beginning with the inability in the tachistoscopic experiment or in a free presentation, to interpret correctly the picture of any single object, and going on up to the inability to decipher difficult painting compositions . . . , graphically presented stories, . . . or of films – all of these faulty reactions are supposed to arise from disturbances in 'total comprehension'. The concepts: picture-detail, picture-portion, picture-element and so on, are used with just as elastic meanings. (p. 190)

In fact, the only fairly tight evidence that could be used to support Wolpert's position was provided at around the same time as Weigl's critique by Kinsbourne and Warrington (1962b). They described four patients who had difficulty interpreting complex pictures and also were letter-by-letter readers. More critically, the patients had a reliable tachistoscopic span of only one item, showing that for reading, at least, an element-by-element account of perception was supported in a more experimental way.[13]

A limit of only one item in what can be recognised in any one visual experience cannot be an adequate general explanation for letter-by-letter reading, however. RAV, when presented with 4 digits tachistoscopically for 100 msec, averaged 3.75

13. In fact, the interpretation of Kinsbourne and Warrington (1962b) was in terms of temporary refractoriness of the relevant perceptual systems.

correct. In general, his level of performance on such tasks was near the mean obtained by a group of patients with localised left hemisphere lesions who Warrington and Rabin (1971) studied and who in the main were not dyslexic. A second reason why letter-by-letter reading is difficult to account for in terms of 'simultanagnosia' is that RAV and ML obtained a high average and an average score, respectively, on the Picture Arrangement subtest of the WAIS, a timed task that requires the interpretation of complex pictures. Thus one supposed component of simultanagnosia (letter-by-letter reading) can occur in the absence of another (complex-picture identification) and be unrelated to a difficulty in perceiving more than one item. As one aspect of a syndrome can occur without the others, we have an example of a syndrome fractionating, discussed in general methodological terms in chapter 2 as the main process for refining the empirical base of neuropsychology.[14] There are, therefore, no good grounds for considering the disorder – simultanagnosia – a unitary (pure) syndrome with any functional relevance.[15]

These findings also suggest that letter-by-letter reading does not arise from a general perceptual impairment. In addition, it is well known that object naming can be relatively well preserved in letter-by-letter readers (Albert, 1979). This was the case for KC and particularly for CH, whose score of 14/15 objects named contrasts strikingly with a 50% error rate on letters. Therefore, another explanation that is implausible is that the disorder is a general one of transmission of information between visual and verbal domains. In letter-by-letter reading, we therefore appear to have a condition in which a system or transmission route specific to reading is impaired.[16] A conclusion of general relevance follows. On the assumption that dissociations provide evidence for modularity, the modular structure of the cognitive system cannot be innately determined.

4.4   Word-Form Dyslexia: Compensatory Strategies and the Locus of the Impairment

The letter-by-letter reader, then, does not read in this strange fashion because of some general restriction of visual perception. Reading letter-by-letter would appear to be a compensatory procedure developed by the patient to circumvent some specifically orthographic-processing difficulty produced by the lesion. Methodologically, there is an important difference between the syndrome being considered here and the STM syndrome, discussed in chapter 3. The behaviour of the patients cannot be thought of as resulting from the normal cognitive system with some components impaired – a subtraction process that produces a 'reduced set' of normally operating subsystems. Normal subjects do not say letter names to themselves when

14. In chapter 10, it is shown that when a syndrome fractionates into more specific ones, it does not necessarily follow that the 'parent' syndrome is not pure. However, there is no apparent way for the alternative possibility considered there to apply in this case.
15. For a recent investigation of the tachistoscopic disorders of the type analysed by Kinsbourne and Warrington (1962b), see Levine and Calvanio (1978). They also reject Wolpert's (1924) hypothesis.
16. It cannot be that reading is in some absolute sense more difficult than object recognition and naming. Some visual agnosic patients cannot recognise and name objects but can read – for example, the patient described by Albert, Reches, and Silverberg (1975).

trying to read. To account for the observed behaviour, we have to assume that the patient has learned a strategy of using some of the relatively intact components of the reading system in a combination not observed in normal subjects.

In general, the detailed understanding of the operation of the compensatory strategy can be important in the diagnostic process and may be of considerable value in the development of rehabilitation procedures (see Beauvois & Derouesné, 1982). However, it will probably not tell us anything directly about the normal organisation of the cognitive system. For that, we need to know the nature of the underlying impairment. For this reason, I will not discuss in much detail the procedure by which the patients read! Indeed, there is no general agreement.[17] But for the discussion of surface dyslexia in section 4.5, a distinction drawn by Patterson and Kay (1982) needs to be outlined. All four of their patients often said letters aloud. MW and CH, who were good spellers, then tried out words, but TP and KC, who had impaired spelling, tried out pronunciations – to use the terms of Patterson and Kay. For instance, TP read *gone* as 'G' 'O' 'N' 'E' . . . 'Joan', which is how it would be pronounced if the *g* were given its soft pronunciation, and KC read *castle* as 'cast-lee'. The type of error that occurs when pronunciations are tried out looks like a surface dyslexia error as will be discussed further in section 4.5.

What, then, is the nature of the impairment of the reading process in a letter-by-letter reader? It has been standard to assume that the deficit is early in the orthographic-processing system, but is there evidence for this? Could it not be that letter-by-letter reading is merely circumventing a problem in, say, reading words aloud? This has been investigated both by Warrington and Shallice (1980) and by Patterson and Kay (1982). The two studies came to similar conclusions, but the evidence obtained by Patterson and Kay was more extensive and convincing. One procedure they used was originally developed for studying semantic access dyslexia, to be discussed in chapter 12. A word is presented to the patient for 2 sec. If the patient cannot read it, a simple categorical decision has to be made about it. If, for instance, *grape* is presented, the decision might be whether it is an *animal* or a *fruit*. In both this test and a second one, in which there was a minor change in procedure, the three patients whom Patterson and Kay tested scored essentially at chance for words that could not be read immediately.[18] Even the grossest aspects of word meaning had not been identified when an exposure duration was used that would be ample for a normal reader and yet is too short to allow the letter-by-letter compensatory process to be completed. This is just what one would expect if the impairment is indeed early in the reading process.[19] In addition, the patients did not employ a rapid sounding-out of the stimulus word despite having intact phonological-pro-

17. For interesting discussions, see Patterson and Kay (1982) and Speedie, Rothi, and Heilman (1982).
18. As the patient knows the categorical decision in advance of the word being presented, the immediate reading rate is higher – often considerably so – than if the same word had been selected at random. This can be simply explained by the patient's guessing based on the categories available and the first one or two letters of the word.
19. It will be seen in chapter 12 that the argument for this conclusion may need to be somewhat more complex. One patient, ML, did not behave in the same fashion as the others.

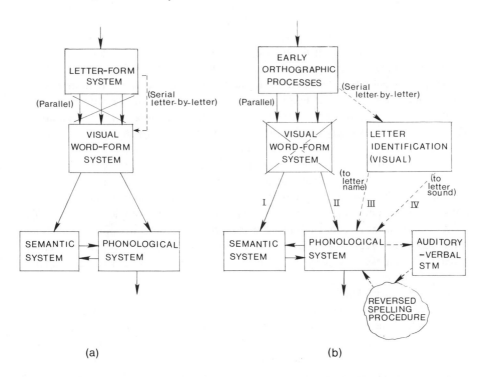

(a)   (b)

Figure 4.4. Two alternative models of the reading procedure used by letter-by-letter readers: those of (a) Patterson and Kay (1982) and (b) Warrington and Shallice (1980). The dotted lines represent the compensatory procedure used by such patients; in (b), III and IV are alternative procedures.

cessing systems, which suggests that the impairment precedes the 'phonological route' too.

Two hypotheses have been advanced as to where in the orthographic-processing system the impairment of these patients lies (Figure 4.4). Patterson and Kay (1982) have suggested a psychological version of the classical disconnection explanation, a pathological limit to the transmission of information from letter-form analysis systems to the systems where words are orthographically categorised – a visual logogen or visual word-form system. The most salient aspect of the syndrome for them was 'that enormous effort was required . . . to identify letters: but, once that had been achieved, moving from letters to words was virtually automatic' (p. 433). As two of their patients could not read all the words they could spell out, the claim that second stage is 'automatic' is not convincing.

The patients with whom Warrington and I (1980) worked had a more pure syndrome, in that their explicit letter identification was more accurate and rapid, and so we were led to prefer an explanation of the impairment as lying after the stage of letter-form processing. We argued that it resulted from damage to the visual word-form system itself. We were impressed by the ability – discussed above – of our patients, particularly RAV, to perform well on reporting digit or letter strings from tachistoscopic presentation. If the transfer of information from the letter-form analysis system was impaired, then this was the case only when the information was being passed to a visual word-form system. If another language-based operation was performed on letters, there was relatively little problem. Any disconnection hypothesised would have to be very specific. In addition, in tachistoscopic presentations, JDC could report as many letters from three-letter non-word strings as from three-letter and six-letter words (2.2 vs. 2.4 and 2.3). The 'wordness' of a letter string gave her no help. It seemed more plausible to attribute the deficit to an impairment within what we called the visual word-form system. As the patients do not sound-out the stimulus word rapidly despite having intact phonological processing systems, it would appear that the impairment precedes the phonological route too. The most parsimonious possibility is that the orthographic processing of both words and orthographically regular non-words is performed in the same system, which we called the visual word-form system. It is this system that we assumed to be damaged in these patients.

The word-form deficit seems the more plausible of the two alternatives for the purer cases. However, no completely compelling argument has yet been presented as to which of these alternatives is correct. Indeed, it may even be logically impossible to distinguish damage to a subsystem from damage to its input if the subsystem is fed by one input route only, unless a detailed model is available of the processing performed by the subsystem itself. This is a conceptual problem that will be met again. Even worse – in this particular example – it could easily be the case that readers who use a compensatory letter-by-letter strategy do not all have functionally identical impairments. It is possible that a common strategy is utilised to compensate for a number of types of impairment!

The analysis of the impairment underlying letter-by-letter reading therefore remains incomplete, since it has not been clearly established which precise part of the reading process has been impaired in the patients who use this strategy, or, indeed, whether the impairment is always the same. The difficulty of pinning down the underlying impairment arises in part because measurable characteristics of the syndrome reflect the nature of the compensatory process and not, as far as is known, the impairment itself. This is true, for instance, for the effects of both word length and script.[20] Thus it is difficult to investigate the impairment itself.

Despite this problem, the situation should not be construed in too negative a fashion. The syndrome corresponds to an impairment of a stage in the reading process that precedes all semantic and phonological processes. Moreover, the im-

20 Some effects, though – for example, the poor performance with restricted stimulus exposure durations – reflect both the underlying impairment and the compensatory strategy. For a fuller discussion of the methodological implications of patients' use of compensatory procedures, see chapter 10. The conceptual problems that compensatory strategies produce for functional analysis appear to have been posed first within the modern dyslexia literature by Marcel & Patterson (1978) with respect to deep dyslexia. The problem is discussed for aphasia in general by Caplan (1981).

pairment appears to be specific to reading. The most plausible explanation for the purer patients remains damage to an orthographic processing stage required for all later phonological and semantic processing of the written word – the visual word-form system.

4.5 Surface Dyslexia

The patient who reads in a letter-by-letter fashion is obviously employing a compensatory procedure. The reading of the surface dyslexic patient, by contrast, appears to reflect the underlying impairment more transparently. 'Surface dyslexia' was the characterisation given by Marshall and Newcombe to the reading difficulties of two patients, JC and ST, they described in their 1973 paper. Each was given roughly 900 words to read. About 50% of the words were read correctly, and 'the vast majority of the errors' were described as 'partial failures of grapheme–phoneme conversion' (p. 183).

During the 1970s, the syndrome was accepted without much debate as theoretically important. People can, in general, read nonsense syllables. So it is plausible that phonological reading – reading aloud without accessing semantics – can occur. The assumption that it was carried out by a spelling-to-sound translation process using grapheme–phoneme correspondences (GPCs) seemed intuitively obvious, theoretically well motivated, and empirically fairly solid (see, e.g., Coltheart, 1978). In so far as empirical evidence was thought necessary, it was quite common to refer to the reading of surface dyslexic patients (see, e.g., Green & Shallice, 1976). Surface dyslexia, therefore, continued to act as a major piece of support for Marshall and Newcombe's two-route model (see Figure 4.2). For these patients, in turn, Marshall and Newcombe's explanation was generally accepted. Surface dyslexia, they argued, resulted from the semantic route being unavailable, leaving the patient 'no option other than attempting to read via putative grapheme–phoneme correspondence rules. . . . The difficulty of this task is shown by the errors' (p. 191).

In fact, relatively little was known about surface dyslexia. The analysis of the reading of the original patients had consisted of little more than the interpretation of error corpuses (Holmes, 1973; Marshall & Newcombe, 1973), and no further patients were to be described in the 1970s. The characteristic noted by Marshall and Newcombe was that the vast majority of the errors could be described as partial failures of grapheme–phoneme conversion. Various types of failure were noted by them. The principal ones were:

1. Assigning the inappropriate sound when a grapheme is ambiguous or its phonemic value depends on the context: *insect* → *'insist'* (hard to soft *c*) and *guest* → *'just'* (hard to soft *g*).
2. Assigning a phonetic value to a silent grapheme: *listen* → *'Liston'* (the boxer).
3. Failing to apply the rule of *e*: *bike* → *'bik'*.
4. Reading only one letter of a vowel digraph: *niece* → *'nice'*.

In addition, two rather different types of errors were to become of theoretical importance. One was stress-shift errors (e.g. *begin* → *'beggin'*). The other, which

Marshall and Newcombe had not drawn attention to, was characterised by Shallice and Warrington (1980) as a 'misapplication of valid correspondence rules' and given the succinct name of a 'regularisation' error by Coltheart (1981). An example in the Marshall and Newcombe corpus is *disease* → *'decease'*. Simpler examples for patients described later are *gone* → *'goan'* and *pint* pronounced with a short *i*. The relevance of these errors is, of course, that they are the type that could be predicted if a GPC procedure was working perfectly but in isolation.

In the 1970s, the detailed relation between these types of error and normal phonological reading – reading by non-semantic means – was not considered. Moreover, no more patients were described. By the early 1980s, more descriptions of the patients with related disorders were beginning to appear (e.g. Shallice & Warrington, 1980; Kremin, 1981; Coltheart, 1982; Deloche, Andreewsky, & Desi, 1982), and the more rigorous critical-variable methodology was starting to be applied. At the same time, though, the predominant theoretical endeavour was to build on an early attempt by Marshall (1976) to characterise in more detail the symptoms that occurred together in surface dyslexia – to describe it as a symptom complex (e.g. Coltheart, 1981).

The most positive part of this attempt was a move away from a total reliance on errors as theoretically relevant data. In particular, it was shown that the reading of certain dyslexics is influenced by the critical variable of the ease of making spelling-to-sound translations of a word. Coltheart, Besner, Jonasson, and Davelaar (1979) had produced matched sets of regular words (e.g. *grill*) and words containing grapheme–phoneme correspondences considered exceptional on criteria derived from Venezky's (1970) theoretical analysis of the GPCs in English (e.g. *gauge*). Dyslexics were found to be differentially sensitive to this variable. Some found the exception words much more difficult than the regular words (see Shallice & Warrington, 1980; Coltheart, 1982). By contrast, deep dyslexics were not influenced by the variable (Patterson, 1981) (Table 4.3). One has a clear difference between the two types of patient. In addition, the patients who showed the effect of spelling-to-sound regularity appeared broadly similar to those reported by Marshall and Newcombe.[21]

The most systematic attempt to characterise the syndrome as a set of symptoms was made by Coltheart (1981). In addition to the partial failure errors and regularisations, Coltheart included the effect of the regularity variable and three other characteristics:

1. Individual letters of words can be read.
2. When a word is misread, it is understood as the response. So, when *gauge* was read as *'gorge'*, is was understood as 'a big dip'.
3. Irregular homophones can be read correctly and yet understood as their homophone complement. So *route* can be read correctly and defined as 'what holds the apple tree in the ground'.

---

21. There was, though, one rather striking exception – the patient, EM, who showed the phenomenon to its greatest extent. Her reading will be discussed in chapter 5. Coltheart (1981) also described another patient, AB, as surface dyslexic; however, the detailed results reported in the appendix of Coltheart, Masterson, Byng, Prior, and Riddoch (1983) do not show a significant regularity effect for this patient.

Table 4.3. *Contrasting performance of two sets of dyslexic patients on reading the matched regular and irregular sets of words of Coltheart, Besner, Jonasson, and Davelaar (1979)*

	Surface dyslexics/phonological readers				Deep dyslexics		
	ROG[a]	EM[a]	KM[b]	EE[b]	DE[c]	BB[c]	PW[c]
Regular words	92	72	74	59	69	72	59
Irregular words	64	13	51	33	69	79	74

[a] Shallice and Warrington (1980)
[b] Coltheart (1982)
[c] Patterson (1981)

Little quantitative evidence was provided for these claims. Somewhat more was provided in Coltheart et al. (1983) but mainly from a developmental dyslexic patient[22] and even then, not for characteristic 3. However, characteristic 2 was clearly supported by results from an acquired dyslexic, AB. Coltheart et al. also extended the list of features of the syndrome to nine. They were separated into one key aspect – regularisations – three essential aspects, and five others, which include characteristics 2 and 3. However, no grounds were given as to why one characteristic was rated 'key' and others were considered 'essential' and 'other'.[23]

One reason for this attempt to refine the syndrome and to differentiate 'essential' from 'other' aspects was that it was becoming clear that not all patients who make surface dyslexic–type errors are functionally identical. In particular, characteristic

22. As developmental disorders raise a whole range of extra conceptual issues, they are not discussed in this book. An impressive treatment of developmental dyslexia from a perspective related to that used in studying the acquired dyslexias but that does not simply reduce the conceptual system for developmental disorders to that for the acquired dyslexias is provided by Seymour and MacGregor (1984). For a detailed analysis of surface dyslexia considered primarily as a developmental disorder, see Temple (1985).

23. Much of the theoretical discussion among those who subscribed to the syndrome-complex approach concerned the origin of the 'partial failure' error, as defined by Marshall and Newcombe (1973). Considerable theoretical disagreements were beginning to emerge within this group of workers. Coltheart (1981; see also Coltheart et al., 1983) argued that instead of being due to a failure of the operation of the GPC route, these errors were better characterised as orthographic ones (letter additions, omissions, and transpositions), since purely visual errors were found to occur in some patients. In fact, no statistical analysis was presented to support this claim. Actually, it would seem that if both the original Marshall and Newcombe account and the Coltheart one could explain an error, then the Marshall and Newcombe account – being a priori less likely to produce an error of the appropriate type by chance – would be the preferable version. For instance, many possible errors involving the word *bike* could be explained by the Coltheart et al. approach – for example, *bake* or *brike* – but only the observed one, *bike* → *'bik'*, is explicable on Marshall and Newcombe's faulty grapheme–phoneme translation account. A powerful later analysis by Saffran (1985b) supports Marshall and Newcombe's view that errors arise in spelling-to-sound translation, at least in the patient being described.

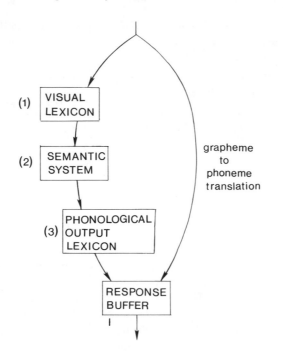

Figure 4.5. Possible points on the semantic route where an impairment can occur and give rise to surface dyslexia, according to the classical two-route theory of reading.

2 does not always apply. Some patients who make surface dyslexic reading errors understand the stimulus word correctly, and not as the response they produce, when tested on comprehension, for example, the patients reported by Kremin (1981, 1985), Goldblum (1985), Kay and Peterson (1985), and Margolin, Marcel, and Carlson (1985). From a theoretical perspective, most of these cases fit reasonably with the characterisation of surface dyslexia as reading by means of the operation of the GPC route when reading by the 'semantic route' is impaired (Figure 4.5). On this account, one would expect the patient to fall back on use of the GPC route if the semantic route were impaired at any point, and, indeed, in all but one of the patients – that of Goldblum (1985) – there is clear evidence of a deficit in accessing output phonology from the semantic system.[24] Thus it is easy to see why characteristic 2 alone should not be treated as an essential part of the symptom complex. The possibility, though, is immediately raised that other aspects may be equally inessential. The symptom complex was beginning to run into difficulties.

The symptom-complex approach to surface dyslexia was hardly ruffled by these

---

24. This account of these patients is rather simplified. As will be discussed in chapter 5, normal subjects have available morphemic spelling-to-sound correspondences. Goldblum (1985) has argued that it is the loss of these correspondences alone that is critical for the occurrence of surface dyslexia.

complications in comparison with the blow it received from the critique put forward by Marcel (1980).[25] Marcel considered surface dyslexia from the perspective of a theory of the normal reading process that was rapidly gaining in popularity – lexical analogy theory (e.g. Baker & Smith, 1976; Baron, 1977; Glushko, 1979). According to this theory, pronounceable non-words (e.g. *dake*) are not read by the use of spelling-to-sound correspondence rules. Instead, they are read aloud by analogy with how similarly spelled words are pronounced.

Marcel analysed in detail the error corpuses of the original surface dyslexic patients (JC and ST) and showed that they did not fit the orthodox two-route approach, in which the phonological route operates by grapheme–phoneme conversion. He went further and showed that many of the characteristics of the reading of JC and ST were what one would expect on the basis of a particular version of lexical analogy theory.

His first point was that only 25% of the errors that the patients made were non-words. They tended to produce words as responses. If, he argued, their errors arise as a result of the application of grapheme–phoneme rules – or even of a flawed application – why were only a minority of the responses non-words? If a word like *colonel* or *yacht* is regularised, the end result is not generally another word. Coltheart et al. (1983) have objected to this argument and pointed out that lexicalisation is not a consistent feature of surface dyslexic reading. However, if lexicalisation errors are not a part of the symptom complex, then patients who make them are qualitatively different, or, more plausibly, their reading cannot be characterised as just GPC reading; other processes must be considered. In either case, the safest procedure would seem to be to exclude such patients from consideration if one is concerned with understanding how phonological-route reading might operate or, at the very least, to consider two sub-types with separable underlying functional explanations. None of the authors using a symptom-complex approach take this step. For instance, the original patients, JC and ST, continue to be quoted by Coltheart et al. as exemplars of the syndrome. The logic of the symptom-complex approach to the dyslexia was beginning to seem somewhat threadbare.

Marcel's second point fits logically with his first. He pointed out that errors that are consistently quoted as exemplars of surface dyslexic errors do not fit with the notion of the application of grapheme–phoneme correspondence rules or even with the idea of flawed application of such rules. Consider *incense* → *'increase'* or *barge* → *'bargain'*. Where does the *r* in *increase* come from, the *-ain* in *bargain;* why not *'inkense'* or *'barg'*, he asked. At the very best, it would appear that the spelling-to-sound relation is embedded in a lexical framework.

In 1982, Marcel's (1980) critique was strengthened theoretically by Henderson. He pointed out that a major theoretical problem for the GPC approach to normal reading is the vast array of contextual rules that would be necessary to support its effective operation. He continued, 'It is therefore inadmissible to cite as evidence

---

25. The critique was developed before the concepts of the regularity effect and of the regularisation error were widely used. However, it remains germane.

for the viability of the GPC route errors which result from the almost total failure to apply contextual rules' (p. 120). On the empirical level, he pointed out that ROG (Shallice & Warrington, 1980), the only surface dyslexic on whom latency data were then available, took an average of 4.2 sec to read a one-syllable word, and from the clinical descriptions available, none of the other patients described seemed to read at anything like normal speed. In one major respect, Henderson differed from Marcel. He did not think that the characteristics of surface dyslexia were relevant to any theory of the normal reading process. He concluded, 'The extremely laboured reading characteristic of surface dyslexia . . . does not suggest at all that a mechanism serving normal reading has been revealed as a consequence of selective damage to alternative pathways' (p. 121).

Later arguments have tended to strengthen yet further the line of argument developed by Henderson.[26] Thus on the model shown in Figure 4.4(b), it is possible that surface dyslexia in its original form might arise from an orthographic-analysis impairment of the type discussed in the context of letter-by-letter reading. As mentioned, Patterson and Kay (1982) differentiated two forms of word-form dyslexic readers. One type of patient – the classical letter-by-letter reader – attempts to circumvent damaged orthographic processing by letter naming and then probably uses knowledge of spelling in a 'reversed spelling' process. In the other type of patient, spelling is impaired, and so a sounding-out procedure is used instead. The sounding-out procedure could be based either on explicitly learned associations between letters and their characteristic sounds (route IV) or on the information that can be passed down a very impaired phonological route (route II). In either case, a considerable amount of guessing based on the known sounds of words would be expected; it is found, as are other aspects of the surface dyslexic error pattern.

Both Marcel (1980) and Coltheart et al. (1983) had, in fact, already argued that surface dyslexia might result from damage to orthographic systems at the morphemic level. The difference between their position and the one being presented is principally metatheoretical. Should the reading process in these patients be viewed as the functioning of certain components of the normal system working under the control of a strategy natural for an adult reader? If so, the disorder should speak to theories of normal function. Alternatively, is it better to see the symptoms as arising from a compensatory procedure that co-ordinates a restricted set of subsystems in an unusual way? If so, the disorder will, as Henderson argued, probably speak little to theories of normal function.

Certain observations of Coltheart et al. (1983) make the compensatory-procedure view somewhat more than just a logical possibility. These authors noted that their patients' spelling was impaired, so that they would indeed have been unable to use a classical letter-by-letter reading strategy effectively. In addition, they claimed that errors similar to those that occur in the reading of surface dyslexic patients occur when the letters are presented auditorially. Such an effect would be expected if in

26. See Shallice and McCarthy (1985) for a detailed version of these arguments.

the reading process, words are indeed built up by the patients laboriously and explicitly from their constituent sounds in the phonological system.

The most plausible conclusion is that surface dyslexia is related to letter-by-letter reading in two ways. First, it arises from a compensatory procedure rather than from the operation of an impaired system operating under essentially normal strategic control. Second, it may well result from damage at the word-form level, at least in many patients so classified.

How should one assess the disorders of reading discussed in this chapter? Positively, there seems good neuropsychological evidence for the existence of a specific orthographic subsystem that has an output that is required for both phonological and semantic processing. No adequate neuropsychological argument has been presented that this subsystem should be divided into a lexical and a non-lexical form, as the concept of a non-lexical GPC route requires. Instead, a visual word-form account seems more appropriate.

There are, though, two negative points to be considered. The move from neuro-psychological evidence to normal function has proved much less straightforward in this area than in the study of short-term memory. In the case of surface dyslexia, the attempt to use a symptom-complex approach to characterise the syndrome was not a success. No set of symptoms that could be effectively related to theory was ever accepted by all workers in the field. In addition, for word-form dyslexia and probably surface dyslexia, there is an unavoidable conceptual difficulty, which is far less important in the case of the short-term memory syndrome – the existence of compensatory strategies.

Indeed, the impasse may not be one for merely the symptom-complex approach. Might the dissociation between, say, surface dyslexics and deep dyslexics concerning the effect of the regularity variable – regular words being easier to read than exception ones – while real enough, be functionally uninteresting? If the regularity effect were to reflect just a rather primitive type of compensatory strategy, then it would not be the signature of the operation in isolation of one major component of the normal reading process. The programme of applying cognitive neuropsychology to reading seems to be in severe difficulties before it has hardly begun.

5   The Central Dyslexias

5.1   The Selective Preservation of Phonological Reading

Chapter 4 began with the programme of understanding dyslexic difficulties using a multiple-route model of the normal reading process. On this programme, the selective impairment of any individual route would correspond to a form of central dyslexia. However, the one candidate reading disorder considered, surface dyslexia, has proved a disappointment. Far from consisting of a selective impairment of the semantic reading route, in its best known form, it seems to consist of compensatory behaviour for an underlying peripheral dyslexic difficulty.

Can an improvement be obtained using the dissociation approach? Can one adapt the method of defining syndromes by dissociations in order to lessen the probability that the dissociation reflects only the operation of a compensatory procedure? One approach is to insist that the better performed task is not merely 'better' than the poorly performed task, but also normal or nearly so on any relevant measure. In the terminology to be developed in chapter 10, this dissociation is a 'classical' or near-classical one. In this case, it would be unlikely to arise as a result of the operation of a laborious compensatory strategy. Having made this distinction, I will, however, immediately relax it. The critical aspects that distinguish the use of, say, a normal phonological reading procedure – if somewhat impaired – from the compensatory strategies discussed in chapter 4 are the speed and fluency of reading. One needs to consider the following question: are there patients who not only show a dissociation between their inability to read aloud by semantic mediation and their ability to read aloud by some phonological means, but also, when they read 'phonologically', do so in a normally fast, fluent fashion?

The answer has come from a somewhat unexpected quarter. Shortly after Marshall and Newcombe (1973) first described surface dyslexia, Warrington (1975) was analysing the semantic memory impairments of certain patients suffering from Alzheimer's disease.[1] Almost incidentally, Warrington noted clinically that the patients read at roughly normal speed, could read regular words reasonably well, and tended to regularise irregular words. The only quantitative evidence available on their reading was obtained for one of the patients, EM: it was shown in Table 4.3. She, in

---

1. The basic disorder of these patients is of great theoretical interest. It will be discussed in chapter 12.

88

Table 5.1. *Basic results on patients with fluent phonological reading*

Patient	Semantics	Spontaneous speech	Reading			Errors on irregular words	
			Regular word (%)	Irregular word (%)	Non-word (%)	Type	Lexicalisation (%)
WLP[1a]	'V. Poor'	'Fluent'	100	95	?	Reg.	0
WLP[2a]	'V.V. Poor'	'Fluent'	85	71	?	½ regs.	46
HTR[b]	P = IQ 57	'Fluent'	79	48	84	Mainly regs.	34
MP[c]	P = IQ 48		100	77	?	Mainly regs.	?
KT[d]	P < baseline	'Empty'	86	41	100	Nearly all regs.	?

P = Peabody test; Regs. = Regularisation error
[a] Schwartz, Saffran, and Marin (1980a)
[b] Shallice, Warrington, and McCarthy (1983)
[c] Bub, Cancelliere, and Kertesz (1985)
[d] McCarthy and Warrington (1986a)

fact, showed much the largest regularity effect of any of the patients discussed there, and hence the most satisfactory dissociation.

Warrington's observations therefore suggest that patients may exist who cannot read by semantic means and yet can read aloud fast and fluently. By now, the reading of four other such patients has been analysed quantitatively: WLP (Schwartz, Saffran, & Marin, 1980a), HTR (Shallice, Warrington, & McCarthy, 1983), MP (Bub, Cancelliere, & Kertesz, 1985), and KT (McCarthy & Warrington, 1986a).[2] A summary of their reading performance is given in Table 5.1 with WLP's results presented for two testing sessions held six months apart; her other cognitive abilities deteriorated over this period.

One striking point illustrated in Table 5.1, is the excellent performance of WLP and the reasonable performance of MP on irregular words. In chapter 4, it was argued that one positive aspect of later research on surface dyslexia was that the effect of spelling-to-sound regularity and the regularisation error had begun to be considered the most important signs of reading by the phonological route. Yet here are patients being introduced as pure phonological readers, and one of them hardly shows the effect at all! However, for the present, this is a secondary issue; the more basic dissociation is the contrast between the ability of the patients to read aloud fluently and their inability to comprehend what they were reading.

2. It is possible that some patients described in chapter 4 as surface dyslexic may be of this type – for example, the patient of Goldblum (1985). However, insufficient information is available on other patients to be sure. Patients of this type who make actual errors in reading aloud have been called semantic dyslexics. WLP has been called a non-semantic reader.

If irregular words can be read, what is the evidence that these four patients do not read by semantic means? For all four, this was fairly apparent clinically. For instance, WLP, presented with *hyena* – a word that if regular in its grapheme–phoneme correspondences would have two syllables only – read correctly, 'hyena . . . hyena . . . what in the heck is that?' The way that this failure to comprehend the written word was demonstrated quantitatively was different in the four cases.

For MP, the procedures adopted were the most stringent. Bub et al. (1985) used a variety of methods – five in all – to show that although MP could read irregular words aloud, she could not understand their meaning. On the Peabody test (Dunn, 1965), a standardised test of word comprehension in which a word has to be matched to one of four pictures, MP's score with written words was at a level equivalent to the (auditory) comprehension of a 2.8-year-old child. In a word–word matching test where an associate of a target word has to be selected from a set of four candidates (e.g., *chair, apple, buy, pen: table*), MP scored at chance (9/26). This is most unlikely to be a failure to understand the task; immediately before, she had been given the equivalent test with pictures and had performed well.[3]

For both WLP and HTR, many of the inferences were indirect. WLP, however, in a task of sorting words into four categories, one of which was *animals,* correctly categorised only 7/20 of the low-frequency animal names, but she read 18 of them correctly, including words as irregular or ambiguous as *gorilla, hyena* and *leopard.* HTR, in her turn, performed very poorly on the written Peabody test, with a score equivalent to an IQ of 57. For KT, the picture was clear. He scored *below* baseline on both the spoken and the written version of the Peabody test and also failed to score on both the Vocabulary and the Similarities subtests of the WAIS, which require word comprehension. When asked what a word meant, he invariably said, 'I do not know the word, I can only read' (p. 363).

The complementary part of the dissociation is the ability of the patients to read words aloud fluently and rapidly. MP, HTR, and KT had reading speeds quantitatively in the normal range; for instance, MP's naming latency for the written word was about 600 msec. Unfortunately, speed of reading was not measured quantitatively for WLP. However, she is reported as being able to 'read aloud with facility' (p. 261) and 'fluently and without effort' (p.261), far from the way that classical surface dyslexic readers are characterised.

From these studies, one can draw inferences both about what is damaged in these patients and about the organisation of phonological reading in general. I will begin with the neuropsychological issue. Even on a simple form of two-route theory, an impairment that leaves the patients reliant on only phonological reading could lie at a number of different points on the semantic route. As a deficit at the level of visual morphemic analysis is a favoured locus for theories of surface dyslexia – and, indeed, it was supported in chapter 4 (see Figure 4.5) – and many theorists do not

---

3. For a critique of the arguments for morphemic correspondences from WLP and MP, see Howard (1985a). Howard discusses each argument in turn. What he does not explain is why so many independent tests on patient MP have converged on the same conclusion.

differentiate between surface dyslexia and the present syndrome, 'semantic dyslexia', one needs to consider whether a deficit at this level could account for any difficulties these patients have.

Such an explanation would not account for the discrepancy, which is very large in some of the patients, between reading aloud and comprehension performance. Could it not provide an explanation of why certain words cannot be read aloud by the patients, in terms of a secondary impairment to a primary semantic one? Bub et al. (1985) elegantly showed that even as a secondary explanation, a visual morphemic problem cannot account for the inability of MP to read certain words aloud. They paired irregular words that she consistently read aloud incorrectly (e.g. *leopard*) with non-words obtained by changing the first letter of another irregular word (e.g. *rubtle*). MP was over 80% correct in selecting the real word. Thus it seems likely that even for words that MP could not read aloud, visual morphemic analysis is reasonably intact. McCarthy and Warrington (1986a) came to a similar conclusion about KT by a different method. KT was presented with 12 cards, on each of which three words were typed without spaces – for example, *picturesunpotato*. He was able to copy them, putting in the correct spaces, and made only 1/24 errors in segmentation. The most plausible explanation for any secondary impairment in semantic dyslexia is that the patients, in addition to a semantic deficit, have a loss of certain spelling-to-sound correspondences.

A much more dramatic inference to normal function can be obtained from the studies of WLP and MP. The preserved reading of irregular words that are not understood – a 'purer' effect in WLP than in MP – shows that morphemic spelling-to-sound correspondences must exist that are independent of the semantic system. Before WLP had been described, it was not standard in either neuropsychology or cognitive psychology to assume that morphemic correspondences existed independently of the semantic system (see, e.g. Coltheart, 1978; Morton, 1979b).[4] It is now a standard assumption.

The most common theoretical response to these findings has been to increase the number of reading routes to three (e.g. Morton & Patterson, 1980) (Figure 5.1). A lexical phonological route is added to the non-lexical one. This three-route model soon became very popular. It has been challenged by two alternatives. One is the lexical analogy approach referred to in chapter 4. However, the support that Marcel (1980) derived for the importance of lexical processes in the origin of traditional surface dyslexia errors cannot be obtained from the errors made by the present set of patients. In all four patients, errors on irregular words tended to be regularisations; lexicalisation was not a major aspect of their performance. Thus MP almost never made an error on 'predictable' grapheme–phoneme correspondences. The

4. A second line of neuropsychological evidence that may also be relevant to the issue is a phenomenon mentioned by Coltheart (1981) as one of the aspects of the surface dyslexia symptom complex – patients who read some irregular homophones correctly but define them incorrectly. For instance, *route* was defined as *root*, even though it was read correctly. If *route* were being read aloud by means of the semantic system, it would presumably not be defined as its homophone *root*. Unfortunately, no quantitative data are presented regarding how often the phenomenon occurred.

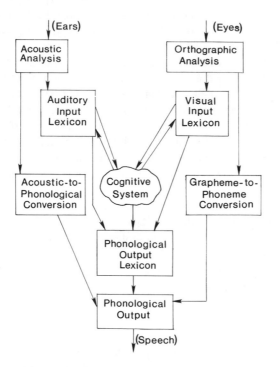

Figure 5.1. Morton and Patterson's (1980) model of the stages of processing single words presented auditorily or visually. In a later version of the model, the non-lexical route can process larger units than graphemes (see Patterson & Morton, 1985).

rule of *e*, for instance, was obeyed on 98% of occasions. The errors that MP made were regularisations. For KT, the effects were, if anything, even clearer. On the occasions when irregular words were read correctly, they did not tend to prime the analogous reading of a similarly spelled non-word that succeeded it – an effect shown by Kay and Marcel (1981) in normal subjects. Yet when the pool of words on which analogy effects can operate is much reduced, then the priming effect of a correctly read irregular word should, if anything, be greater. Instead, the vast majority of KT's error responses continued to reflect the utilisation of standard spelling-to-sound correspondences. Lexical analogy theory, while not refuted by findings on patients, receives no support.[5]

The second alternative was suggested by the way one of Warrington's original patients, EM, read, but it is also present in HTR's performance. According to the three-route model, shown in Figure 5.1, if a word cannot be read by the GPC route,

5. A variety of arguments can be presented against lexical analogy theory, with respect to both its empirical account of normal subjects and its computational plausibility (see Patterson & Morton, 1985; Shallice & McCarthy, 1985).

Table 5.2. *Performance of HTR and KT on three different sets of words*

	Levels of regularity			Vowel pronunciation	
	Regular (e.g. *boost*)	Mildly irregular (e.g. *crow*)	Very irregular (e.g. *vase*)	Regular (e.g. *peach*)	Mildly irregular (e.g. *head*)
HTR[a]	74	49	29	78	65
KT[b]	70	40	24	92	63

[a] Shallice, Warrington, and McCarthy (1983)
[b] McCarthy and Warrington (1986)

then its degree of irregularity will not affect whether it is read by either of the other two routes. Such a model treats the regularity variable dichotomously, words being either regular, in which case they can be read by the GPC route, or exception, in which case they cannot be so read. For EM, though, mildly irregular words seemed to be read more easily than very irregular words. This was demonstrated quantitatively in both HTR and KT. In one experiment, so-called 'mildly' irregular words were used. These are words that involve a single grapheme–phoneme correspondence that Venezky (1970) called 'minor', one that is quite common but not the most frequent in the language, as in *crow* (the *ow:* contrast with *how*) or *dread* (the *ea:* contrast with *beat*). Such words were read at a level roughly midway between regular and very irregular ones (e.g. *colonel, yacht, area*), all three groups being matched for frequency (Table 5.2).[6] Indeed, in a second experiment, performance with mildly irregular words (e.g. *soul*) was not significantly worse than with regular ones (e.g. *mouse*) for HTR.

Analogous findings have been obtained with normal subjects. Parkin (1982) investigated words whose pronunciation is given in the *Oxford Paperback Dictionary* (*OPD*), which lists the pronunciation of a word if it is held to be 'difficult to pronounce'; thus it lists *marine, chute,* and *subtle*. Parkin discovered that in previous studies that had contrasted the reading of regular and 'exception' words, only 30% of the exception words in the study of Coltheart, Besner, Jonasson, and Davelaar (1979) and only 10% of those in the study of Baron and Strawson (1976) were in the dictionary. Parkin compared the processing of these *OPD* words with the processing of regular words and with ones that contain a minor correspondence (MC) and are not listed in the dictionary (e.g. *double, bugle, steady*). Lexical decision time was slower for the *OPD* words (741 msec) than for either of the other two

6. It has been objected by a number of authors – for example, Kay and Lesser (1985) and Derouesné and Beauvois (1985) – that this result could be due to a lack of consistency in the grapheme–phoneme correspondences used by a patient. Maybe on occasion the minor correspondences would be utilised, which would increase performance on mildly irregular words but not on very irregular ones. This effect seems likely to be too small to account for the difference (see Shallice & McCarthy, 1985).

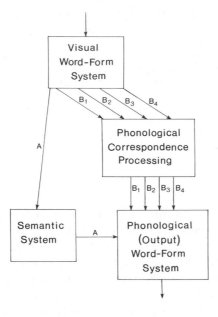

Figure 5.2. The word-form model of the reading process. A is the semantic route; B_1 to B_4 represent different-size units being transmitted by the phonological route.

groups (MC: 668; R: 709), and a similar result was obtained for reading speed.[7] Only very irregular correspondences produced difficulty.

The correspondence between the phenomena obtained with patients and with normal subjects is even more impressive if word frequency is considered. Seidenberg, Waters, Barnes, and Tanenhaus (1984) investigated the interaction of frequency and regularity on naming latency for visually presented words in normal subjects. For low-frequency items, there was an effect of mild degrees of regularity; their 'regular inconsistent' words – similar to mildly irregular ones – were read 30 msec more slowly than regular words. For high-frequency items, however, there was no latency difference between the two types of word. The stimuli in the Levels of Regularity lists, with which an analogous difference was obtained with HTR, were also mainly of low frequency. The Vowel Pronunciation lists, with which no such difference was obtained with her, consisted primarily of high-frequency words.

An alternative approach stimulated by these findings is to assume that phonological correspondences exist for a range of sizes of units, as suggested, for instance, by Smith and Spoehr (1974). When applied to the acquired dyslexias, it was assumed that a 'broad' phonological route existed that could be distinguished from a semantic one. Correspondences were held to be available at the graphemic, sub-

---

7. Parkin & Underwood (1983) have shown that these effects cannot be attributed to any purely visual irregularity.

syllabic (e.g. the rhyme), syllabic, and morphemic levels (e.g. Shallice et al., 1983; Shallice & McCarthy, 1985) (Figure 5.2).[8] Sub-syllabic or, at most, syllabic correspondences would be sufficient for the reading of mildly irregular words, but very irregular words would require morphemic correspondences. It was also assumed that in neurological disease, correspondences based on larger units are more vulnerable than those based on smaller units; a progressive disease, such as that suffered by EM and WLP, would increasingly restrict the range of correspondences available to the patient.

A second relevant effect was obtained with HTR. Minor correspondences were divided according to the most frequent pronunciation of the spelling pattern (i.e. their rhyme) in which they were contained. In some words – those with 'typically irregular' pronunciation – the spelling pattern was most commonly pronounced with the minor correspondence (e.g. *ead* in *tread,* compare with *bread, dread*). In others – atypically irregular words – the spelling pattern normally took the major correspondence (e.g. *owl* in *bowl,* consider *fowl, owl*). The former type were read considerably more satisfactorily than the latter (75% vs. 42%). This effect would fit well with the multiple-levels account of the phonological route, since the former words but not the latter could be read correctly at the sub-syllabic level.[9]

There is, though, an alternative explanation of these last two phenomena. Consider again the standard three-route model (see Figure 5.1), but assume that the routes operate on activation principles, as in so-called 'cascade' models (e.g. McClelland & Rumelhart, 1981); transmission of information is not all-or-none, and activation in the phonological system must exceed a certain threshold for output to occur. In a semantic dyslexic patient, morphemic correspondences might produce sub-threshold degrees of activation for less frequent words. Indeed, HTR made errors that seemed to reflect partial morphemic activation. For instance, *yacht* was read as 'yat' and *suede,* as 'swede'. In these two examples, one does indeed see the influence of an (irregular) morphemic correspondence: the pronunciation of the *ch* in *yacht* and the *u* in *suede,* respectively. Yet the activation was insufficiently strong to determine the complete pronunciation of the word; regularisation tendencies also operated. Assume further that the effective difference between a major and a minor

8. In the first account of this approach to the acquired dyslexias (Shallice & Warrington, 1980), it was assumed that the correspondences had an upper limit of 'short words'. There was, however, no principled reason for the restriction. It was soon forgotten, except by critics!

9. PT, a patient of Kay and Lesser (1985), did not show the typicality effect at all. Yet with respect to both his performance on different levels of regularity and his errors, the patient behaved in a similar fashion to HTR. However, PT read very much more slowly that HTR, taking an average of 3.49 sec to read a word, whereas HTR took an average of 1.03 sec. PT's reading speed was no faster than that of certain letter-by-letter readers – for example, BY and RAV – described in chapter 4. It is therefore likely that PT was using a careful but conscious reading strategy that emphasises graphemic over subsyllabic effects. Considering KT does not help to resolve the issue. He did read typically divergent words better than atypically divergent ones (55% vs. 26%). However, in this patient, the effect appears to be restricted to a subset of vowel–consonant cluster combinations. His performance on irregular words indicates, though, that his phonological route is less intact than that of HTR.

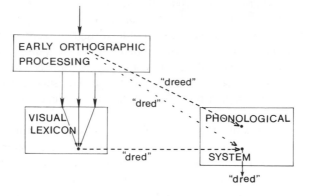

Figure 5.3. The possible combination for the reading of the word *dread* of sub-threshold activation transmitted over separate lexical and non-lexical phonological routes, in which the latter operates by multiple grapheme–phoneme correspondences. The "dreed" line represents the major correspondence; "dred" represents the minor correspondence. The strength of the hatching denotes the strength of activation (see text).

correspondence is just that they produce different levels of activation in the phonological system. If this were the case, then a minor correspondence could still produce sufficient sub-threshold activation to sum with sub-threshold activation coming from morphemic correspondence and so exceed threshold (Figure 5.3).[10] Thus it seems possible to explain the characteristics of semantic dyslexia by a more elaborate version of the GPC theory as well as by the multiple-levels position.

One final theory should be mentioned because it has certain similarities with the word-form theory and has characteristics related to cascade ones. It has, though, a very different conceptual basis. Sejnowski and Rosenberg (1986) have simulated a three-component system for spelling-to-sound translation in which the input units correspond to letter parts, and the output units, to distinctive features (the 'elements' of phonemes) (Figure 5.4). The central subsystem consists of many neuron-like units, so-called hidden units. There are connections between all pairs of units in neighbouring levels, each having a 'weight' that can be modified by learning. The system undergoes a training procedure that mimics reading text aloud; a reinforcement schedule is used that operates after every attempt to 'read' a letter or phoneme. This model is therefore an activation one in which all levels of correspondences (grapheme through to morpheme) are conveyed by the same set of neuron-like units. If 'lesioned', it seems likely to show both levels of regularity effect

10. The typicality effect may well be explicable on this approach as an example of the so-called gang principle (see McClelland & Rumelhart, 1981). In another elaboration of the standard theory, produced by Patterson and Morton (1985), the nonlexical route utilises sub-syllabic units as well as GPCs. The difference between this version of the standard model and the multiple-levels position is mainly terminological.

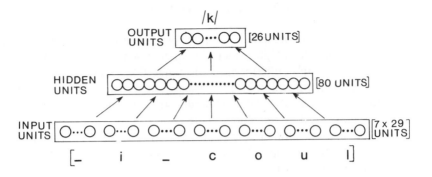

Figure 5.4. The groups of units in Sejnowski and Rosenberg's (1986) model of the operation of the phonological route.

and the typicality one, although this has yet to be done. Indeed, it can be seen as a concrete realisation of the word-form approach.[11]

The conclusions that can be drawn from the study of these phonological-reading patients are much more positive than those obtained from the patients described in chapter 4. First, some support is indeed provided for the modular approach to reading. Patients exist who cannot use a semantically mediated method of reading and yet whose ability to use spelling-to-sound correspondences is more or less satisfactory. Indeed, the neuropsychological approach has gone one stage further. It has shown that morphemic spelling-to-sound correspondences that are not mediated semantically do exist. Coltheart et al. (1983) argued that at the time they were writing, it was not possible to draw this inference from the normal literature.

If, however, one asks how the phonological route or routes actually works, the evidence from the phonological-reading patients is much less clear. At least three theories seem capable of explaining most of the findings on semantic alexia. Whether they are all equally good at explaining the characteristics of another dyslexic syndrome – phonological alexia – will be discussed later in the chapter. Yet what can be made of the evidence from studies of normal subjects? Patterson and Morton (1985) rather sadly said,

In the 1970s, the only major variables which seemed germane to research on assembling phonology from print were the distinction between words and nonwords and, for words, the distinction between regular and irregular (or 'exceptional') spelling-to-sound correspondences. In the mid-1980s, we are sadder but wiser. (p. 338)

They then listed five complicating variables or phenomena that led them to echo Cutler's (1981) title 'Making up Materials Is a Confounded Nuisance, or: Will We

11. This theory is an example of a 'distributed-memory' model (see Hinton & Anderson, 1981). Models of this type will be considered in chapter 11. A related approach has been suggested by Seidenberg (1985). One result obtained on KT may well present difficulty for most current theories; he was remarkably good at assigning stress correctly in multi-syllabic words.

Be Able to Run Any Psycholinguistic Experiments at all in 1990?' The problem is not unique to neuropsychology.

A final point should be borne in mind. From a neuropsychological perspective, in asking how the phonological route (or routes) actually works, we are in part descending – in Marr's (1982) terms – from questions about the modular level to those about the algorithmic level. In consequence, one would expect the power of the approach to be less. It is therefore hardly surprising that after a very few years of neuropsychological investigation of the phonological route, many possibilities on the detail of its operation are still open. It is on the broad brush strokes, not on the finer detail, that neuropsychology needs to be judged, and in this respect, its record on phonological reading is good.

5.2 Deep Dyslexia

The other major reading disorder described by Marshall and Newcombe (1973) was deep dyslexia. It provided them with the neuropsychological evidence for the existence of a semantic reading route from orthographic analysis systems to the semantic system that was unrelated to phonology (see Figure 4.2). In terms of the interest it has generated over the past 10 years or so, deep dyslexia must stand in the first rank of neuropsychological disorders, alongside, say, agrammatism and amnesia. It has the advantage of containing an intuitively fascinating primary symptom, the semantic error – such as, to quote an example of Patterson and Besner (1984), the patient reading *muddy* as *quagmire* – and it was given, when initially described, an alliterative and mysterious name![12] A large literature has come to exist on it, and the publication of the book on that topic alone (Coltheart, Patterson, & Marshall, 1980), discussed in chapter 2, is often considered a critical point in the early history of cognitive neuropsychology.

As soon as one begins to ask simple questions about the disorder, though, it becomes apparent that research on it has not produced any consensus of views. What defines deep dyslexia? What variables affect the patients' performance? How should one explain it? What does the explanation tell us as far as theoretical inferences to normal function are concerned? For only the second of these questions is there even a modicum of agreement. Moreover, the issues raised in the attempts to answer these questions are diverse and complex.

The syndrome presents two additional difficulties for the approach being taken in this book. One is conceptually trivial. There are now too many well-described cases for the characteristics of all the patients being considered to be worth listing. Coltheart (1980a) discussed 16 cases and Kremin (1982), another 8; by 1982, at

12. In the mid-1970s, a rather puritanical attempt was made to replace the vague but attractive term *deep* with a term considered more functionally correct, *phonemic* (see Shallice & Warrington, 1975). However, with the discovery of another syndrome for which the word *phonological* seemed more suited, *phonemic* has been generally dropped as an alternative to *deep*.

least 3 other cases had been described in the literature.[13] Since excellent reviews exist (e.g. Coltheart, 1980a; Patterson, 1981; Kremin, 1982), I shall not present the empirical information on the syndrome in as much detail as was given for the short-term memory syndrome and the peripheral dyslexias.

The second difficulty is one familiar from the discussion of surface dyslexia in chapter 4. Deep dyslexia is the disorder *par excellence* for which the symptom-complex approach has been used in cognitive neuropsychology. For other syndromes, such as Broca's and conduction aphasia and possibly even surface dyslexia, the appeal of the symptom-complex approach has grown weaker at a theoretical level. For deep dyslexia, it remains vigorous. To force the literature into a dissociation mould would be to prejudge an issue that is still being debated.

It is simplest to begin with a description of the patient in whom the condition was first described, GR (Marshall & Newcombe, 1966, 1973). GR had sustained a left parieto-temporal bullet wound roughly 20 years before his reading was first systematically analysed. Non-verbal abilities were demonstrated to be intact; but GR had some comprehension difficulties, and his spontaneous speech was telegrammatic and halting.

The basic corpus used to investigate his reading consisted of his responses to 2,000 individually presented words. Two very interesting aspects of his reading performance were noted. The first concerned the errors he made, which were of various types. Prime among them – both in number (more than half) and because they are so counterintuitive – were *semantic* errors where the response had only a semantic relation to the stimulus: *ill* → *'sick'*, *bush* → *'tree'*, *cheer* → *'laugh,'* and *bad* → *'liar'*. Semantic errors were critically important for Marshall and Newcombe; they provide strong support for the existence of a semantic route that is presumably operating in isolation in GR, as even minimal phonological information would allow him to eliminate the errors. However, GR also made two other types of error: *visual*, such as *life* → *'wife'* and *sword* → *'words'*; and *derivational*, such as *card* → *'cards'*, *fleeing* → *'flee'*, *entertain* → *'entertainment'*, and *beg* → *'beggar'*.[14]

The second phenomenon was that the chance of a word being read correctly by GR was greatly affected by a variable other than word frequency (or familiarity); this was assumed to be syntactic class. Thus 46% of nouns were read, but only 16% of adjectives and 6% of verbs. Of 54 function words (closed class items such as prepositions and pronouns), he read only two: *I,* which can, of course, be produced

---

13. See Shallice and Coughlan (1980), Nolan and Caramazza (1982), and Friedman and Perlman (1982). There is insufficient detail to base functional inferences on a number of the patients included in the reviews, but there are still an ample number of well-described cases.

14. A criterion relatively frequently used for visual errors is that 50% of the letters must be shared by the stimulus and the response. The phrase 'derivational error' is used to cover cases in which the stimulus and the response have the same root morpheme or the two are different inflectional forms of the same irregular morpheme.

Table 5.3. *Performance of four deep dyslexic patients on reading aloud*

	Concrete	Abstract	Adjective	Verb	Functor	Regular non-word
GR[a]	50*	10*	16	6	1	0
KF[b]	73*	14*	32	7	10	—
PW[c]	67	13				0
DE[c]	70	10				10

*Nouns
[a] Marshall and Newcombe (1966)
[b] Shallice and Warrington (1975)
[c] Patterson and Marcel (1977)

merely by letter naming; and *and!* An ordering of noun > adjective > verb > function word was obtained.

GR is far from being unique. As mentioned earlier, there are a considerable number of well-reported patients whose reading has these characteristics. Thus Coltheart (1980a), in his review, described 16 patients who make semantic errors in reading and for whom a 'reasonable' amount of detail about other symptoms is available. In 13 of these patients, both the other types of error and the word-class effects occur, and in his discussion of 2 patients, Coltheart seemed to be making a polite genuflection towards inadequately recorded cases from the prehistory of the topic. Table 5.3 illustrates the characteristic effects in four of the earlier patients described.[15] In only one case he considered – to be discussed later – did the conjunction of symptoms not hold.

The word-class effects also have the comforting property that they fit with the critical-variable approach discussed in chapter 4. The ability of many deep dyslexic patients to read pronounceable letter strings is strongly affected by at least two other stimulus variables. The first of these has not been mentioned so far, but it should not be surprising. As can be seen from Table 5.3, the reading of function words presents an almost insuperable problem to deep dyslexic patients. Moreover, many function words, such as *on, if,* and *it,* are regular. Therefore, the early investigators argued that if the phonological route were operative, the patient should be able to read words such as these. Since they cannot, the route must be inoperative, which supports the conclusion derived from the presence of semantic errors. This was

15. One of the patients listed in the table, KF (Shallice & Warrington 1975), is the same patient whose impaired short-term memory was described in chapter 3. It is possible for a patient to have more than one impairment of theoretical interest, provided that the deficit is specific in any particular domain and the deficits in other domains introduce no awkward confoundings. For any one disorder, it may be possible to treat the patient as a pure case. Three pure syndromes, each previously unknown, have in fact been reported in the same patient, RG (Beauvois, Saillant, Meininger, & Lhermitte, 1978; Beauvois & Derouesné, 1979, 1981)!

shown more directly by Patterson and Marcel (1977), working with patients PW and DE. These patients read 0% and 10% of pronounceable single-syllable non-words, compared with 53% and 63% for content words classed as 'highly imageable'.[16]

The effect of word type also appears to involve more than the syntactic class of the word. The position of the word on an imageability or concreteness versus abstractness scale is important. Thus GR read 45–50% of concrete nouns, but only 10% of abstract nouns, and for KF, the effect was even stronger. Attempts to determine whether there is any influence of part of speech when imageability or concreteness differences are removed do not all agree (see Allport & Funnell, 1981). The most detailed data were, however, provided by Allport & Funnell (1981) themselves. They reported one deep dyslexic patient they examined and four tested by Patterson, for all of whom the reading of nouns and verbs of matched imageability was of an equal level. However, to assume that part of speech, per se, has no effect would, in my opinion, be premature.

It seems particularly inappropriate to consider the function-word deficit as just an effect of the low imageability or concreteness of the words. Thus Patterson and Morton (1980) showed that 'semantic' decisions about function words could be made reasonably well. Their patient, PW, was asked to place one function word with whichever of two other words 'goes with' it. When there was a semantic basis for the decision (e.g. Does *we* go with *I* or *he?* Does *next to* go with *beside* or *apart?*), he generally scored over 80% (7 series out of 10). But if the decision had to be based on purely syntactic criteria (e.g. Does *her* go with *he* or *him?* Does *that* go with *this* or *thus?*), he was at chance or below.[17] To summarise these findings in terms of imageability conceals the implication that syntactic information is not available to the patient. However, the overall pattern of results on imageability and part of speech make clear that a critical operational variable in deep dyslexia is imageability or concreteness.[18]

5.3 In What Does Deep Dyslexia Consist?

A patient like GR has more than just a reading problem. He is an aphasic who would be termed a Broca's aphasic in the clinical classification stemming from the diagram-makers' syndromes (chapter 1), spontaneous speech being much more impaired than comprehension. In Broca's aphasia, the prototypic symptoms as far as

---

16. As mentioned in chapter 4, both letter-by-letter readers and, more particularly, semantic dyslexics can read non-words as well as words (see, e.g., Warrington & Shallice, 1980; Kremin, 1981; Table 5.1). Thus an assumption of greater non-specific task difficulty for non-words would be a most implausible way of explaining the effects of lexicality found in PW and DE.

17. A related finding has been made for the auditory comprehension of function words by agrammatic aphasics (see Schwartz, Saffran, & Marin, 1980b).

18. Letter-by-letter readers can show no effect of imageability (e.g., Warrington & Shallice, 1980). The variable has been less adequately studied in patients with phonological reading. Other patients will be discussed later who contrast with deep dyslexia in this respect.

expressive speech is concerned are awkward articulation and prosody, a much reduced maximum length of utterance and a restriction of grammar to, at most, its simplest forms but with a relative sparing of content words (see, e.g., Goodglass & Kaplan, 1972; Berndt & Caramazza, 1980). In addition, GR's auditory–verbal STM performance was very poor, he had an agraphia, and he made semantic errors in auditory as well as visual word–picture matching.

GR is far from unique in these respects. Of the patients listed in Table 5.3, PW and DE also have effortful non-fluent spontaneous speech of this general type. Moreover, the difficulty that the deep dyslexic has with function words and the relative preservation of content words are characteristic of Broca's aphasic speech. In the typical deep dyslexic, the reading difficulty is just one of a variety of impairments. This raises a number of questions. Is deep dyslexia – or, at least, some of its elements – merely the effect of a more basic language problem on reading? Given the number of subsystems that must be damaged in these patients, does 'deep dyslexia' really correspond to the same functional deficit in each patient, or is it a label for damage to different but overlapping sets of subsystems in different patients? If the locus of impairment is the same for all deep dyslexias, is it a single-component pure syndrome or a multi-component one?

First, could deep dyslexia just be what happens when a Broca's aphasic attempts to read?[19] Such an attempt to reduce a novel symptom complex to an apparently familiar entity would be multiply misguided. Broca's aphasia is a standard operational category to modern neurolinguists, but it seems most unlikely to correspond to a disorder of a single functional system (see, e.g., Berndt & Caramazza, 1980). Second, some deep dyslexic patients do not have the expressive speech difficulties of a Broca's aphasic. The clearest example is probably WS (Schwartz, Saffran, & Marin, 1977), who had a 'profile' over the subtests of the Boston Aphasia Battery of Goodglass and Kaplan (1972) that was very different from that attributed to the prototypic Broca's aphasic and yet who showed both the word-class and error pattern results characteristic of deep dyslexia.[20] Finally, patients diagnosed as Broca's aphasic on the Boston Aphasia Battery do not necessarily show a deep dyslexic reading pattern. For instance, a group of four such patients tested by Caramazza, Berndt, and Hart (1981) read nouns, verbs, and adjectives roughly equally well (73%, 78% and 74%, respectively); in addition, one (BD) could read function words fairly well and made no semantic errors.

What, then, are the essential aspects of deep dyslexia, the defining group of

19. This point has been discussed by Coltheart (1980c) and Friedman and Perlman (1982). For a more detailed consideration of Broca's aphasia, see chapter 7.
20. It should be noted that WS was only 13 years old when his lesion occurred. However, there are other such patients, including LEC (Kremin, 1981), who had normal spontaneous speech and a mild but typical deep dyslexia, and NT (Howard, 1985a), who has fluent grammatical spontaneous speech and a severe deep dyslexia. The example of KF (Shallice & Warrington, 1975), which is often quoted in this context, is less convincing. His spontaneous speech, while not of a classical Broca's aphasic type, was still halting, and he made many syntactic errors (see Shallice & Butterworth, 1977, Table 3).

symptoms? The standard move on the symptom-complex approach has been to argue that the semantic error is the key defining feature and that if it is present, a variety of other characteristics are also found (see Coltheart, 1980a; Marshall & Newcombe, 1980).[21] Yet Coltheart pointed out that there is at least one patient who appears to spoil the scheme, AR (Warrington & Shallice, 1979), who made 5% semantic errors and 12% errors with both a visual and a semantic similarity to the stimulus word (e.g. *paper* → *page*). He read 49% of function words correctly, compared with 51% of content words – insignificantly different. Coltheart's response to this exceptional case was principled. He did not just ignore AR as a statistical freak. His position was that if deep dyslexia does reflect damage to a single functional entity, then all patients in whom there is damage to that system should show all characteristics of the disorder. If a patient with the key defining feature fails to show all the other characteristics, then the specific pattern shown by the patient requires explanation. Coltheart (1980a) argued that AR differs from other deep dyslexia patients in having some limited ability to derive phonology from print:

On some theories of the semantic error, this residual ability would reduce the rate of semantic errors: if the patient is unsure whether to read *bush* as 'bush' or 'tree', even a limited amount of phonological information from the printed word would allow him to rule out 'tree' as a possible response. Since function words are in general shorter and phonologically simpler than content words, residual phonological ability might selectively favour function words, thus closing the gap which normally exists between the two types of words in deep dyslexia. (p. 45)

AR did make a smaller number of semantic errors than, say, GR. However, this explanation would require that, in general, AR should have found shorter words easier to read than longer ones. In fact, he showed only a small effect of the word-length variable. Thus on the one word pool where the effects of word length were investigated, the mean length of words correctly read was 5.4 letters, compared with only 5.9 letters for words not read. Moreover, it is hard to see how this 'residual phonological ability' would explain AR's relatively good performance with adjectives (63% correct, compared with 54% for nouns).[22]

Thus it seems that the word-class effects most frequently found are not an inevitable concomitant of the occurrence of semantic errors. It would be possible to delete word-class effects from the properties of deep dyslexia in order to try to maintain the logic of the 'psychologically strong syndrome', discussed in chapter 2. No one, as far as I know, has yet made this suggestion. The reason is clear. The once ample symptom complex would by analogous arguments be reduced to a relatively uninteresting wraith, composed, say, of semantic and visual errors and with little potential theoretical clout. The alternative is to assume that AR has a functionally different disorder that also results in semantic errors. The logic of how

21. This uses the strong symptom-complex approach (see chapter 2).
22. AR is, in fact, different in many respects from a typical deep dyslexic patient. His 'semantic access dyslexia' is discussed in chapter 12.

one defines the functionally critical cluster of symptoms for deep dyslexia is, however, left in tatters.

One approach – the purist one – would be to ignore the similarity among deep dyslexic patients and just consider individual deep dyslexic patients. An alternative is to concentrate on the dissociation aspects of the disorder as the defining characteristic. At least two stimulus variables strongly affect the reading of certain central dyslexic patients, including the deep dyslexics: lexicality and imageability or concreteness. As there are other patients whose reading is not affected by these variables, changes to these variables do not just make the reading process generally more difficult; the effect of the variables presumably reflects a stressing of some sub-part of the reading process.[23] This aspect of the individual deep dyslexic's reading disorder is therefore both replicable and an appropriate starting point for a functional explanation.

This procedure has not, however, proved popular. The approach that is now most frequently seen is to *define* deep dyslexia as some combination of characteristics – in particular, as the existence of various error types and certain word-class effects (e.g. Friedman & Perlman, 1982). Ironically, this grouping was initially made as a rough-and-ready shorthand for communication purposes by those who did not believe in the syndrome as a unitary functional entity (Morton & Patterson, 1980; Shallice & Warrington, 1980). It is now increasingly used without the original caveats. Yet no justification is given as to why this combination of characteristics should reflect damage to a unitary functional entity.

One possibility is that the methodological problem can be solved by an elegant theoretical account that explains why a particular set of characteristics have a common functional origin. Does such an account exist?

5.4 Simple Explanations of the Deep Dyslexia Symptom Complex

The complexity of the pattern of symptoms found in deep dyslexia is matched by the variety of accounts put forward to explain it. The simplest type of explanation has been to take a model like any of those shown in Figures 4.2, 5.1, and 5.2 and to assume that deep dyslexia is, in essence, reading by the semantic route alone.

One aspect of this explanation – that the operation of the phonological route or routes is very impaired – is widely accepted. The basis for Marshall and Newcombe's (1973) classic explanation for semantic errors was that if any phonological information were available, it would allow the patient to eliminate such errors by means of a checking procedure. A number of other results also fit this view. For instance, the deep dyslexic patient VS was unable to perform rhyme judgements satisfactorily for visually presented words, although she was almost perfect with auditory presentation (Saffran & Marin, 1977); this effect has been observed in

---

23. See chapter 10 for discussion of this inference. Whether all patients who show, say, strong effects of word imageability also show the error-type effects is unclear.

other patients with a similar set of symptoms (see Coltheart, 1980a).[24] One possible explanation for such phenomena is that it is not the route that is impaired, but the output phonological word-form itself. This alternative can be most easily rejected if there are conditions under which the output word-form system operates normally. For instance, PW and DE could repeat single-syllable words perfectly but could not read all of them aloud (Patterson & Marcel, 1977).[25]

How is the semantic route itself thought to operate in deep dyslexia? A number of authors have argued that deep dyslexia is, in essence, reading by means of the semantic route alone in a relatively normal fashion (see, e.g., Saffran, Schwartz, & Marin, 1976; Newcombe & Marshall, 1980a). Others, however, have argued that there is also some impairment to the semantic route; this has been assumed to be a quantitative one by Nolan and Caramazza (1982) and a qualitative one by Morton and Patterson (1980) and Shallice and Warrington (1980). Finally, a radically different hypothesis has been suggested by Coltheart (1980b) and Saffran, Bogyo, Schwartz, and Marin (1980) – that deep dyslexic reading is, in essence, reading by the right hemisphere, which is assumed to lack any equivalent of the phonological route or routes.

The idea that deep dyslexia involves reading by a 'normal' semantic route unassisted by any form of phonological information is clearly the simplest hypothesis. If it gives a plausible account of the data, then more complex alternatives can safely be relegated to historical footnotes. The explanation entails that some form of phonological route is needed to read certain classes of word aloud. Saffran, Schwartz, and Marin (1979) and Jones (1985) have presented arguments about why this should be the case. Saffran et al. express it in the following fashion:

The gist of our argument is that the mechanism that mediates oral reading performance in deep dyslexia is designed for the *comprehension* of written words, not their production. It is in the nature of comprehension mechanisms, we believe, that a word will elicit a broad representation, rather than a narrow specification of its meaning. On this view, the oral reading task presents the patient with the following problem: he has no information about the target other than the semantic representation that it evokes; his task, then, is to produce the

24. Another example is the absence in the lexical decision performance of deep dyslexic patients of the so-called 'pseudo-homophone' effect, the interference produced in normal subjects by non-words that sound like words (see, e.g., Patterson & Marcel, 1977; Coltheart, 1980a).

25. The possibility that *some* information is available for deep dyslexics from 'direct' non-semantic morphemic correspondences has been suggested by Friedman and Perlman (1982), Howard (1985a), and Goldblum (1985). Thus Howard shows that some deep dyslexics – for example, Patterson's (1978) PW – perform well on a fairly difficult picture–word matching test, suggesting that object recognition is intact. Yet reading aloud is better than picture naming in some. Howard attributes this reading superiority to the use of additional information from a non-semantic route. However, although PW and the other deep dyslexics considered by Howard performed at 90% or above on the picture–word matching test, they still appear to have performed the test at a level below the normal range, suggesting that there might be some problem in accessing the semantic system from pictorial input; in addition, the difference in performance between reading aloud and picture naming is not dramatic (e.g. PW: 90% vs. 77% correct). Moreover, the explanation has some difficulty in explaining why semantic errors were much more frequent in reading than in object naming for PW (Patterson & Besner, 1984)!

word on the basis of his self-generated definition, which (the aphasic not being Webster) is likely to be less than perfect. One can imagine, further, that the difficulty of this task will vary with the nature of the stimulus word. A concrete word – a reference term like 'rose' – has a core meaning that is little altered by context (a rose *is* a rose). . . . The meanings of abstract words, on the other hand, tend to be more dependent on the contexts in which they are embedded. Consider a word like 'phase', for example; the meaning that is elaborated for it will be radically different depending on whether we read 'phase of development in the child' or 'phase of the moon'. A representation for the isolated word 'phase' is likely to be rather vague and difficult to lexicalise, particularly for an aphasic subject. A similar problem will occur with functors, which carry little meaning in themselves but, rather, function in the language as modulators of meaning. (Saffran et al., 1979; unpublished)

That it is more difficult to achieve the name of an abstract word than that of a concrete word from its semantic representation is supported by the findings of Barnard, Hammond, MacLean, and Morton (1982) of the relative ease of providing a word from a definition. Thus 77% of subjects were able to give *barrel* for 'a round wooden container for liquids, usually bulging in the middle', but only 23% gave *betray* for 'to break trust or allegiance by double-crossing, revealing secrets or spying'. Overall, low-frequency concrete nouns were 78% correct, and low-frequency abstract verbs were 38% correct. In addition, it has been shown that a related explanation accounts neatly for the effects of word class found in at least one deep dyslexic – the original patient, GR. Barry (1984) used the 'ease of predication' measure developed by Jones (1985), which assesses how easy it is for a person to think of factual statements about a word, a measure that appears conceptually relevant for the theoretical position of Saffran et al. (1979) and of Jones himself. It was as satisfactory a measure as concreteness in separating out the groups of words to which GR made different types of responses (correct, semantic errors, omission).

Would an explanation of this type be able to account for the existence of semantic errors? One suggestion that is compatible with Saffran et al. and Jones's position is that made by Newcombe and Marshall (1980a) – that the semantic system is intrinsically unstable unless it is 'corrected' or 'checked' by its various peripheral devices. They assumed that very little information from peripheral devices is sufficient to eliminate semantic errors.[26] There are a number of major problems for this suggestion. Most simply, as Saffran (1984) has pointed out, the degree of intrinsic instability would have to be very great indeed to account for errors such as *turtle* → *crocodile* and *genealogist* → *babies*. Second, because normal subjects can name objects without making semantic errors, Newcombe and Marshall would be forced to postulate a phonological route to stabilize object naming as well as one for word reading.[27] Whether or not it is plausible to assume that a separate phonological route exists for naming objects, it can hardly do so for responding to questions. It seems unlikely that normal subjects would show much variability in responding to ques-

---

26. In fact, semantic errors are made by patients who can read some non-words – for example, AR (Warrington & Shallice, 1979), PS (Shallice & Coughlan, 1980), and BL (Nolan & Caramazza, 1982).

27. Ratcliff and Newcombe (1982) put forward such a suggestion. However, as we will see in chapter 12, there are problems in making this assumption.

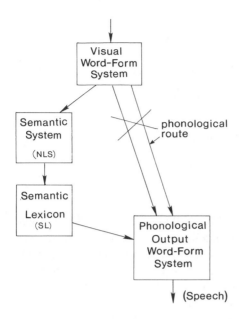

Figure 5.5. The locus of the impairment in deep dyslexia based on the concept of the semantic lexicon. The cross represents the hypothesised locus of the impairment. The phonological route is the 'broad' type, illustrated in Figure 5.2.

tions such as 'What is the name for the period of time between two days when it is dark?' Yet this lack of variability can hardly be due to any 'checking' by peripheral devices. It seems unlikely that the question specifies *night* any more adequately than the visual stimulus *night*. Patterson's patient, DE, however, read *night* as *sleep*.

A more adequate explanation of semantic errors within this broad class of theory can be seen if one elaborates a little the account of the naming process. It is now frequent in theorising on spontaneous speech to presuppose that the highest level of representation of an utterance is based on units more abstract than individual lexical items (e.g. Miller & Johnson-Laird, 1976). Selection of lexical items, to fit particular semantic and syntactic requirements, therefore represents one sub-process in the determination of the form of the utterance (see, e. g., Butterworth, 1980; Garrett, 1980); this can go wrong even in normal subjects, giving rise to rare semantic errors in spontaneous speech, as in 'He rode his bike to school *tomorrow*' (instead of *yesterday*), (Garrett, 1980).

Assume that in deep dyslexic reading, the 'deeper' non-lexical semantic representation (NLS) has to be used as the stage prior to a semantic lexical item (SL) being selected (Figure 5.5).[28] Then the more abstract the representation at stage

28. A related model has been suggested by Howard (1985a). However, he argues that the SL stage precedes the NLS as well as following it, so that reading by semantics by-passes the latter stage. It is unclear how this approach accounts for the difficulty that deep dyslexics have with abstract words.

Table 5.4. *Contrasting performance of two deep dyslexic patients on the Peabody Picture-Vocabulary test*

	Visual	Auditory
VS[a]	124	129
PS[b]	57	108

[a] Saffran and Marin (1977)
[b] Shallice and Coughlan (1980)

NLS, the wider the variety of lexical items that might be used to express the idea in 'normal' spontaneous speech. It would then follow, as suggested by Barry (1985), that there would be wider but weaker activation of individual lexical items at stage SL. Semantic errors would occur if an incorrect response were both sufficiently strongly activated and activated by chance more than the correct response. This would be expected to arise most often for words intermediate in abstractness between those giving rise to sharply peaked activation profiles across candidates (concrete stimuli) and those having low, flat activation profiles (abstract stimuli). This has been shown to be the case statistically for semantic errors in both KF (Shallice & Warrington, 1975) and GR (Barry 1985; and personal communication; see also Jones, 1985).

5.5   The Inadequacy of the 'Normal Isolated Semantic Route' Theory

A major problem still exists for the theory that deep dyslexia reflects the operation of a normal semantic route, with the phonological route or routes grossly impaired. Deep dyslexic patients are not functionally identical. It seems possible to locate their impairments at different places on an input–output dimension (Shallice & Warrington, 1980; Friedman & Perlman, 1982). Thus some deep dyslexics, such as VS (Saffran & Marin, 1977) and PW (Patterson, 1979), perform almost as well on quantitative tests of comprehension, such as the Peabody picture–word matching test, when written words are the stimuli, as they do when the words are presented auditorily. Others, however, such as PS (Shallice & Coughlan, 1980) and KF (Shallice & Warrington, 1980), perform much more poorly on the written version (Table 5.4). All four patients, though, showed qualitatively similar word-class and error-type effects.

There is another aspect of the disorder that fits with the existence of a functional distinction between deep dyslexic patients of an 'input' type, in whom the impairment affects the visual modality specifically, and those of an 'output' type, in whom the disorder is modality-independent. This is the ratio of semantic to visual errors, which varies widely across patients, as can be seen in Table 5.5. None of the

Table 5.5. *The proportion of different types of error made by certain deep dyslexic patients (in percentages)*

Patient	Semantic	Visual and/or semantic	Visual	Derivational	Other
PW[a]	54	4	13	22	6
GR[b]	56	?	22	11(?)	11
DE[a]	23	6	35	32	4
WS[c]	21	17	35	4	23
VS[d]	19	16	48	10	7
PS[e]	10	7	51	9	23
KF[f]	4	10	61	19	6

[a] Patterson (1978)
[b] Marshall and Newcombe (1966)
[c] Schwartz, Saffran, and Marin (1977)
[d] Saffran (personal communication)
[e] Shallice and Coughlan (1980)
[f] Shallice and Warrington (1975)

patients who make the higher proportion of semantic errors are of the input type, whereas the last two patients in the table are both of that type.

Could it be that patients low in the table, like KF and PS, have not only a pure deep dyslexia, but also a pre-semantic visual impairment? For instance, could one explain their reading characteristics by adding a partial impairment to the visual word-form system in the model illustrated in Figure 5.5? An extra visual difficulty would explain both the auditory–visual difference and the high rate of visual errors. Any visual deficit would presumably be independent of the semantic and syntactic factors. If this were the case, then the overall performance of input deep dyslexics across different classes of words should be qualitatively similar to that of output patients, but scaled down across the whole concrete–abstract dimension. The concrete–abstract and word-class differences of such patients should therefore be weaker than those of the more pure output patients. Comparable figures are difficult to obtain. However, the abstract–concrete and word-class differences of patients like PS and KF (see Table 5.3) seem to be at least as high as those obtained in patients who on the criterion of the ratio of semantic-to-visual errors should be much more 'pure' – for example, GR, FD (Friedman & Perlman, 1982), and BL (Nolan & Caramazza, 1982).[29] Thus the argument runs into a difficulty.

Second, if visual errors do arise from an additional impairment at a pre-semantic visual level – for example, in the visual word-form system – why are there no deep

29. DE and PW may, however, show larger concrete–abstract differences – 70–10 and 67–13, respectively (see Patterson, 1981).

Table 5.6. *Rate of visual errors made by three deep dyslexic patients on different types of words*

GR[a]	Nouns 4%; adjectives 13%; verbs 10%
PS[b]	High concrete 4%; low concrete 14%
KF[c]	High concrete 11%; all words 23%

Note: Errors occur less frequently on the word classes that give better reading performance.
[a] Marshall and Newcombe (1966)
[b] Shallice and Coughlan (1980)
[c] Shallice and Warrington (1980)

dyslexic patients who do not show them? More important, since the process that produces them would precede the semantic system, they should occur equally at all points on the abstract–concrete dimension. In fact, they tend to occur predominantly on the types of word that the patient cannot read – the more abstract words (Coltheart, 1980b; Morton & Patterson, 1980; Shallice & Warrington, 1980) (Table 5.6). This suggests that visual errors do not reflect an impairment of some pre-semantic system, but a process dependent on the failure of the stimulus word to access an adequate semantic representation.[30]

It is therefore more plausible that 'input' deep dyslexia is not a pure deep dyslexia *plus* a visual deficit, but a primary deficit consisting of an inability to access the semantic representation of abstract words, given visual input. By contrast, a patient such as PW – a relatively pure 'output' deep dyslexic – can access the semantic representations of abstract words but cannot produce their names. If this were the case, the symptom complex would fractionate into separate functional entities, with many patients having a combination of both difficulties.

Differences within deep dyslexic patients are not limited to the input–output dimension. Some patients show semantic errors in other situations, such as writing to dictation and picture–word matching – GR (Newcombe & Marshall, 1980b) – or both these tasks and individual word repetition – VS (Nolan & Caramazza, 1983). But in other patients, there are tasks where semantic errors do not occur, or at least are far more rare than in reading aloud – for example, word–picture matching in PW (Patterson & Besner, 1984). This suggests that there is a third sort of

---

30. A complex debate exists on the mechanism by which visual errors occur in deep dyslexia; for discussions, see Shallice and Warrington (1975, 1980), Morton and Patterson (1980), and Nolan and Caramazza (1983). It has been suggested by Goldblum (1985) that the errors classically assumed to be visual errors in deep dyslexia are phonological. Strangely enough, this question does not appear to have been considered empirically in any patient since KF. Everyone working in the field just treated the issue in scientific paradigm fashion as obvious. However, in an error such as *was* → *saw*, made by KF, every letter that occurs in both has a different phonological representation in the stimulus than the response. Related examples are *choice* → *choir* and *ever* → *even* (except for *v*).

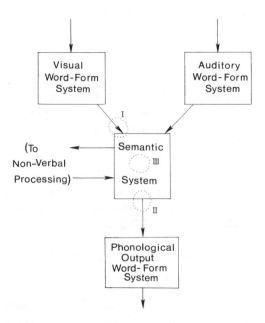

Figure 5.6. Varieties of deep dyslexia; the three possible loci of the secondary deficit are discussed in the text. (Only the semantic route is represented. The phonological route is assumed to be totally inoperative.)

deep dyslexic who has a central disorder within the semantic system (Figure 5.6). Thus the view has been increasingly widely expressed that the symptom complex found in deep dyslexia can arise from a number of types of impairment. One consequence of this is that the most famous symptom – the existence of semantic errors – could itself arise from a number of impairments: as an inaccuracy in semantic access, an instability of the semantic representation, or a consequence of a difficulty in attaining the precise lexical semantic representation in the speech output system.[31]

A fairly obvious general type of explanation of the word-class effects that would apply roughly equally well to the different loci of impairments also seems to be available. The semantic processing of abstract words may just be more difficult or less overdetermined than that of concrete words and so more affected by impairment at any stage of operation of the semantic route (see Nolan & Caramazza, 1982). In fact, this explanation may well underestimate the degree of modularity within the semantic system. To assess this possibility, another form of central dyslexic disor-

31. For a more detailed discussion of the types of semantic errors that occur in deep dyslexia, see Coltheart (1980c). The 'semantic lexicon' has not been considered in this argument. An implication of this section is that such a subsystem is not entailed by the facts of deep dyslexia; to consider it would complicate further an already complex argument.

der needs to be considered. There remains, however, a further type of explanation of deep dyslexia – of a very different type from those so far considered.

5.6 Deep Dyslexia: The Right Hemisphere Theory

A much more dramatic challenge exists to the Marshall and Newcombe (1973) theory of deep dyslexia. Perhaps deep dyslexia does not result from the operation of the normal reading system, within which certain components have been damaged. A much more radical theory is that the reading of deep dyslexic patients depends on subsystems in their right hemispheres that are not normally used. It is standard to assume that speech production is controlled by the left hemisphere, so the right hemisphere locus would apply at least up to the stage of word comprehension. The properties of the syndrome would then reflect those of right hemisphere language-processing systems (Coltheart, 1980b, 1983; Saffran et al., 1980; Zaidel & Peters, 1981).[32]

The attraction of this idea stems from two sources. The first is that one can draw analogies between the characteristics of deep dyslexia and the properties of right hemisphere language, as inferred from split-brain studies and visual-field studies. The second is that deep dyslexia arises from large and deep left hemisphere lesions that affect much of the areas of the left hemisphere classically associated with language (see Coltheart et al., 1980, appendix 1).[33]

The strongest arguments for the 'right hemisphere reading' position stem from the similarity in reading pattern between deep dyslexics and right hemisphere reading in a small sub-group of so-called split-brain patients – a famous set of patients in whom the corpus callosum and the anterior commissure have been sectioned for the relief of epilepsy, thus cutting all cortical connections between the two hemispheres.[34] The right hemisphere of the split-brain patient seems to be incapable of deriving phonology from print, as are deep dyslexics, and makes semantic errors in word–picture matching, as did, say, GR (Zaidel & Peters, 1981; Zaidel, 1982). For instance, the right hemisphere of split-brain patients cannot match two words or a word and a picture on the basis of rhyme, although their left hemispheres can.

Coltheart (1983) also argued for the theory from a comparison of deep dyslexic

32. Deep dyslexia is only one of a set of syndromes for which it has been suggested that the right hemisphere takes over functions that, prior to the patient's illness, were presumably the responsibility of the left hemisphere. Others include deep dysgraphia (chapter 6) and the auditory parallel to deep dyslexia (chapter 7). Such explanations, if valid, present a grave conceptual problem for the whole enterprise of making theoretical extrapolations from abnormal to normal function. These problems will be considered in chapter 10.

33. The multiple-deficit theory would also predict that deep dyslexic patients have large lesions, so this is not a very compelling argument, especially given our present ignorance about the relation between anatomy and function for cognitive processes.

34. Other aspects of the split-brain syndrome – in particular, its relevance for information-processing theories of consciousness – are discussed in chapter 16. For the present purposes, an important point is that the properties of the split-brain reading described here arise from a small sub-group of split-brain patients, who are probably atypical.

performance and visual-field studies in normal subjects, particularly with respect to the abstract–concrete difference. Early studies on normal subjects had shown that there is a special difficulty in recognising abstract words presented to the left visual field (e.g. Ellis & Shepherd, 1974; Hines, 1976). However, between 1979 and 1984, numerous experiments were reported on the topic, and only one (Day, 1979) – which had a very high error rate – showed a significant interaction between visual field and concreteness; 11 others did not (see Lambert, 1982; Patterson & Besner, 1984). It appears now that the earlier positive reports were artefactual. Perhaps the failure to find an interaction should count as a refutation of the right hemisphere hypothesis? It may be, though, that visual-field studies cannot tell us anything subtle about the lateralisation of function.[35]

Even if visual-field studies are ignored, the analogies drawn between deep dyslexic reading and right hemisphere split-brain processing seem powerful. But a number of major difficulties have become apparent for the theory that deep dyslexia involves right hemisphere reading. The first is that, as already discussed in chapter 4, letter-by-letter readers in general have an entirely intact right hemisphere. Why, then, do they not at least produce the same sort of reading responses as the deep dyslexic when they cannot read letter-by-letter? Coltheart (1983) has argued that the right hemisphere of the letter-by-letter reader can indeed comprehend, say, concrete words, but the information cannot be transferred to the left hemisphere because of a functional disconnection at the semantic level between the hemispheres (Figure 5.7). This disconnection (to C) is in addition to the one that, following the traditional theory of the syndrome, he assumes to exist at a much earlier level of visual processing (chapter 4). He presented no evidence for the existence of this high-level disconnection. In chapter 4, it was pointed out that such patients can obtain information about the semantics of objects given left visual-field presentation; Coltheart's suggestion seems an unacceptably ad hoc prop for the theory.

On the whole, the proponents of the right hemisphere theory of deep dyslexia share the general subtraction assumption – that the deep dyslexic can be understood merely in terms of a loss of mechanisms available to the normal subject and that right hemisphere reading mechanisms can operate in the normal subject (e.g. Coltheart, 1980b; Zaidel, 1983a). However, if one abandons this assumption, an alternative response is available. Letter-by-letter readers have normal fluent speech, but most deep dyslexic patients do not. It could be that only when there is release from left-hemisphere control or inhibition does language effectively relateralise, and this occurs only when expressive speech is impaired (for a discussion, see Nielsen, 1946).

This is yet another ad hoc assumption. Moreover, it, too, is faced with difficulties. Some deep dyslexics retain fluent speech – for example, WS (Schwartz, Saf-

---

35. Coltheart (1983) also argued extensively from visual-hemifield differences in Kanji and Kana recognition in Japanese readers. Such studies are, however, doubly remote from those of deep dyslexia. To accept them as relevant evidence presumably means that the results of visual-field studies in normal alphabetic-language readers should be accepted as relevant disconfirming evidence.

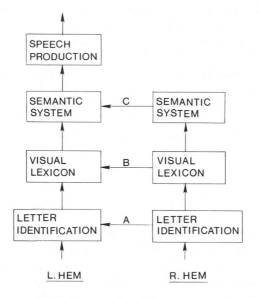

Figure 5.7. Hypothesised connections between the hemispheres involved in the discussion of the right hemisphere theory of deep dyslexia. In letter-by-letter reading, route A would remain at least partially intact.

fran, & Marin, 1977) – and some patients with unilateral left hemisphere strokes show no evidence of any form of relateralisation – severe global aphasics. For instance, the patient VER (Warrington & McCarthy, 1983) more than a year after having suffered a massive left hemisphere stroke, only occasionally used single words, either spontaneously or in response to a question, and was unable to carry out the simplest verbal instructions. She received a scaled score of 0 on all tests involving verbal functions; for instance, on the Peabody word–picture matching test, she was unable to achieve the so-called basal level, scoring only 15 out of the first 25 very easy items. She was even worse at comprehending written material.[36] In other words, in VER a total loss of left hemisphere language did not lead to any development of right hemisphere language. Therefore this defence of the right hemisphere hypothesis would be forced to assume individual differences in relateralisation potential. The right hemisphere hypothesis is becoming almost completely irrefutable.

As a final argument, which is apparently clinching, Patterson and Besner (1984) have directly compared test performance levels in deep dyslexics with those in the supposed analogue – the split-brain right hemisphere patient. The most impressive comparison consists of the visual version of the Peabody word–picture matching

36. Her impairment will be discussed further in Chapter 12.

Table 5.7. *Performance on Peabody Word–Picture Matching (Dunn, 1965) from two deep dyslexics and two split-brain patients for whom stimuli were lateralised to the left visual field*

	Deep dyslexics		Split-brain (Rt Hem)	
	DE	PW	NG	LB
Raw score	102	116	23	76
Age scaled (Years: months)	15.11	18+	6.6	10.2

From Patterson and Besner (1984)

test using written words (Table 5.7). Their deep dyslexic patients DE and PW performed far better than NG and LB, split-brain patients reported by Zaidel (1978). Yet NG and LB are known to produce the best right hemisphere performance of 40 or so split-brain patients tested, except for two in whom language lateralisation may well have shifted in early childhood due to early brain damage (see Gazzaniga, 1983).[37] The performance of NG and LB therefore represents the very best that could be expected from the isolated right hemisphere. Yet it is still considerably inferior to that of the deep dyslexic patients studied by Patterson and Besner.[38]

In fact, the right hemisphere theorists can wriggle, for some deep dyslexic patients do have much lower 'visual' Peabody scores than PW and DE and, indeed, very much in the range of scores obtained by the right hemispheres of NG and LB – for example, PS: 57 (Shallice & Coughlan, 1980) and WS: 54 (Saffran, 1980). So one cannot say that all deep dyslexics are better than all split-brain patients on the visual version of the Peabody test. However, this response just raises another problem for the right-hemisphere theory. Deep dyslexia, as pointed out in section 5.5, is probably functionally heterogeneous, which is, in turn, something that the right hemisphere theory would not predict.

The right hemisphere theory of deep dyslexia has not been conclusively refuted. However, it has the appearance of a scientific theory in what the philosopher of science Lakatos (1970) called its 'degenerating problem shift' stage. Problems for the theory keep arising. As soon as one leak is temporarily plugged, another bursts through. Since none of the salvage operations has turned into a fruitful source of

37. Gazzaniga's (1983) paper makes fairly dismal reading. It suggests that the whole edifice of right hemisphere language capacities inferred from split-brain performance over the past 20 years may well be an artefact of concentrating on the odd patient with abnormal lateralisation in early childhood. For further discussion of this point, see chapter 16.
38. There is a metatheoretical aspect to the argument of Patterson and Besner (1984). The type of argument – that of comparing two syndromes – would not be legitimate on the metatheoretical position of opposition to syndromes, discussed in chapter 2.

facts in its own right, the arguments to preserve the theory become increasingly ad hoc.

5.7 Deep Dyslexia: Conclusions

The attempt to produce a unitary functional account of deep dyslexia seems to be suffering the same fate as the attempt to characterise the disorder rigorously using a symptom-complex methodology. It is most plausible that the patients so labelled are functionally heterogeneous. They have in common a severe impairment of phonological reading, but vary in the locus of secondary damage to the semantic route. Deep dyslexia, then, is probably neither a pure syndrome nor a homogeneous one. Does this mean that it can add little to our understanding of normal function? Surprisingly, this would be too pessimistic a conclusion. The range of disorders covered by the label fits well with the two-route theory, and unless the right hemisphere theory is correct, they would be very difficult to explain on a single-route theory. Moreover, even if a disorder does not illuminate normal function directly, it may be applied indirectly to assist in the solution of some problem concerning normal function.

An excellent example is the work of Saffran (1980). Saffran was interested in whether word reading is appropriately characterised as 'ideographic'. Do we read words as visual wholes? Normal subjects when presented with information in distorted format (e.g. mixed-case *AdMiRe*) show no qualitative changes in performance (e.g. McClelland, 1977). This suggests that the visual word-form system receives its input from a system that detects 'abstract letter identities': *A* and *a,* say, are the same. However, normal subjects may merely switch from semantic-route reading to some other strategy, such as phonological reading. Such alternative strategies are not available to deep dyslexic patients. They are unable to transform a visually presented letter string into phonological form and are, in general, unable to spell. If, then, words are read as Gestalts, presenting words in a mixed-case form should lead to the patient's being unable to read them.

Saffran presented four deep dyslexic patients with 35 words they had previously read. Each word was presented (in different lists) in three forms: normal lower case, mixed case, and vertical. The patients made 10% of errors in normal lower case, but only 5% in mixed case and 6% in vertical presentation. This, therefore, provides strong evidence that orthographic analysis in word reading can be based on an ordered set of abstract letter identities or, at least, is not necessarily ideographic.[39] This illustrates that plausible inferences about normal function can be made even if the syndrome under investigation is far from being a 'pure' one!

---

39. It is conceivable that this is an emergent property of some hypothetical right hemisphere reading system, but is not available to the normal left hemisphere reading system. Although this is a logical possibility, it is more the argument of a pedant than a realist. Even if deep dyslexic reading were a right hemisphere process, why should just that hemisphere and not the left use abstract letter identities? For neuropsychological arguments that visual recognition can use sources of information other than abstract letter identities, see Howard (1987).

Table 5.8. *CAV's performance on matched abstract and concrete words on four testing sessions over a period of one week*

	Concrete words correct $n = 36$	Abstract words correct $n = 36$
I	5	15
II	9	21
III	9	25
IV	26	29

From Warrington (1981) with permission

5.8   The Exceptional Case: CAV

Of all central dyslexic patients so far studied, one patient, CAV (Warrington, 1981), is in a certain respect unique. He provides an important contrast with the deep dyslexic patients in being able to read abstract words more easily than concrete.

Most dyslexic patients who have been studied have been stroke patients. CAV, however, was suffering from a tumour affecting the left parieto-temporal region. After the diagnosis was first made, his tumour responded to treatment, and he showed an improvement that unfortunately proved to be only temporary; during this period, the study took place.

When first seen, CAV appeared to be totally unable to read. He failed to read any of the easiest 10 words on a standard reading test (the Schonell); these are mainly highly concrete words, such as *milk* and *tree*. However, it was incidentally observed that he could read the occasional highly abstract word, such as *applause, evidence,* and *inferior.* On four different days, he was asked to read a set of 36 abstract and concrete words matched for length and frequency. He gradually regained some of his reading ability, but an abstract–concrete difference remained clear (Table 5.8). On a much larger set of words, which was attempted at a time when his reading had progressed somewhat, he was correct on 55% of words more abstract than the median, but only 36% of more concrete ones. This may not seem a large effect, but performance on high-frequency (A or AA) concrete words (44%) was no better than that on abstract words of a lower frequency range (1–50 per million) (44%).

Although CAV made very few semantic errors, it appeared that he was using the semantic route, at least in part, for reading aloud. His reading was helped considerably by his being given a word's category. Warrington (1981) therefore suggested that there is some form of categorical specificity within the semantic system, and in CAV, the regions within it responsible for abstract-word comprehension were more easily accessed.[40] In fact, his better processing of abstract words was not limited to reading. CAV showed a parallel deficit in picture–word matching when the words were presented auditorily. He could match abstract words to pictures at a much more satisfactory level than he could concrete words.

If one considers Warrington's findings on CAV as a whole, the argument that the abstract-word superiority is an artefact is not strong. Yet there remains the problem of the uniqueness of CAV. Why should one give theoretical weight to this one set of findings when the vast bulk of patients who read by the semantic route are better with concrete words. At the core of this objection are the metatheoretical issues concerning the uniqueness of individual cases and replication in cognitive neuropsychology. I will return to these questions in chapter 10. There are, however, specific factors that should be borne in mind when considering why only one patient of this type has so far been reported. The patient had a different aetiology from that usual in deep dyslexic patients and had fluent spontaneous speech, which is also rare in deep dyslexics. There was also a difference in the type of study. Most patients analysed as individual cases are observed in the chronic phase of their illness. These are the only patients to whom many research workers have access. It is also technically easier to work at a slow pace, gathering evidence on a weekly basis, than in a highly concentrated period. Detailed case studies with patients in the acute stage of their illness are much more difficult to carry out and are sufficiently rare that we have no way of knowing how well the pattern of syndromes observed maps onto the chronic syndromes.[41] Theoretically, acute syndromes should represent more adequately what is now called a 'reduced set' of the normal subsystems, since less time has been available for compensation and neurological reorganisation to occur. It would therefore be dangerous to ignore CAV just because no similar patient has yet been observed.

In chapter 12, I will return to the general issue of categorical specificity within semantic systems. It is, though, worth pointing out that although no other dyslexic

---

40. Coltheart (1983) has challenged this interpretation. He analysed the results of the main experiment in more detail and showed that the relation between probability of being correct and concreteness does not show a gradual change, as one might expect a priori, but a step function at roughly the median. In fact, Warrington's (1981) main result was highly significant, and without a theory of how and why and where abstract–concrete divisions should occur, it is premature to rule out results because they conform to a pattern that seems a priori unlikely. More critically, this result is only one of a number that support the same position.

     Non-word reading was very poor although not completely impossible, in CAV. Little contribution therefore seems likely to have been made by the use of non-lexical spelling-to-sound correspondences. It is, however, possible that non-semantic morphemic correspondences may have been used to read some words. If CAV was reading primarily by the semantic route, why should he have made such a small rate of semantic errors (2%)? In fact, patients who read by the semantic route and have an input central dyslexia tend to make low rates of semantic errors. KF is an example of this (see Table 5.3).

41. In many acute neurological conditions, the testing involved in, say, reading words in no way harms the patient. Many patients prefer the interaction with the clinician or research worker to the monotony of the hospital ward, where they often cannot carry out the activities that fill their daily life. An acquired dyslexic patient, for instance, cannot read books or newspapers.

patient has been described who has an abstract-word superiority in reading, as does CAV, two patients with preserved auditory comprehension for abstract words and impaired concrete-word comprehension are on record. Therefore, from other aspects of CAV's disorder and the parallel that can be drawn with syndromes in other modalities, the most plausible interpretation of Warrington's (1981) findings on CAV is, indeed, that there is some form of categorical specialisation within the semantic systems.

The argument that deep dyslexia represents merely a quantitative impairment of the semantic route, as argued by Nolan and Caramazza (1982), becomes less convincing.[42] The alternative possibility (see Shallice & Warrington, 1980), that it can arise from damage specific to the semantic processing of certain classes of words (i.e. abstract words, function words), thus becomes more plausible.[43]

5.9 Phonological Alexia: A Distinct Syndrome?

The central dyslexic disorders discussed so far, in which the operation of the phonological route is impaired, seem likely to be multi-component syndromes. Is it possible to fractionate deep dyslexia, say, and obtain a more selective impairment of the phonological route? This was the rationale for the early investigations of phonological alexia (Beauvois & Derouesné, 1979; Shallice & Warrington, 1980; Patterson, 1982).

A strict dissociation methodology was employed in the first study of this syndrome, with the result that the patient described, RG (Beauvois & Derouesné, 1979; Beauvois, Derouesné, & Saillant, 1980), who was French, now appears to be a pure case. The disorder, as initially described, was characterised in terms of a set of three dissociations. Non-lexical 'phonological' reading was impaired, although

1. Lexical reading was nearly intact
2. There was no deficit of the visual processing of letter strings
3. There was no problem in producing pronounceable non-words

The basic phenomenon was that 4- to 5-letter pronounceable non-words were read by RG at only a 10% level, while 94% of 320 nouns of 3 to 14 letters were read successfully. The intact visual processing was demonstrated by RG's being perfect at matching a single letter with one of the letters of a letter string in a different case (e.g. *f* ↔ *LOUFREVANT*) and at detecting the difference between letter strings in a different case (e.g. *ZANROLIER* and *sanrolier*). On the production side, repetition of eight-phoneme non-words was perfect. Indeed, apart from a naming disorder

---

42. The finding of an effect of abstract-word superiority in reading has implications for deep dyslexia. It provides yet another difficulty for the right hemisphere theory. If the subsystems involved in comprehending concrete words are duplicated in the two hemispheres, how can abstract-word superiority occur with a unilateral lesion? As CAV had fluent speech, a similar response could be made to that raised in response to the letter-by-letter reading objection (see section 5.7).
43. It may well be that the deep dyslexics who have been described vary in the degree to which damage specific to certain classes of words is present.

for tactile stimuli – bilateral tactile aphasia (chapter 12) – and a reduced digit span (four items), neither of which was relevant for the reading of the individual words, the patient was not aphasic. The selective nature of the disorder and, in particular, the intact visual and phonological processing make the attribution of the syndrome to a difficulty of non-lexical spelling-to-sound translation much more solid than the accounts of the multi-component disorders discussed earlier in the chapter.

Since the analysis of RG's reading disorder was described, a considerable number of apparently similar cases have been reported. Indeed, Sartori, Barry, and Job (1984), in an extensive review, listed 16 cases! In many of these papers, however, phonological alexia is treated as simply a superiority of word over non-word reading.

There are two reasons why the use of this criterion alone is an insufficient basis for effective theoretical inferences to normal function. The first is that the use of this definition treats the syndrome as merely a single dissociation, not a set of dissociations. One needs to be confident that the dissociation cannot be attributed to more basic disorders outside the domain in question. For instance, an apparent agnosia would be of no theoretical interest if the patient was almost blind. Much the safest procedure for analysing phonological alexia is that adopted in the initial study – namely, to investigate the syndrome only in patients with little or no expressive aphasia. This is important, since it is known that many aphasics have more difficulty repeating non-words than words; this was so for nearly 60% of a large series of aphasics studied by Dubois (1977). A non-word reading deficit in such an aphasic patient could clearly be totally unrelated to any process specific to spelling-to-sound translation and reading.

An investigation by Marcel and Patterson (1986) makes clear how critical this factor is. They studied six phonological alexics selected only because they showed a word–non-word difference in reading. None of the six was capable of performing perfectly the purely phonological task of producing a three-phoneme non-word from its separately pronounced phonemes (e.g. /k/ /ae/ /g/ → *cag*).

Second, in a number of the patients described, the difference in performance between the reading of words and of non-words was not very great. Yet as discussed in chapter 2, any dissociation, by itself, is potentially explicable in terms of the two tasks differing merely in their quantitative demands on the same subsystem. This danger is clearly greater when the difference in level of performance on the two tasks is not dramatic, when the better performed of the two is a priori the easier, and when it still is performed far from perfectly so that the subsystems that undertake it must be impaired. I will therefore consider only patients who show a large word–non-word difference and are, at most, mildly aphasic (see Table 5.9).

The principal dyslexia syndrome discussed so far, in which the dissociation between the reading of words and of non-words occurs, is deep dyslexia. Is it appropriate to think of deep dyslexia and phonological alexia as qualitatively distinct? The rare word-reading errors that phonological alexics make are nearly always visual errors. This has led Newcombe and Marshall (1980a) to argue that the impairment of phonological recoding might simply be less severe in phonological dyslexia

Table 5.9. *Performance (percent correct) of four phonological alexic patients in reading words and non-words (of no more than 6 letters)*

		Reading	
	Speech	Word	Non-word
RG[a]	'Good'	100	10
GRN[b]	'Relatively Intact'	98	8
AM[c]	'Somewhat Hesitant'	83–95	0–37
LB[d]	Normal	87–99	48

Note: Where a range is given, it corresponds to values in different tests.
[a] Beauvois and Derouesné (1979)
[b] Shallice and Warrington (1980)
[c] Patterson (1982)
[d] Derouesné and Beauvois (1985)

Table 5.10. *Comparative performance of one phonological alexic (P) and three deep dyslexics (D) on auditory–visual non-word matching*

		% correct	
Patient	Type	Distant distractors	Similar distractors
AM[a]	P	79	60
PW[b]	D	75	36
DE[b]	D	80	44
VS[c]	D	100	70

[a] Patterson (1982)
[b] Patterson (1978)
[c] Saffran and Marin (1977)

than in deep dyslexia, and so the patient can obtain sufficient phonological information from the letter strings to eliminate potential semantic errors.

Deep dyslexics and phonological alexics cannot, though, be clearly distinguished on measures of phonological reading ability. In one test, the patient is presented with a single written non-word on a card while listening to three non-words that are either very distinctly different (e.g. *fleb, trean, mide*) or similar (e.g. *pabe, pame, pake*). The patient's task is to decide which of the three spoken items corresponds to the written word. Table 5.10 shows the performance of one phonological alexic, Patterson's (1982) patient AM, and three deep dyslexics. There is no evidence that there is a severity difference between the two types of patient.

Second, phonological alexics, in general, show little or no effect of abstraction or part of speech, with the exception of a difficulty on function words in some cases. Thus AM performed perfectly on a test of reading abstract words, and there was no effect of concreteness on RG's reading. It is difficult to see how a slight improvement in the phonological route from totally impaired to merely grossly impaired could provide sufficient information to increase abstract-word reading from, say, 20% to 90%. Phonological alexia would appear to differ qualitatively, not merely quantitatively, from deep dyslexia.

5.10   Phonological Alexia: What Processes Are Impaired and Intact?

What problem do phonological alexic patients have with non-words? Derouesné and Beauvois (1979) were not content with merely isolating a new syndrome. In addition, they proposed that it can exist in at least two distinct forms, depending on the stage of the phonological route that is impaired. They compared four French phonological alexic patients on two complementary tests of non-word reading. In one, the graphemic complexity of non-word reading was varied. Patients had to read non-words that were composed of simple grapheme–phoneme correspondences – for example, *iko* – in which each of the three graphemes is a single letter, or ones in which more complex correspondences were required – for example, *cau,* in which the *au* is a unit corresponding to a single phoneme. In the second test, half the non-words were homophonic with real words, but visually very different from them – for example, *kok* (for *coq*). In this test, the subjects were told that the homophones sounded like a word.

All four patients performed perfectly in reading nouns, and their spontaneous speech was normal or nearly so; in particular, syllables and non-words could be repeated perfectly. However, they showed a very different pattern of performance on the two experimental tests (Table 5.11). Two patients showed a major effect of graphemic complexity, and one of them, JA, did not show a significant effect on the homophony test.[44] By contrast, MF and RG showed little effect of graphemic complexity and yet roughly doubled their score on the homophony test. Derouesné and Beauvois (1979) therefore argue that one can distinguish two sub-varieties of phonological alexia, with impairments at the graphemic level and in phonological conflation respectively, although it should be noted that the latter does not correspond to an aphasic disorder.

The instructions used in the second type of test were most unconventional for the time it was conducted. They were intended to induce a particular strategy, on the assumption that one can determine whether a patient has the capacity to perform a particular manipulation only if the conditions are optimal.[45] Patterson (1982) has, however, argued that the subjects who benefitted from homophony may have made use of a visual-approximation strategy; if they induced visual errors in themselves,

44. The other patient, M, was at ceiling on the homophony test. It should be noted that the non-word reading of the three patients other than RG was not as poor as that of the phonological alexics discussed individually in section 5.9.
45. This strategy-induction procedure is discussed in chapter 10.

Table 5.11. *The effect of two different critical variables (graphemic complexity; homophonic with a real word or not) on the ability of three phonological alexics to read non-words (% correct)*

	Graphemic		Phonological	
	Simple (e.g. *iko*)	Complex (e.g. *cau*)	Homophone (e.g. *kok*)	Non-homophone (e.g. *fuj*)
JA	92	50*	78	65
MF	75	62	76	43*
RG	65	55	78	36*

*Significant effect of the variable
From Derouesné and Beauvois (1979)

then some of them could have been homophones. In a later investigation with another phonological alexic patient, LB, Derouesné and Beauvois (1985) found that when the degree of visual similarity to words was controlled, homophonic non-words were still read better than non-homophones. Moreover, LB is the only phonological alexic who has been given the test described in section 5.9 – an articulatory conflation of a non-word from a set of auditorily presented phonemes – and shown no deficit on it. Thus the homophone superiority effect can be accepted as non-artefactual and not secondary to a speech production problem.[46]

How is phonological alexia, or, to be more specific, its two sub-varieties, to be explained? The different theories of phonological reading discussed in section 5.1 are relevant again. Marcel (1980) attempted to explain phonological alexia from the standpoint of lexical analogy theory. He sees it arising as a problem in segmentation and argues that, referring to the findings of Derouesné and Beauvois (1979), 'the distinction between impairments at the graphemic and phonological stages would map rather well onto segmentation impairments at the two stages' (p. 255). As far as the phonological stage is concerned, it is unclear why segmentation is theoretically critical and not its inverse, conflation of elements. For the graphemic stage, the argument again seems rather thin. Non-words like *iko* require more segmentation than non-words like *cau*, but they are easier for the phonological alexic patients with the graphemic deficit. This is what one would expect if the difficulty arises from the complexity of the individual graphemes themselves or their lower frequency and not from the problem of separating them from their neighbours.

46. Partial corroboration of this second type of phonological alexia has come in a surprising way. Denes, Ciplotti, and Semenza (1987) studied an Italian patient who, in addition to Italian, spoke a dialect called Friulano, which is never written down. The patient was a phonological alexic in Italian. However, she read Friulano words written in Italian – which, of course, she had never seen – much better than Italian non-words. Thus the existing phonological form of the Friulano word assisted reading. The patient could repeat non-words, but it is unclear whether she could perform the articulatory-conflation task.

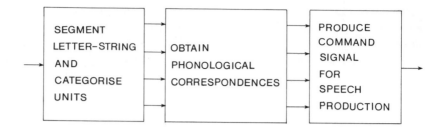

Figure 5.8. Three stages in spelling-to-sound translation of non-words.

On the more standard approach, non-word reading would need to have at least three stages in addition to those in common with word reading and speech production (Figure 5.8) (for a related analysis see Coltheart, 1985).

1. The segmentation of the letter string into an ordered set of units, each of which has a phonological correspondence, and (visual) identification of the units. The segmentation and identification processes would need to operate together.[47]
2. The obtaining of the phonological correspondences of the graphemic units, maintaining information about their order.
3. The integration of these activated ordered sets of phonological units into a form suitable to act as a command signal for controlling speech production.

Of these stages, the only one that is not self-explanatory is the third. However, it is now frequently argued that the control of speech output depends on phonological organisation at the level of the syllable; speech is not just a concatenated string of phonemes, but requires a syllabic structure (see, e.g., Kahn, 1980; Crompton, 1982). On this position, the process of reading a non-word by using spelling-to-sound correspondences at a lower level than the syllable must include this third stage, too. Even a model as simple as this produces five possible locations for a functional lesion. Theoretically, as many as four or five varieties of phonological alexia are possible! Impairments before the second stage would correspond to Derouesné and Beauvois's graphemic deficit. Ones after it are possibilities for producing difficulties similar to those exhibited by their phonological stage patients. Their homophone-superiority effect would arise once the correct phonological units are achieved; it is easier to construct the 'speech command signal' if the overall utterance corresponds to a word.[48]

Derouesné and Beauvois's (1985) patient, LB, also provides evidence about the type of unit on which these subsystems in the phonological route operate, an issue

47. It is theoretically possible for this segmentation and identification process to operate on more than one level – for example, graphemes and demisyllables (see, e.g., Shallice & McCarthy, 1985). This paper also discusses the possible mechanisms by which order might be coded. Stage 1, like stage 3, was discussed in the context of the lexical analogy model by Marcel (1980).
48. The claim that the graphemic-complexity sub-variety could arise from a disconnection depends on the assumption that more complex graphemes have lower frequency correspondences than the simpler graphemes. Whether the third stage is a candidate location depends on whether this subsystem is in any way specific to the reading-aloud process.

discussed in section 5.1. Derouesné and Beauvois compared LB's performance on reading syllables like *bre*, which contain consonant clusters that are present in French written words, with syllables that were matched for *spoken* frequency but are virtually never written, such as *jra*. Thus the beginning of *je ramene* tends to be pronounced like *jra* in spontaneous speech, although it would be two distinct words in reading aloud. There are no differences in the speech organisation characteristics of the two types of syllable. So if the information transmitted by the phonological route consists of three graphemes – *b, r, e,* or *j, r, a* – there would be no reason to expect any difference in LB's ability to read them. In fact, he read 83% of the *bre* type and only 10% of the *jra* type. The obvious explanation is that information about units larger than graphemes is transmitted by the phonological route and is easier to use than information about graphemes. This supports the multiple-levels position.[49]

It seems possible to explain phonological alexia if one asks what processes must be damaged. It is not, though, apparent which processes are intact. It is often argued that phonological alexia provides one key piece of evidence for the three-route model of reading illustrated in Figure 5.1; the phonological alexic is held to read aloud by direct input–output logogen connections, with the non-lexical phonological route impaired (e.g. Coltheart, 1985). This seems in conflict with the multiple-levels position, which has just received support.

These issues were not addressed directly in the study of the earlier patients described. However, some indirect evidence is available. The one type of word for which RG, AM, and LB had a deficit in reading was function words. RG read 93% of nouns and adjectives correctly, but only 69% of 'meaningless' function words – for example, *ceux* (those) and *comme* (as). AM read only 72% of function words correctly, compared with 92% of content words, and for LB the values were 82% and 94%. On the assumption that the patient's word reading is mediated by the semantic system, the difficulty with function words is entirely comprehensible, since 'meaningless' function words could not be expected to be represented there. If, however, they are read solely by the third route, why should there be a difficulty with function words? One would have to argue that they are not represented in either the visual logogen system or, more plausibly, the phonological-output lexicon system. It might be possible to argue that in the speech production process, function words are supplied from a different lexicon. This is, however, far less straightforward than the first possible explanation.[50] Phonological alexia does not help to

49. Whether a model like that of Sejnowski and Rosenberg (1986) discussed in section 5.1 can explain phonological alexia has yet to be investigated.
50. Strong claims have been made from a phonological alexic patient, WB, studied by Funnell (1983), that there must be separate lexical and non-lexical routes (e.g. Coltheart, 1985). Funnell's patient, however, appears to have had quite a severe expressive aphasia and performed poorly on Marcel and Patterson's (1986) test of conflating auditorily presented phonemes into a non-word. The non-word reading difficulty therefore seems likely to have been secondary to a speech production impairment (see also Howard, 1985a). Overall, any attempt to argue for separate lexical and non-lexical routes on the basis of phonological alexia is fraught with difficulties. Inference problems, discussed in chapter 11, are relevant, as are the purity of the disorder and the stage of the impairment.

discriminate the rival theories of the operation of spelling-to-sound conversion processes.

Phonological alexia contains an extra wrinkle. Why do a number of phonological alexics have a specific difficulty reading function words? One possibility suggested by Patterson (1982), following an idea put forward theoretically by Allport (1979), is a restricted version of a hypothesis considered earlier in the chapter. Function words and affixes, Patterson argued, may differ from content words in requiring the phonological route in order to be read aloud. She also noted the beguiling fact that in Japanese, function words and affixes are read using Kana, the syllabic script. There is, however, a major difficulty for this theory. Some phonological alexics do not show the function-word effect; for instance, GRN was 94% correct on reading individual function words. However, as the conflation of auditorily presented phonemes test was not carried out with GRN, it remains possible that her phonological alexia was secondary to a subtle speech production deficit. The issue remains open.[51]

It is, then, clear that there remain a considerable number of unanswered questions about phonological alexia. This is hardly surprising, given the youth of the concept. It is apparent, though, that if one compares the syndrome with deep dyslexia, the nature of the theoretical questions posed by it are much more clear. This is a testimony to the value of working with a highly selective impairment.

5.11 The Acquired Dyslexias and Modularity

Do the characteristics of the network of dyslexic syndromes discovered in the past two decades or so help us to understand the normal reading process? It should be obvious from the lengthy and complicated discussions presented in this and the preceding chapter that the cognitive neuropsychology project cannot be achieved in a simple transparent fashion. The history of research on acquired dyslexia illustrates clearly that if one is concerned with extrapolation to normal function, empirical traps have to be avoided and major theoretical complexities may need to be confronted.

Much of chapter 4 was concerned with traps that occur in the interpretation of findings. Patients develop strategies for coping with the practical difficulties that their cognitive impairments produce. As in normal experimental psychology, the effects of the operation of specific mechanisms and of the control processes that operate on them must therefore be distinguished; in general, the control-process aspects of patients' performance are not relevant for extrapolation to normal function. Sometimes, the strategic aspects are fairly obvious, as in letter-by-letter reading. But in other cases, as in the disputes over the nature of surface dyslexia, the proper empirical basis for theoretical generalisation to normal function has in practice proved difficult to determine. Finally, there is the danger of generalising inappropriately from associated deficits in a patient with multiple impairments, as has probably occurred in research on a number of the central dyslexias.

51. If Patterson's argument is correct, then the hypothesis of Saffran, Schwartz, and Marin (1979) and Jones (1985) that the reading aloud of abstract words requires the use of the phonological route can hardly be valid. Such words could be read satisfactorily by RG and AM.

Theoretical complexities arise because the set of subsystems that the patient is using may not be any simple subset of the components of the normal system. To explain some syndrome, one might, for instance, need to postulate additional cognitive systems not relevant or present in normal functioning, such as systems in the hemisphere not used by normal subjects when performing a particular task. The right hemisphere theory of deep dyslexia is the obvious example of this difficulty in this area. Also, theories on the algorithmic or even the mechanistic level of explanation may be necessary to give more than a superficial account of some types of behaviour; thus convincing explanations of semantic errors seem most likely to come from these levels. They should, however, not be crucial as far as the overall modular organisation is concerned.

It would seem from the detailed analysis of the syndromes presented in this chapter and chapter 4 that these difficulties can in general be circumvented or overcome. What, then, can we learn from the findings on the dyslexics as far as normal function is concerned?

The fundamental positive point is that the very existence of a number of clearly dissociable syndromes is just what one would predict if the reading system is modular and cognitive neuropsychology can assist in mapping the functional geography. If one wants to assess the accuracy with which neuropsychology can map the modular system, one runs into a problem. There are a very large number of models of the normal reading process, and the vast normal literature is widely held to be rather inconclusive. To take one example, Henderson (1982), in his definitive and exhaustive review of the reading literature, says, when discussing the basic question of the role that phonological recording plays in semantic access, 'We must take care to distinguish the volume of claims made from the actual weight of evidence' (p. 331). He concludes that only one of many techniques 'seems capable of supporting strong conclusions, and even here, there is room for doubt' (p. 331). Testing the cognitive neuropsychology approach by checking whether it gives the same conclusions as normal experimental methods runs the danger that one extracts from the normal literature the experiments that fit best with neuropsychological findings. However, there is another internal check. Inferences from different syndromes should support one another.

The fundamental common thread running through all cognitive neuropsychological theorising about the acquired dyslexics is that there are alternative functionally distinct procedures for reading words and that one of these allows information to reach semantic systems without phonological mediation. The earliest modern advocates of the two-route position were Marshall and Newcombe (1973), who were motivated by the neuropsychological evidence, and certainly when they wrote, single-route positions, such as that of Rubinstein, Lewis, and Rubinstein (1971), were the most widely believed (see Henderson, 1982, p. 324).[52] While it might prove possible to explain the characteristics of any individual central dyslexic syn-

---

52. It is ironic that Henderson (1982), who had earlier (1981) argued that the research on acquired dyslexia was conceptually parasitic on that on the normal reading process – ignoring the great difference in the amount of work in the two fields – dates the dual-process theory from Meyer, Schvaneveldt, and Ruddy (1974).

drome without assuming more than a single type of reading process, it would be an extremely daunting task to attempt to explain the whole gamut of central dyslexic disorders in this way. The variety of dissociations that exist would have to be explained. No one, to my knowledge, has even attempted it.[53]

The distinction between phonological and semantic routes in reading was not produced as a post hoc account of the neuropsychological evidence. The patients who fit well the characterisation of reading by a phonological route alone were first described after the theory was current. The same applies to demonstrations that similar patterns of symptoms can occur as a result of interruptions at different stages of one of the routes (see sections 4.5 and 5.5). Indeed, the existence of a set of such subsyndromes fitting the 'surface/semantic dyslexic' reading pattern was specifically predicted before they were discovered.[54]

Of course, despite the doubts raised by Henderson (1982), there are strong pointers to the same conclusion from the normal literature. For instance, a secondary phonological task (shadowing) creates much less interference for semantic judgements about pairs of words than for rhyme judgements (Kleiman, 1975). In complementary fashion, substituting non-word homophones for words creates much more difficulty for semantic judgements than for rhyme ones (Green & Shallice, 1976). Forcing phonological mediation makes semantic decisions harder, suggesting that an independent orthographic-to-semantic route exists.

A more subtle inference from the neuropsychological literature is that morphemic spelling-to-sound correspondences exist independently of the semantic system. This can be inferred from the characteristics of patients such as WLP (Schwartz et al., 1980a) and MP (Bub et al., 1985).[55] It seems much more difficult to obtain direct evidence for this inference from the normal literature because any experimental manipulation would have to isolate the effect of morphemic spelling-to-sound correspondences both from effects mediated semantically and from ones mediated by non-morphemic spelling-to-sound correspondences. Thus this would appear to be an inference that it may be possible to validate internally to neuropsychology, but for which corroborating evidence from the normal literature is likely to be difficult to obtain.

53. The existence of semantic errors in reading is not conclusive. One of the earliest explanations of deep dyslexia including semantic errors, that of Morton (1970), was based on a *single* lexicon system and separate thresholds for semantic access and output. It is, however, much simpler to explain on the separate visual and auditory lexicons position. Another line of argument is that if phonological mediation is obligatory, then patients should show the same pattern of comprehension difficulties *across semantic variables* in the two modalities. For instance, a difficulty with abstract words in one modality should coexist with the same difficulty in the other. Input deep dyslexics do not show the same pattern. (This argument depends on the conclusion obtained earlier that all patients who cannot read by means of the phonological route do not differ just quantitatively in any additional impairments to the semantic route. Complementary arguments can be obtained from auditory analogue to deep dyslexia, discussed in chapter 7.)
54. See Shallice and Warrington (1980).
55. A potential corroboration internal to neuropsychology is the way that certain surface dyslexic patients are said to understand an irregular word as its homophone (see footnote 4).

Finally, certain inferences about the operation of particular components map onto those from the normal literature. One example stems from Saffran's (1980) analysis of the non-ideographic nature of whole-word reading in deep dyslexia.[56] Another concerns the nature of the units involved in non-morphemic spelling-to-sound correspondences; Shallice et al. (1983) and Derouesné and Beauvois (1985), from a neuropsychological direction, came to a conclusion similar to that of Patterson and Morton (1985), using evidence from normal subjects – that units larger than individual graphemes are involved.[57]

It would appear, then, that the cognitive neuropsychology approach is indeed working within the acquired dyslexia field. Modules seem to have been isolated, and the pattern of modular organisation that the syndromes suggest looks fairly consistent both internally and within the normal literature. In addition, a rich vein of empirical evidence has been tapped, whose existence earlier generations of neuropsychologists and experimental psychologists never even suspected.

56. For an interesting, but not compelling, neuropsychological criticism of this inference, see Howard (1987).
57. A third inference, which remains more controversial, concerns the presence of morphological-decomposition processes at the visual word-form or visual lexicon level (see, e.g., Job & Sartori, 1984).

6   The Agraphias

6.1 Do Specific Agraphias Exist?

Ten years of work on the acquired dyslexias has been basically positive as far as the broader cognitive neuropsychology research program is concerned. However, the overall picture is complicated as the use of the syndrome-complex approach and the large variety of syndromes and sub-syndromes that have been isolated have led to the natural lines of functional cleavage in the domain being not too clearly visible. As a counterpoint, it would be useful to take another domain where the correspondence between syndromes and normal function is simpler. The complementary set of disorders – the agraphias, impairments in the writing process – provides an excellent example in this respect.[1]

Before 1980, agraphia was treated by neuropsychologists as a poor relation of aphasia. Writing was viewed as a highly complex secondary skill, with forms of breakdown of little theoretical interest. Most work was concerned with the pattern of the concomitant aphasic or apraxic disorders that occurred with agraphic difficulties (see, e.g., Marcie & Hécaen, 1979).[2] One influential view was that cases of agraphia that appeared to be pure were not the result of damage to specific mechanisms concerned with writing, but were the secondary effect of a confusional state characterised by a reduction and/or ready shifting of attention (Chedru & Geschwind, 1972). Writing, it was argued, was affected because it is a complex skill that is rarely overlearned. But it was convincingly shown by Basso, Taborelli, and Vignolo (1978) that pure agraphia could not always be explained in this way. Specific disorders of the writing process itself do exist.

These authors described two patients who were not confused and who had a writing problem that was not secondary to either aphasia or apraxia. Neither patient had much of an aphasic difficulty or any apraxic one, as measured by quantitative test batteries. Thus their word repetition was at least 95% correct, and oral naming was 85% correct or better. However, written naming was very poor – 0% and 35% correct, respectively. Moreover, both patients copied and transcribed from upper to

---

1. For simplicity, I will concentrate on the writing process and the role that spelling plays in it and, in general, ignore other methods of spelling, such as spelling aloud, until the last section.
2. Apraxia is the name given to disorders of action resulting from neurological disease. The apraxias remain one of the most poorly understood regions of neuropsychology.

130

lower case considerably better (65 to 95%), so that the difficulty could not be attributed to a motor problem; it appeared to be of a relatively central origin. Basso et al. also observed two patients with a selective preservation of written over oral naming in whom word repetition was relatively spared.

The work of Basso et al. (1978) provided solid quantitative evidence that isolated disorders specific to writing can occur, although they were very rare – only two out of the 500 patients in their series.[3] However, the principal advances in the study of the agraphias that have taken place since about 1980 have been a result of the application of an information-processing approach. The syndromes uncovered seem to fit neatly with the somewhat tentative theories of the normal writing process that are beginning to be developed.

Like the acquired dyslexias, agraphia syndromes may usefully be subdivided into central and peripheral types. In the central, or linguistic, agraphias, there is a breakdown in the process by which the sequence of 'abstract letter identities' is obtained. The patient can no longer spell as effectively as before. In the more peripheral varieties, which correspond to what were known traditionally as the apraxic agraphias, there is the complementary problem of an impairment in the concrete realisation of a sequence of letters – for instance, as a series of pen strokes on the page.

6.2 The Central Agraphias

In languages with an alphabetic orthography, a word is represented as a sequence of letters – its spelling. If the spelling of a word is required, one procedure that can be used is to segment its sound and use some form of sound-to-spelling correspondence for each of the component sounds. Support for this intuitively obvious claim can be derived from the results of a study carried out by Frith (1980). She showed that 12-year-old children have little difficulty in obtaining a spelling for simple nonwords that is compatible with accepted English sound-to-spelling correspondences. How this procedure operates is a subject of some debate, as we will see later. For the present, I will assume that the phonological components are elements such as phonemes or the type of sub-syllabic units discussed in chapters 4 and 5.

Certain authors have assumed that this process is basic to the way that words are spelled by normal subjects. Thus Luria (1970a) argued that the writing process involves several steps, with speech being broken down into individual sounds, each of them being represented by letters, and finally, the individual letters being integrated to produce the written word. Luria was presumably basing his intuition on Russian. A language such as English, however, contains many irregular words. Therefore, an additional assumption is required to give the procedure any chance of being able to realise English spelling; this is that the irregular portions of irregular

---

3. One reason why selective impairments of writing were so rare in the series of Basso, Taborelli, and Vignolo (1978) is that their patients were Italian and the Italian language is almost entirely regular in its spelling-to-sound correspondences. As we will see, this makes a selective central deficit of writing difficult to detect.

words are added after the sound-to-spelling correspondences have been used (e.g. Dodd, 1980; Frith, 1980).

As Ellis (1982a) has pointed out, even such a modified proposal is implausible for a language such as English because of the sheer number of alternative graphemic renderings of common phonological forms. In English, the acceptable sound-to-spelling correspondences used in writing are far more numerous than the spelling-to-sound ones utilised in reading. Thus for the phonological form /rid/, theoretically acceptable graphemic forms would be *read, rede, reed, wread, wrede, and wreed* – not to mention *reade, reid, wreade,* and so on. To obtain a correct spelling, a large amount of the graphemic information would therefore have to be specified after the correspondence procedure had been applied. It seems simpler and more plausible that in normal writing, use is made of representations of the complete graphemic structure of all words in a person's spelling repertoire. Morton (1980a), in making this suggestion, called the structure in which they were stored the 'graphemic output logogen'. I will use the phrase 'graphemic output lexicon'. On this approach, if the spelling of a word is not in the subject's repertoire, then the sound-to-spelling correspondence process is available as a back-up, but is otherwise not required (see Ellis, 1982a).

One can therefore make a plausible a priori case that lexical and non-lexical procedures for spelling should exist. The first two central agraphia syndromes isolated – lexical agraphia and phonological agraphia – speak directly to this position. Both syndromes were initially described in a fairly pure form, so that the inferences that can be made to normal function are much more straightforward than those discussed in chapters 4 and 5, on the dyslexias.

6.3   Lexical Agraphia

Lexical agraphia was first described by Beauvois and Derouesné (1981) in a French patient, RG, whose dyslexia was discussed in chapter 5.[4] Before his operation for a left parieto-occipital angioma, RG spelled and wrote well. His position, that of sales manager, entailed frequent correspondence. After his illness, his ability to write a word correctly, whether from dictation, in object naming, or in spontaneous writing, was critically dependent on how regular and unambiguous were the sound-to-spelling correspondences involved in the word's spelling. Thus non-words, even long or complex ones, were written perfectly (110/110) from dictation. The spelling of a word, by contrast, depended on the number of phonemes it contained that had an ambiguous or irregular correspondence. There was a very systematic relationship. Completely unambiguous words (e.g. *madame*) were written correctly on 93% of occurrences; if one phoneme was ambiguous (e.g. *en* in *mental*), RG was 67%

---

4. The syndrome has also been referred to as phonological spelling and surface dysgraphia. The latter name is unfortunate, in view of the complexities over the functional basis of the reading syndrome from which the label is derived.

Table 6.1. *Results of lexical agraphic patients on writing non-words and words of different levels of ambiguity (percent correct)*

		Level of ambiguity (words)		
	Non-words	Low (e.g. *hotel*)	Medium (e.g. *brain*)	High (e.g. *city*)
RG	100	93	67	36
PT	—	93	—	38[a]
LA 1	90	100	90	30
LA 2	90	100	88	70
LA 3	100	100	100	90
JG	100	90	—	70
MW	100	100	—	88
KT	95	86	—	19
Controls[b]	90	100	100	98*

Note: The word sets differ across authors.
[a] For PT, the high-ambiguity results refer to irregular sound-to-spelling correspondences.
[b] Brain-damaged patients of Roeltgen and Heilman (1984).
From reference papers on the syndrome (see p. 133)

correct in writing the word; if two or three phonemes were ambiguous (e.g. *an* and *s* in *anchois*), he was correct on 36% of occasions. The effect of the degree of ambiguity of a word's spelling – the number of possible alternative versions – was stronger for lower frequency words; this parallels results obtained by Seidenberg, Waters, Barnes, and Tanenhaus (1984) on the reading of normal subjects, which were discussed in chapter 5. As one would expect with this pattern of correct performance, errors almost always consisted of a phonologically correct spelling, but with an inappropriate sound-to-spelling correspondence being used: *'église' → aiglise*) and *'rameau' → ramo*. Analogous errors in English from the patient PT of Hatfield and Patterson (1983) are *'spade' → spaid* and *'flood' → flud*.

The impairment was not caused by an inability to comprehend the word. For instance, RG performed at the average level on an auditory synonyms test. And the difficulty was not specific to written output. In his spelling aloud, RG showed the identical characteristics.

RG's impairment is by no means unique. Other patients with a similar deficit have since been described – PT (Hatfield & Patterson, 1983), LA 1–3 (Roeltgen & Heilman, 1984), JG and MW (Goodman & Caramazza, 1985, 1986a), and KT (Baxter & Warrington, 1987) – although most had impairments that were less severe or less pure than that of RG (Table 6.1). For a number of these patients, as for RG, the deficit could not be attributed to a difficulty in recognising or understanding the word. For instance, Goodman and Caramazza's patient JG provided an adequate definition for 98% of the words she was given to spell. The errors of those patients

Table 6.2. *Repeating and writing of words and non-words by relatively pure phonological agraphic patients (percent correct)*

	Aphasia	Word		Non-word₁		Non-word₂	
		Repeat	Write	Repeat	Write	Write	Repeat after[a]
PR	Mild conduction	100	94	94	18	27	77
MH	Mixed expressive	?	70	100	5	6	100

[a] Repetition of non-words after an attempt to write them.
From reference papers on the syndrome (see p. 134).

for whom an error analysis has been reported – PT and JG – were on the whole similar to those of RG (e.g. *'subtle'* →*suttle*).[5]

The interpretation of lexical agraphia seems straightforward, probably because of the purity of the initially described patient. Spelling by any lexical means is impaired – in some cases, severely – with the most plausible locus being the graphemic output lexicon. However, the use of the procedure based on sound-to-spelling translation is intact. Before discussing the interpretation in more detail, it is helpful to present the complementary syndrome.

6.4 Phonological Agraphia

Phonological agraphia provides a neat double dissociation with lexical agraphia. In phonological agraphia, non-words cannot be written or spelled aloud at anything like the same level as words, but irregular words can be spelled and written as well as regular ones. Like lexical agraphia, phonological agraphia was first described in 1981: PR (Shallice, 1981a). Since then, a second reasonably pure case has been analysed: MH (Bub & Kertesz, 1982a).

As can be seen from Table 6.2, both PR and MH demonstrated a dramatic difference between their ability to write a word and to write a single phonologically acceptable non-word of two to four letters. For a disorder to be considered an agraphia, it must not be merely secondary to some non-writing problem. For phonological agraphia, this is a more complex matter than for lexical agraphia. It is necessary, for instance, to know that the patient can perceive and remember the

5. PT displayed another type of error, which Hatfield and Patterson (1983) argued occurred when the patient went through the procedure of making a phonological segmentation and then applying correspondence rules but segmented in a slightly inappropriate fashion. For instance, *cute* was spelled *quet,* which, it was argued, was due to the /kju/ being spelled as *que* and the /t/ left as *t*. The patient is therefore making a minor segmentation error, in separating the terminal consonant cluster from the syllable onset (initial consonant cluster plus vowel) rather than separating the initial consonant cluster from the rhyme.

non-word while attempting to write it. In fact, both patients could repeat a non-word far better than they could write it (see Table 6.2). Thus perception of the non-word cannot be the problem. However, if the trace of the non-word were at all fragile, attempting to decompose the non-word into more elementary sounds and translating each of them into an orthographic form might have an effect analogous to that produced by the intervening task in a Brown-Peterson short-term memory procedure (chapter 3) and lead to the loss of the trace. It is therefore necessary to test the ability of the patient to remember the non-word *after* the failure of an attempt to write it. In both PR and MH, repetition of a non-word after an attempt to write it was significantly more accurate than the writing itself. Therefore, the difficulty that they have in writing non-words is, indeed, an agraphia.

As far as the writing of words is concerned, the two patients performed well within the normal range. For high-frequency words, PR was 96% correct and MH, 85%. For lower frequency ones, the values fell to only 88% and 66%, respectively. PR's errors in writing words were mainly derivational – *'ascend'* → *ascent* – and a type that Ellis (1979b), in a study of writing slips in normal subjects, called 'completion errors' – *'absorption'* → *absolve*. Only one of PR's errors in writing over 600 words was a 'misspelling' – *'apprehension'* → *apprension*. MH made rather more misspellings, but otherwise showed a similar error pattern.[6]

The obvious explanation of the writing difficulty of these patients is that the non-lexical writing procedure is impaired, but the lexical one is intact. Further evidence for this was obtained from PR. He could neither segment words phonologically (e.g. *cat*→/k/ /ae/ /t/) nor write accurately the single letter corresponding to their syllabic sounds. In addition, when writing non-words, he produced a rather bizarre type of error; it seems that when trying to write a non-word, he tended to use a word as a mediator and then added or subtracted letters in a rather haphazard fashion. Thus in attempting to write *'na'*, he wrote *gn*, which he explained was through using the word *gnat* as a mediator.

Lexical writing seemed to be based on the operation of the semantic route. PR would say that he could not understand a word such as *amenable,* and so could not write it. The meaning could come to him suddenly a little later, and only then would he be able to write it. There was, indeed, a strong correlation between the occasions when PR could not write an abstract or a function word and those when he could not understand it. The writing response seemed to act as an indication that he had accessed the precise semantic representation of the word. Moreover, when the representation was accessed, the word was written correctly; no pure semantic error ever occurred in his writing of more than 600 words.

A number of other patients have been described as phonological agraphic (Roeltgen, Sevush, & Heilman, 1983). However, they differed from PR and MH in var-

---

6. There was one clear difference between the patients, in the effect of word class. PR showed a mild effect of the abstractness of words and a decided effect of content as opposed to function words (97% vs. 62%). MH showed neither of these effects. This difference between the two patients resembles that found in patients with phonological alexia; it will be discussed in section 6.6.

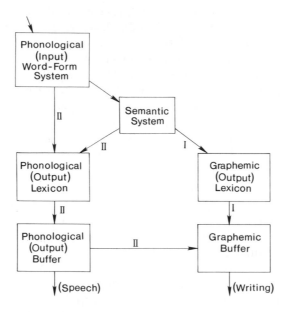

Figure 6.1. A simple-two route model of the spelling process. I is the lexical/semantic route; II is the phonological route using sound-to-spelling transformations.

ious respects: word writing was well below normal; non-word repeating was unimpressive (in two patients); and the critical test of non-word repetition after attempting to write the non-word was not performed. They did, however, show differences between word writing and non-word writing.

6.5   The Double Dissociation

These two syndromes form a clean double dissociation. In both disorders, the preserved task can be performed at a normal or virtually normal level, while the impaired task is very poorly performed. The existence of a normal or near-normal level of performance on the preserved task in both syndromes, together with the sharpness and complementary nature of the dissociations, make it very difficult to explain them other than as two functionally distinct processes that are being separately impaired. What processes could these be? It seems clear that the process preserved in phonological agraphia and damaged in lexical agraphia is the lexical-spelling procedure (procedure I). The high level of performance on words that can be achieved in phonological agraphia suggests that, as Morton (1980a) argued, the procedure can be used for all words (Figure 6.1).

What is the process complementary to the lexical-writing procedure? The obvious candidate is a non-lexical procedure based on segmenting the word-sound and using sound-to-spelling correspondences for each component sound (procedure II).

This, indeed, has been the standard explanation (e.g. Beauvois & Derouesné, 1981; Shallice, 1981a; Ellis, 1982a).

An alternative has been suggested by Campbell (1983). She argues that the process is better understood in terms of the lexical analogy theory originally developed by Glushko (1979) and Marcel (1980) for reading. Her position is that the writing of non-words occurs through the use of the spelling of similar-sounding words as an analogy. So *prain* is spelled by use of the knowledge of the spelling of *brain*. On this theory, if nearly all word-forms were lost in the graphemic output lexicon, this would lead to the patient not being able to spell non-words. There would be an inadequate number of word-forms available for the analogy process to work on. Campbell assumes that this is why certain surface dysgraphic patients have difficulty spelling both irregular words and non-words.[7] This, though, can hardly account for the writing of KT (see Table 6.1). He wrote only 17% of three- to six-letter 'high ambiguity' words correctly, which indicates that few morphemic correspondences were still available. Yet he wrote correctly 95% of two- or three-phoneme nonsense syllables.[8]

Campbell does not discuss phonological agraphia. The natural explanation of the syndrome, following her theory, is that it results from a failure of the analogy process, with the stock of word-forms being intact. This is not, though, a particularly plausible account of the spelling of, say, the phonological agraphic patient PR. PR normally attempted to spell non-words by explicitly using a word as a mediator. He then added or subtracted letters in a rather haphazard fashion. This inability to manipulate a word's subcomponents led to glaring errors, such as *na→gn,* which, as discussed earlier, seemed to involve mediators. He therefore appeared to use an analogy process and had the correspondences for words as wholes, but not for their subcomponents. There was no evidence that the analogy process itself was impaired.

On Marcel's (1980) account of the lexical analogy theory, it is assumed that the spelling-to-sound correspondence is available for each subcomponent of each word in the language. Thus it might be argued that phonological agraphics have lost these

7. Campbell (1983) illustrates this by a discussion of a patient, EE. Unfortunately, the only information presented on EE's spelling is the result of one rather special test, so it is unclear what precise characteristics are being predicted. The primary evidence that Campbell produces for lexical analogy theory comes from an experiment on normal subjects analogous to that devised by Kay and Marcel (1981) for reading. She shows that the way that normal subjects write a non-word is influenced by the spelling of a rhyming word presented 2 or 5 sec beforehand. However, it seems likely that in this situation subjects notice the rhyming relation and make use of it explicitly to reduce the cognitive effort required in what must be a demanding session.

8. KT could comprehend very few words (see chapter 5, where the patient's reading is discussed). Indeed, Baxter (personal communication), after a detailed analysis of individual spelling patterns, considered that in only 3% of one set of 160 words was the existence of a lexical component of the spelling performance reasonably convincing. Therefore, the semantic route was on the whole unavailable. This, however, makes inferences about lexical analogy theory simpler, since only the phonological route(s) need(s) be considered. In fact, it is not at all clear theoretically on Campbell's (1983) approach how much impairment could exist in the graphemic output lexicon and yet provide sufficient raw material for the lexical analogy process to operate satisfactorily.

word-specific correspondences. Yet one can question whether individual spelling-to-sound correspondences are known independently of generally applicable ones, even in normal subjects. For words with regular correspondences, there are obviously no simple grounds for assuming that one knows the individual spelling-to-sound correspondences of the word directly and not indirectly as an instance of a more general rule. What, though, is known about the correspondences in irregular words? Consider *colonel*. What corresponds to the first vowel? Is it *o, ol,* or *olo?* In *through,* is the *gh* silent or part of the vowel, as is *r* in *part?* Unless one can explain how the system could infer component spelling-to-sound correspondences in words from the overall spelling-to-sound correspondences *for that word alone,* it seems most implausible that spelling-to-sound correspondences for the components of particular words are utilised in spelling independently of the general correspondences that seem to be required in order to obtain the individual ones.[9] If general spelling-to-sound correspondences exist, why not assume that they can be used and are what are lost in phonological agraphia?

Campbell's (1983) approach does not seem satisfactory for either lexical or phonological agraphia. The standard view that non-words are written primarily by the use of a non-lexical route, which is separable from a semantic lexical one, seems more natural, empirically more solid, and theoretically sounder. The basic central dysgraphic syndromes fit well with a simpler model of normal writing that can be defended on a priori considerations.

6.6   Other Central Agraphia Syndromes: Writing via Semantics

In the acquired dyslexias, single-component disorders of the semantic and phonological routes are not the only disorders that exist; there are also multi-component ones. The situation is analogous for impairments of written spelling. Putative central agraphia syndromes other than lexical agraphia and phonological agraphia have been described – deep dysgraphia (e.g. Bub & Kertesz, 1982b) and semantic agraphia (Roeltgen, Gonzalez-Rothi, & Heilman, 1986).

In order to discuss these syndromes, it is appropriate to elaborate the simple two-route approach used so far in this chapter. Consider the model illustrated in Figure 6.2, which is the analogue for writing of that developed for reading in chapters 4 and 5. It is closely similar to that suggested by Morton (1980a) – also based on an analogy with the reading process – which is illustrated in Figure 1.2. The stages of the speech output process explicitly distinguished include the phonological output lexicon, which contains representations of phonological word-forms, and the phonological output buffer, to store a string of phonemes prior to output. Damage to this buffer would lead to classical conduction aphasia (see chapter 3). The model

---

9. A related point is made by Patterson and Morton (1985). On certain versions of lexical analogy theory, it is not assumed that the spelling-to-sound correspondences of individual words are used (e.g. Henderson, 1982). However, such theories, too, have problems (see, e.g., Shallice & McCarthy, 1985).

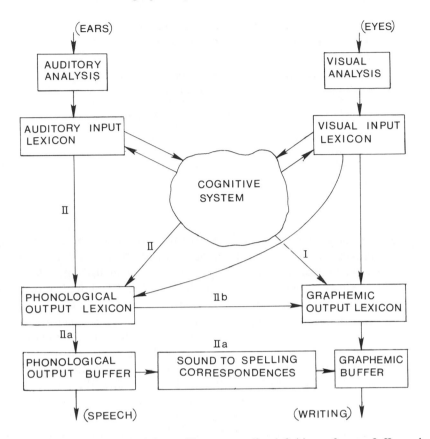

Figure 6.2. A three-route model of the spelling process (for definitions of routes I, IIa, and IIb, see the text).

contains three possible routes by which words may be written. Route I is the semantic route; route IIa is the non-lexical phonological route; and route IIb is the lexical phonological route.[10] Separation between routes IIa and IIb is not meant to imply that these routes are necessarily functionally distinct. This representation, however, allows the question of the existence of different types of sound-to-spelling correspondences to be most simply discussed.

A number of syndromes can be situated on this more complex model. The first is writing by means of a partially impaired semantic route, with phonological writ-

10. The discussion of agraphia does not depend critically on the oversimple assumptions implicitly made about the speech output process in the model. An additional route could be added. The graphemic output lexicon could theoretically be accessed from the auditory input lexicon. However, for the sake of simplicity, this possibility will in general be ignored in this chapter because it is very difficult to distinguish the operation of this route from that of route IIb; the operation of route IIb can, however, be assessed separately as in written naming.

Table 6.3. *Percentage correct performance of GA on repeating and writing from dictation short sentences*

	Word type	
	Content	Function
Repetition	17	60
Writing	38	11

From Patterson and Shewell (1987)

ing being no longer possible. This syndrome was first noticed because of an interesting contrast between speech and writing. It used to be assumed that writing was necessarily more impaired than speaking, unless the patient had a peripheral speech production problem. Then Lhermitte and Derouesné (1974) described two patients – one with classical conduction aphasia and the other with so-called Wernicke's aphasia – in whom written output was much better preserved than spoken.[11] The relative preservation of writing in Wernicke's aphasia has since been described by a considerable number of authors (e.g. Hier & Mohr, 1977; Basso et al., 1978; Michel, 1979; Assal, Buttet, & Jolivet, 1981; Bub & Kertesz, 1982b; Ellis, Miller, & Sin, 1983; Patterson & Shewell, 1987). Of these studies, the classic case is the patient AF of Hier and Mohr; his speech was fluent, but he could not name objects. By contrast, he could write the names of the objects very much better (52% correct). As his spontaneous speech was fluent and did not contain paraphasias, it seems likely that the naming deficit lay at or above the level of the phonological output lexicon in the speech output process (see Figure 6.2).[12] This implies that written naming was supported by use of the direct route from the semantic system to the graphemic output lexicon, which by-passes all phonological processing (route I).

In fact, AF's spontaneous writing was agrammatic and so contrasted strikingly with his spontaneous speech. Written production was asyntactic but contained content words, and yet speech was fluent and empty. The patient GA of Patterson and Shewell (1987) showed a similar pattern. Table 6.3 shows GA's success in reproducing the content and function words in 35 auditorially presented short sentences

11. In Wernicke's aphasia, the patient has impaired comprehension and speaks fluently but with a loss of content words. Neologisms – non-words apparently unrelated to any intended word – can occur, as can literal paraphasias – phonological approximations to the intended utterance.
12. Impairments at lower levels would be expected to manifest themselves differently. For instance, a deficit in the response buffer should lead to phonemic-ordering errors of the sort found in classical conduction aphasia (see, e.g., Lecours & Lhermitte, 1969; Shallice & Warrington, 1977a; chapter 3).

by speaking or by writing. Thus when reproducing 'Come into the garden', she said, *Come into the /roudǝn/,* but she wrote it as *I was up garden.*[13]

It remains unclear whether the converse pattern – of fluent empty writing and contentful asyntactic speech – occurs. I do not know of any such case. If such cases do not exist, then this would suggest that the grammatical construction involved in writing is parasitic on the syntactic processors used in speech production. Cognitive neuropsychology is, however, still too young to base a theoretical argument on the failure to observe a particular type of case.

The syndrome of so-called deep dysgraphia also appears relevant in this respect. This was originally described by Bub and Kertesz (1982b). They based the concept deep dysgraphia on deep dyslexia, since the writing of their patient JC had characteristics analogous to those most widely associated with deep dyslexic reading. As in the syndrome of phonological agraphia, JC had great difficulty writing non-words (1/20), even though all could be repeated. In addition, concrete words could be written better than abstract ones (29/35 vs. 14/35), and function words were poorly written (6/20). Semantic errors also occurred in his written output.[14]

There is, though, a danger in the use of this analogy. In chapter 5, we saw that the interpretation of deep dyslexia is at present far from clear, and it is widely accepted that the patients so labelled do not form a unitary functional group. It therefore provides a shaky foundation on which to base an analogy. There is a second problem. Earlier in this chapter, it was noted that a difficulty in producing a written response does not by itself constitute an agraphia. The writing difficulty may be a secondary consequence of some more basic problem. One possibility that must be considered is whether the pattern of deficits seen in deep dysgraphia arises from a difficulty in the attainment of the semantic representation of the word from the auditory input.[15]

The writing difficulty of patient GOS, reported by Baxter and Warrington (1985), does not seem explicable in this way. Apart from a moderate span deficit and some naming problems, GOS was no longer aphasic a few weeks after a left-hemisphere stroke, but had a phonological alexia. Her spelling of irregular words was above the normal median level on a graded difficulty test developed by Baxter (1982).

---

13. The interpretation of some of the other patients (e.g., those of Lhermitte & Derouesné (1974); Ellis, Miller, & Sin, 1983) needs to be more complex, since they made paraphasic errors in spontaneous speech and produced neologisms. Thus one cannot immediately rule out an impairment at, say, the response-buffer level. In fact, it seems plausible that their deficits, too, lay at or 'above' the level of the phonological output lexicon (see Ellis et al., 1983). If this were the case, then the preserved writing in these patients must be dependent on the direct semantic-to-graphemic output lexicon route, since the phonological writing route would not be accessible.

14. Somewhat related patients have been described by Assal, Buttet, and Jolivet (1981) and Patterson and Shewell (1987).

15. Bub and Kertesz (1982b), in their discussion of JC, did not favour an explanation of this type, but they failed to report any relevant results. Consideration of the phonological agraphic patient PR indirectly makes this possibility more plausible; when PR could not write a word, it was usually because at that time he failed to understand it.

However, GOS did have difficulty in spelling both high-frequency function words and verbs. Thus adjectives were written 78% correctly, verbs, 58%, and function words, 50%; in another series, nouns were 90% correct and matched verbs, 67%. For a set of high-frequency words of various parts of speech, 97% of the high concrete ones were written correctly, but only 69% of the abstract ones. Nonsense words of more than two phonemes could not be spelled. In addition, she made a few semantic errors. GOS therefore presents with a mild but pure deep dysgraphic spelling pattern. However, she had no comprehension difficulties. She scored at just above average level on the Vocabulary subtest of the WAIS, and in the spelling tests could almost always define the stimulus words correctly. A deep dysgraphic pattern cannot therefore always be explained away as a secondary effect of comprehension problems.

The other possible explanations of the deep dysgraphic pattern are analogous to those given for the output forms of deep dyslexia in reading.[16] The most plausible is related to the theory of Saffran, Schwartz, and Marin (1979) and Jones (1985), discussed in section 5.4; it is that the pattern stems from the greater difference in the specificity of the semantic representations of concrete nouns by comparison with those of abstract words and verbs.[17] Alternatively, some specialisation within the orthographic output lexicon could provide an explanation.

6.7   The Capacity of the Phonological Writing Route(s)

In chapter 5, it was argued that the phonological route in reading carries information about a variety of different sizes of units from graphemes through sub-syllabic units to morphemes. Less is known about the phonological route in writing.[18] The most basic question is whether a writing syndrome exists that is analogous to that of reading without semantics, described in patient WLP by Schwartz, Saffran, and Marin (1980a) and discussed in chapter 5; in such a syndrome, writing could be based on sound-to-spelling morphemic correspondences. There is as yet no description of a patient with these characteristics, who, say, writes words that are not understood as well as WLP reads them or as PR writes them. However, a number of attempts have been made to establish the existence of a lexical non-semantic route (route IIb) (e.g. Roeltgen et al., 1986; Goodman & Caramazza, 1986a; Patterson, 1986; Kremin, 1987).

16. For instance, an analogy can be made with Newcombe and Marshall's (1980a) theory that deep dyslexia and phonological alexia differ only on whether the phonological route is completely damaged or not. Indeed, Margolin (1984), in a perceptive review, has suggested that the lack of semantic errors in PR's writing by comparison with that of JC might arise from the greater sparing of the lexical non-semantic route in PR. There is, though, a problem. Why, if PR has a relatively intact route IIb, should he have difficulty writing function words? They are surely frequent enough to be well represented in it.

17. PR presents some problem for this explanation, for the reason related to those discussed in footnote 16. Partial damage to the route from the semantic system to the graphemic output lexicon might, however, produce this pattern.

18. For an initial attack on the question, see Baxter and Warrington (1987).

Table 6.4. *Writing of homophones and of high-frequency regular and irregular words by three semantic agraphic patients of Roeltgen et al. (1986)*

	Homophones		Words	
	Correct	Incorrect mate	Regular	Irregular
SA 1	44	42	72	38
SA 2	40	37	58	31
SA 4	31	33	58	25

The difficulties involved in establishing an independent route of this sort are very considerable. They are well illustrated by considering the work of Roeltgen et al. (1986) on semantic agraphia. They described patients for whom semantic mediation does not appear to contribute to lexical writing. On aphasia tests, the impairments of all the patients were classified within the transcortical group of aphasia syndromes.[19] The experimental investigation of these patients by Roeltgen et al. was not extensive. It consisted basically of a single test of spelling homophones. The homophone was dictated and followed immediately by a sentence – for example, 'Spell *not,* as in "He is not here"'.' As can be seen from Table 6.4, three of the patients produced the spelling of the homophonic mate as frequently as that of the correct word; this showed that semantic mediation was not important in their spelling.

Roeltgen and his colleagues argued that this effect cannot involve the use of just the non-lexical route (IIa), since even irregular words could at times be spelled. However, for all three patients, spelling of non-words was far better than that of 'irregular' words (80% vs. 30%; 80% vs. 30%; 70% vs. 17%, respectively); the criterion for irregularity was that a less common spelling of component sounds was required – for example, the *ight* in *might* (contrast with *ite*). Thus if one ignores the fact that the words used in the experiment were homophones, the three patients would be classified as lexical agraphics. However, the less frequent spelling correspondences are occasionally produced as an error in lexical agraphic patients (Beauvois & Derouesné, 1981; Goodman & Caramazza, 1986a; Baxter & Warrington, 1987). The 17 to 30% correct performance of the semantic agraphic patients on irregular words could therefore have been entirely non-lexically mediated (use of route IIa).

A clearer case of semantic agraphia has been reported in the literature. However, because it predated the recent work on agraphia and because the patient's writing

19. These disorders, first described by Lichtheim (1885), were discussed in chapter 1. The defining characteristic is that repetition is more intact than one or both of speech comprehension and production, the original theory being that it is caused by damage to one or both of the pathways to and from the 'centre where concepts are elaborated' (see Figure 1.1).

skills were not the focus of the investigation, it appears to have been ignored. In an analysis of the language functions of the patient WLP, whose corresponding reading syndrome was discussed in chapter 5, Schwartz, Marin, and Saffran (1979) were interested in demonstrating the relative preservation of her syntactic abilities by contrast with her grossly impaired semantic skills. One technique they used involved the presentation, a word at a time, of each of 30 pairs of homophones for writing from dictation. The words were presented auditorily in a number of different types of context, two of which will be discussed here. In one situation, the context was syntactic; for example, for the phonological form /noz/, a 'nose' was dictated on one trial, and 'he knows' on another. On this test, *both* members of the homophonic pair were spelled correctly for 17/30 pairs, a result well above chance and within the normal range (of 12–30 mean 24).[20] However, if the context was semantic, as in *priest – pope* – /nʌn/ (*nun*) and *some – many* – /nʌn/ (*none*), WLP performed extremely poorly, with only 4 pairs correct in comparison with the normal mean of 25.

How is one to explain this striking contrast? That context can work in one situation implies that the failure to obtain semantic facilitation in the other is not due just to a failure to perceive or remember the context. The contentless speech of the patient and her gross difficulties in picture–word matching make it most plausible that there is indeed a deficit in the semantic representations themselves, which would mean that they could not support writing-to-dictation by a purely semantic route.[21]

In the condition where both members of a homophone pair are frequently written correctly, lexical mediation seems to be required. This supports the existence of morphemic sound-to-spelling correspondences, which are independent of the semantic system, although their use can be influenced by syntactic information.[22] More globally, it supports the separability of semantic processes from a cluster of syntactic, phonological, and orthographic ones.

The model illustrated in Figure 6.2 is not the only one compatible with the existence of morphemic sound-to-spelling correspondences. An alternative, which is analogous to the reading model illustrated in Figure 5.2, is shown in Figure 6.3. As this particular reading model is, in my view, the more satisfactory of the two reading alternatives, and also would be more compatible with a parallel distributed processing approach, I prefer it to that shown in Figure 6.2. However, the discus-

---

20. Note that chance performance would be 7.5/30.
21. More support for this conclusion is presented in chapter 12.
22. Support for the existence of non-semantic morphemic correspondences in sound-to-spelling translating can be derived from analysis of the agraphic patients studied by Patterson (1986), Goodman and Caramazza (1986a), and Kremin (1987). However, two of these patients had a complex pattern of impairments, and the impairment of the third was mild. This makes the inferences much more delicate than for WPR. Both Patterson's patient, GE, and Kremin's patient, M, had virtually no spontaneous speech; GE had a severe STM impairment, and so probably did M. Retention of the nonsense syllables would therefore be difficult for them, so poorer performance on writing nonsense syllables cannot be taken as cast-iron evidence that it is the non-lexical correspondences that are damaged.

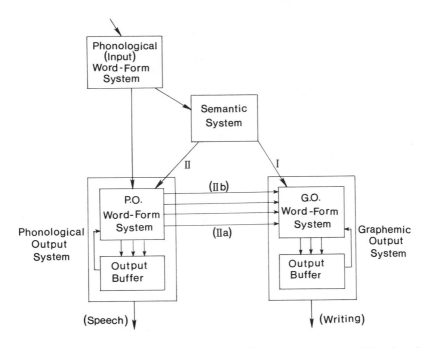

Figure 6.3. A word-form model of the spelling process. I is the semantic route; II is a broad phonological route, with IIa and IIb corresponding to the procedures by which the smallest and the largest units are transmitted by the route – phonemes and morphemes, respectively.

sion that has taken place over the corresponding choice of models in the acquired dyslexias (chapter 5) has yet to occur for agraphia.

The existence of morphemic non-semantic correspondences helps to explain a surprising result in the normal literature. People can write words to dictation at the same time as they are reading aloud for meaning (Spelke, Hirst, & Neisser, 1976). Presumably, they are using morphemic spelling-to-sound correspondences. The relation between dual-task performance in normal subjects and a neuropsychological dissociation is an issue to which I will return in the next chapter. It provides indirect support for the validity of the inferences from the neuropsychological findings.

6.8 The Writing Process and the Peripheral Agraphias: Impairments of the Graphemic Buffer

Ellis (1979b, 1982a) has developed a model of the part of the writing system concerned with the concrete realisation of the spelling of a word into pen strokes as a series of transformation processes between different types of representation, which

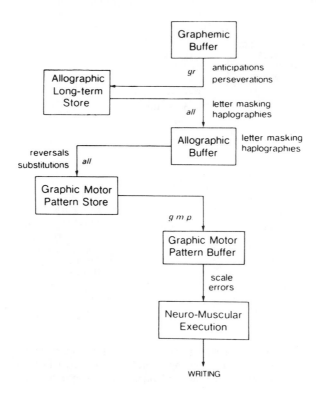

Figure 6.4. Ellis's (1982) model of the processing stages involved in the act of writing following the accessing of a word's spelling. *All* stands for allographic code; *g.m.p.,* for graphic motor pattern code; *gr,* for graphemic code. Reprinted from Ellis (1982a) by permission of Academic Press.

are temporarily stored in a number of buffers (Figure 6.4).[23] His framework depends on differentiating a hierarchy of levels of abstraction, each of which appears to correspond to a functional stage in the writing process. Graphemes are distinguished from allographs, which, in turn, are distinguished from graphic motor patterns. Graphemes are abstract letters, the stuff of which our knowledge of spelling is made. Allographs are the concrete forms they can take, not just capitals and lower case, but also variants (Figure 6.5). Graphic motor patterns specify the sequence, direction, and relative size of strokes, but not their absolute size and duration, or how they will be effected.

One valuable line of evidence for a model of this type comes from the studies of spontaneous lapses by normal writers (e.g. Ellis, 1979b; Hotopf, 1980; Wing & Baddeley, 1980). Different types of lapse seem to result from failures at different levels of the writing process. Using a very large corpus of errors of a normal subject – himself – Ellis showed that different types of error have different characteristics. Some, such as letter transpositions, do not respect the allographic form with which

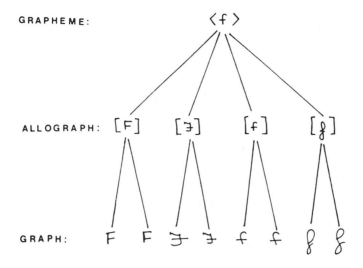

Figure 6.5. Different level units in the writing process. Reprinted from Ellis (1982a) by permission of Academic Press.

the letters are realised: *J. Neurol. Neurosurg.→J. Seuro,* and *Pye Cam-bridge→Pyce.* Ellis argued that this type of transposition (of the *s* and *c*, respectively) occurs at a processing level before the letter has been realised as an allograph – in other words, at the level of selection from the graphemic buffer. By contrast, errors such as so-called haplographies – the omission of one of a pair of repeated letters and all the letters lying between them – occur only when the two repeated letters have the same allographic realisation. Thus when *Depending* is the intended output, an error based on the repeated letters *e* or *n* can occur, such as *Dending,* but not one based on the repeated *D/d*, such as *Ding.* Finally, there are letter substitutions, which seem to depend on similarity at the graphic-motor-pattern level, as in *within→mi,* and *from→str* (of *m* for *w* and *st* for *f*, respectively).[23] Thus the letter transpositions are assumed to occur in retrieval from the graphemic buffer; the hap-lographies, in retrieval from the allographic buffer; and the letter substitutions, in retrieval from the graphic-motor-pattern buffer.

In my view, this evidence does not require the assumption that an allographic stage must be accessed between the graphemic and the graphic. Allographs could be alternative graphic-motor-pattern representations; selection between them would

23. A related theoretical approach was suggested by Margolin (1984). Ellis (see Miller & Ellis, 1987) would now replace the buffers in his framework by patterns of activation across distributed memory units at different levels of the spelling system. This is analogous to the position adopted by Allport (1985) for auditory–verbal short-term memory (chapter 3). At the present stage of knowledge of the agraphias, these alternative means of conceptualizing storage processes are not empirically distin-guishable. I will use the 'buffer' terminology for ease of communication.

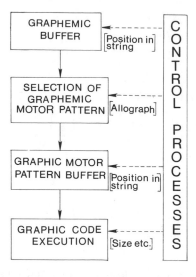

Figure 6.6. An alternative model of the processing stages involved in the act of writing a letter. 'Control Processes' refer to all processes additional to those in the set of writing subsystems specified. The bracketed labels refer to aspects of the output of each subsystem, which are dependent on these external processes. For instance, the first letter of the sentence affects the selection of allographs.

depend on factors such as context and position in the string. An alternative model is that shown in Figure 6.6. Haplographies would then arise from errors of selection from the graphic-motor-pattern buffer.[24]

Can converging evidence be obtained for a model of this type, as it was for Morton's (1980a) model of the central agraphias? On this view, there should be at least three types of peripheral agraphia. They would stem from problems at the graphemic-buffer level, the graphic-motor-pattern level, and the graphic-code level, respectively. Can converging evidence be obtained from the agraphias for a model of this type? The prospects are promising, but as relevant patients are only just beginning to be reported, conclusive evidence is not yet available.

The initial attempt to analyse an agraphic in terms of an impairment at the graphemic-buffer level was made by Nolan and Caramazza (1983). In fact, their patient had multiple deficits, so the results are difficult to assess. Two much purer patients whose writing impairments have been investigated with this hypothesis in mind are two Italians: FV, studied by Miceli, Silveri, and Caramazza (1987); and LB$_2$, studied by Caramazza, Miceli, Villa, and Romani (1987).[25]

24. General support for the assumption that the different types of errors do not all result from problems on the same level comes from Wing and Baddeley's (1980) analysis of the serial position curves of the letters within a word at which different types of errors occur. They are not at all the same.
25. The $_2$ in LB$_2$ is used to distinguish the patient from the different patient LB discussed in chapter 5.

Table 6.5. *Types of error produced in writing to dictation by two graphemic buffer patients (percent)*

	FV[a]		LB$_2$[b]	
	Words	Non-words	Words	Non-words
Substitutions	46	46	37	36
Insertions	16	10	8	9
Deletions	7	10	34	37
Transpositions	3	—	21	19
Mixed	27	34	—	—

[a]Miceli, Silveri, and Caramazza (1987)
[b]Caramazza, Miceli, Villa, and Romani (1987)

FV had a particularly pure impairment arising from a stroke that had produced a small lesion involving only a part of the angular gyrus region of the left parietal lobe. He seemed to have no difficulties outside the writing sphere. Indeed, he continued to practice as a lawyer. His Wechsler Full Scale IQ was 119, and Wechsler Memory Scale performance was 132. His spontaneous speech was quite normal, and no comprehension, naming, or repetition difficulties were apparent on standardised tests. He made only one error in reading 220 words and 110 non-words. By contrast, he made errors in writing 20 to 30% of words or non-words. He made the same sort and rate of errors in typing. As he had no deficits in visually guided reaching, one can presume that the typing deficit is due to a specific agraphia, which implies, in turn, that the writing deficit presumably does not lie in the motor execution of the graphic patterns.[26] Indeed, he wrote rapidly and fluently.

LB$_2$ had a somewhat more widespread deficit; for instance, he had a phonological alexia, which was attributed to a phonological output buffer deficit. His writing was also more impaired than that of FV; he made 41% errors on words and 58% on non-words, the difference being explicable by his minor phonological output buffer problem.

A striking aspect of the writing difficulty of the two patients is that apart from the somewhat greater number of errors with non-words made by LB$_2$, the errors occurred in very much the same fashion for non-words as for words (Table 6.5). In fact, the clear quantitative parallel between the results with the two types of stimuli means that one can apparently confidently exclude the graphemic output lexicon as the source of the errors, since it is not involved in the writing of non-words.[27] Otherwise, it would have to be assumed, implausibly, that the lexical and non-

26. As Italian is a regular language, spelling aloud – a task that is standard for English-language agraphic patients – is not a natural one to use with these patients.
27. The impressive quantitative parallel also means that this is one of the occasions on which it is possible to use an association between deficits as theoretically relevant evidence.

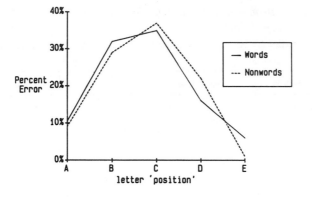

Figure 6.7. Relative positions within the letter string where LB_2 makes errors. Reprinted from Caramazza, Miceli, Villa, and Romani (1987) by permission of Elsevier Science Publishers, North Holland.

lexical routes are independently impaired in such a way as to produce the same error patterns. A locus within the domain of the peripheral agraphias seems to be required.

If one considers the nature of the errors made by FV and LB_2 in terms of an analysis that Ellis (1979b) gave of the lapses made by normal subjects – some of the errors, such as anticipations (e.g. *'pudure'* → *purdode*), would fit on Ellis's analysis, with the impairment being at the level of selection from the graphemic buffer. However, many of the errors were substitutions, which Ellis argued can occur in stroke selection, a much more peripheral stage of the writing process. Yet stroke-selection errors are held by Ellis to be visually similar to the intended letters. This appears not to be the case in general for the substitutions made by both FV and LB_2. Moreover, many of the substituting letters occur earlier in the input – such as *'sopreva'* → *sopresa* (FV) and *'esentule'* → *esensunte* (LB_2) – and the substituted letter can also occur elsewhere, as in *'racchetta'* → *ranchecca* (LB_2). Both these effects are to be expected if the errors arise in selection from the graphemic buffer; thus a substituted letter will presumably remain undeleted to compete with the following letters. The qualitative nature of the errors therefore fit well with a deficit of selection from a graphemic buffer.

This account is closely related to that given by Caramazza et al. (1987) for the writing difficulty of LB_2 – selective damage to the graphemic buffer. They supported this explanation by examining where in the word LB_2 made errors and showing that they occurred in medial positions (Figure 6.7). Following Wing and Baddeley (1980), they argued that such a serial position curve is to be expected in 'read-out' errors from the graphemic buffer; end letters are more adequately 'anchored' to end positions and so less easily confused with others, as in general span tasks.

Ironically, Miceli et al. (1987) argued that in FV's case, the deficit may be more central. Their principal argument is that if a word or non-word is presented to the patient and 10 sec after it has been removed, he has to copy it, he performs almost flawlessly (47/48 correct). For a patient with a graphemic-buffer deficit, this might well seem as difficult a task as writing a word from dictation, and, indeed, LB_2 did find it so (36% errors with words). Miceli et al. therefore argue that an alternative explanation is required for FV and that despite the similar pattern of performance on word and non-word stimuli, the patient has a partial impairment at a more central level – namely in the non-lexical route (route IIa) (see Figure 6.2). Why, then, cannot FV write words lexically? The difference, they argue, between FV and PR – the phonological agraphic patient discussed in section 6.4 as an example of a pure non-lexical-route impairment – is one of individual differences in the degree to which the lexical routes (routes I and IIb) were used premorbidly. Miceli et al. suggest that this difference may stem from FV's writing in Italian, which has an orthographically regular script; so he might rely more on the nonlexical route, IIa, even though it is impaired, and less on lexical routes than would someone writing in English.

The explanation presented by Miceli et al. for FV's errors seems suspect for a number of reasons. Many errors that FV produced resemble the writing lapses of normal subjects, as has been discussed. They differ from those that would arise from the use of an impaired phonological route and are of types that Ellis (1979b) plausibly ascribed to the writing process itself. Thus an anticipation error like the *l* in *'sonaglino'* → *solanglino* appears to be a purely orthographic error with no phonological component because in Italian, *l* is pronounced differently when in *gli* than in *la*. It would not be expected in someone making use of an impaired phonological route. Moreover, there are patients who show phonological alexia and agraphia in Italian (e.g. IGR of Caramazza, Miceli, & Villa, 1986). Thus a total reliance on the non-lexical route is not a consequence of reading or writing Italian.

The strong part of the case made by Miceli et al. is that if the problem of these patients lies in the *selection* of graphemes from the graphemic buffer or in rapid decay in the buffer, then under certain conditions, any refreshing of the buffer from the graphemic output lexicon or the phonological system would not avoid the patient's difficulty. This would apply if the use of these routes *necessarily* leads to information about more than one letter being entered into the buffer in parallel or more rapidly than the writing system can use it. There is, though, an alternative procedure. Visual attention processes (see Duncan, 1987) could be used to allow information to be fed into the graphemic buffer from the orthographic part of the reading system grapheme-by-grapheme (Figure 6.8).[28] Thus a difficulty arising from a number of letters being in the graphemic buffer at the same time could be by-passed in copying, and probably even when copying was from visual short-term memory, too. As this effect would depend on the adoption of a particular strategy by the patient, it is not surprising that the effect is shown in LB_2, but not in FV.[29]

One should not be too surprised by the complexity of these rival arguments and

28. Visual attention is discussed in chapter 13.
29. The problems in interpretation created by the strategy that patients use is discussed in chapter 10.

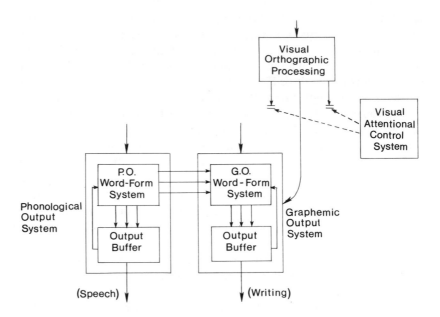

Figure 6.8. A model for the copying process in FV. Three arrows between boxes represents transmission about multiple letters occurring in parallel; one arrow represents serial transmission.

the difficulty of giving a definitive answer even for a well-analysed patient. With multiple routes and multiple stages needing to be considered, a dissociation analysis necessarily becomes much more complex. Moreover, to produce a functional conclusion from an error analysis is in general an order of magnitude more difficult than from dissociations, since one needs to theorise on more than one of Marr's (1982) conceptual levels simultaneously rather than just on the modular level. The most plausible account of FV is, though, that like LB$_2$, he has an impairment in selection from the graphemic buffer.

6.9   Selecting and Realising the Graphic Motor Pattern

All the patients discussed so far can write individual letters normally. There are, though, patients who have a specific difficulty in this task. For them, the problem lies in the selection or the execution of the appropriate graphic motor pattern.

Patients with a difficulty in selecting the appropriate graphic motor pattern rather than in executing it physically have been described clinically (e.g. Kapur & Lawton, 1983). However, none had been extensively investigated quantitatively until the description of patient IDT by Baxter and Warrington (1986). Although suffering from a bilateral parieto-occipital tumour, IDT performed well on intelligence, perceptual, and language tests. He retained his ability to spell aloud, scoring at the 60th percentile on Baxter's (1982) graded spelling test. However, his writing, even

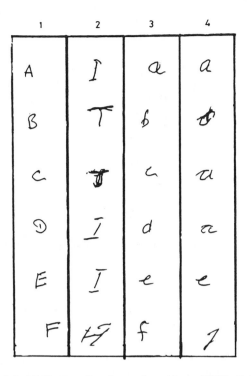

Figure 6.9. Writing to dictation and copying of IDT. Columns 1 and 3 are copying, and 2 and 4 are writing to dictation. The stimuli were the letters *A* to *F* in capitals and lower case. Reprinted from Baxter and Warrington (1986) by permission of the *Journal of Neurology, Neurosurgery and Psychiatry*.

of individual letters, was very poor. He was 42% correct at writing individual capital letters to dictation, and 29% correct at writing lower-case letters. His level of performance for transforming lower case to capitals and vice versa was quite similar (31% and 27%, respectively). By contrast, he could copy both capitals and lower-case letters almost perfectly (each 98% correct). His error responses were quite variable, but the most frequent were letter-like substitutions (Figure 6.9).

The intact copying performance supports the idea that the impairment lies at the level of selecting the appropriate graphic motor pattern. Interestingly, the disorder seems to be restricted to the writing domain. He was virtually error-free at using objects, producing gestures, and carrying out complex action sequences like tying a bow. In addition, he was able to draw from memory – a much more difficult task than writing a letter – and produced recognisable versions of 62% of items such as *apple, shoe, pipe,* and *car*.

A contrast is the patient RB (Margolin & Binder, 1984) a left-handed man who had had a large right hemisphere stroke. He, too, had intact language functions (verbal IQ 111) and could spell aloud normally (30/30 words correct), but was

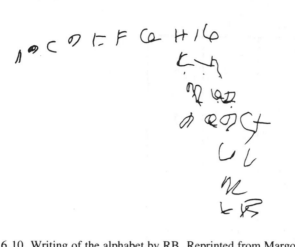

Figure 6.10. Writing of the alphabet by RB. Reprinted from Margolin and Binder (1984) by permission of Academic Press.

impaired on perceptual tasks (performance IQ 76). His spontaneous writing and his writing to dictation were severely impaired, with most letters being too poorly formed to be legible (Figure 6.10). While better at copying than at unguided production, even this was still poor (about 10/26 correct), and many attempts were grossly distorted. In addition, RB could not draw. In the terms of the model presented in Figure 6.6 RB would have difficulty in implementing the graphic motor code.[30]

Although this was not conclusively demonstrated, there were strong suggestions that IDT's impairment was specific to the writing process. It remains possible, though, that the agraphic motor code impairment of RB would occur with any task requiring fine temporal and spatial control; it may not be specific to the writing process. Overall, the model presented in Figure 6.6, which is a descendent of one originally suggested by Ellis (1979b), seems to have considerable promise for explaining the more peripheral agraphias.

6.10   A Few Complications

The picture that is beginning to emerge for the agraphias seems fairly clear and satisfactory. The two domains – that of producing a word's spelling and that of realising it as strokes of the pen on a page – seem to be conceptually fairly distinct. On a modular specialisation position, one might expect the two processes to be mediated by subsystems distinct both from each other and from other cognitive

---

30. One problem is that RB was originally left-handed, but had to be tested with his right hand because of a hemiparesis. However, a patient described by Roeltgen and Heilman (1983) appears similar to RB, except that copying was somewhat more spared. He was right-handed and had a right hemisphere lesion. Relatively little quantitative information is available on this patient. The patient described by Kapur and Lawton (1983) appears similar to IDT.

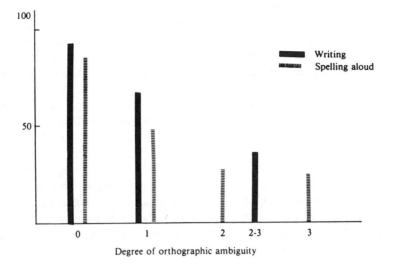

Figure 6.11. Spelling aloud and writing of words of different degrees of ambiguity by RG. Reprinted from Beauvois and Derouesné (1981); *Brain 104*:30; by permission of Oxford University Press.

systems. The evidence available from the agraphias on both points is accumulating rapidly, if somewhat more so for the central agraphias than for the peripheral ones. Also within both domains, we are beginning to see the emergence of sub-syndromes that fit with the functional divisions one would expect from a priori considerations and, to a lesser extent, from the analysis of the errors made by normal subjects.

There are, however, a few skeletons lurking in the neuropsychological cupboard. To start with, the spelling of a word can be produced not only by writing, but also by printing, by using letter blocks, and by spelling aloud. Some people can also type and use Morse code and semaphore. So far in this chapter, such methods for producing a word's spelling have been almost entirely ignored. However, spelling aloud, in particular, is frequently used clinically, so it is natural to ask whether the same system is being used – at the more central level – for spelling aloud as for writing.

Particularly clear evidence appears to come from the first patient considered in this chapter, the lexical agraphic patient RG (Beauvois & Derouesné, 1981). Figure 6.11 shows RG's attempts to spell aloud words of different degrees of ambiguity. There is a roughly similar quantitative effect of this variable as for writing (see Table 6.1). The writing performance is somewhat better, but the difference can be simply explained by the added memory factor involved in spelling aloud; thus spelling aloud was significantly affected by word length, but writing was not. There is not merely an association between the impairments in writing and spelling aloud; the two deficits also have relevant quantitative properties in common. It therefore seems more plausible that the two effects have a common functional origin than that they arise from damage to functionally distinct systems that are anatomically close. In fact, Beauvois and Derouesné come to a different conclusion. They attribute the impairments of writing and spelling aloud in RG to two separate deficits. Their argument depends on the existence of patients whose ability to write and spell orally dissociates.

The first modern example of an acquired dysgraphia syndrome that was analysed quantitatively was that of preserved writing with impaired spelling aloud. The syndrome consists in being able to say letters perfectly adequately and to write words to dictation, and yet to be unable to spell words aloud. This was the case for JP, a patient studied by Kinsbourne and Warrington (1965).[31] Following a stroke, JP had some expressive difficulties, but he could write words virtually normally (93% correct). Yet he was grossly impaired at spelling aloud words shorter than or equal to his span of five letters (7% correct). Moreover, he could name visually presented letters almost perfectly (24/26). So the difficulty could not be attributed to any simple impairment of realising letters in a spoken form.

How is one to explain the pattern of results across JP and RG? There seem to be three possibilities:

1. A single graphemic buffer is indeed used for both output modes; JP has a particular difficulty in transmitting information from it to the letter-name system, but RG does not. Possibly, letter naming from a basically non-phonological source of information is sufficiently demanding that it acts like a Brown-Peterson intervening task, and JP forgets where in the word he is or what he is trying to spell.
2. There are two quite distinct systems for writing and spelling aloud; RG has parallel impairments of the two, and JP of only one.
3. There are two separate representations of the spelling of a word, one basically for writing and the other – a relic of teaching in childhood – basically for spelling aloud, but with the second also being able to control writing, if less efficiently. According to this view, one can write a word directly without 'thinking' (or, rather, speaking) about it, and, conversely, one can write it by explicitly naming the letters to oneself one at a time. In this case, JP has an impairment of the second system only, but lexical agraphics, including RG, must have an impairment of both so that they need to fall back on a further procedure – the use of the non-lexical route (IIa).[32]

To adjudicate among these three alternatives does not seem possible at present.

There are analogous problems concerning phonological agraphia. PR, the first such patient described, claimed to write by transcribing off an inner screen. GOS seemed to be doing something similar; at times, she would write correctly from right to left across the page (Baxter, personal communication). A related example, which is even more dramatic, will be considered in chapter 13. Possibly, the contents of the graphemic buffer can be fed by a process related to imagery into a visual

---

31. The complementary disorder also exists; see Kinsbourne and Rosenfield (1974).
32. The spelling aloud store would not be available in a language like Italian, since Italians do not learn to spell. Hence, the second procedure would not be available for a patient like FV.

short-term store, held there, and transferred back, at least by some subjects.[33] We know far too little about the writing process in normal subjects to be able to assess whether this is possible. Such an account would explain why PR, despite his experience of transcribing off an inner screen, still showed an error pattern similar to that found by Ellis (1979b) in his analysis of his own lapses. One side effect of recent investigations of agraphia seems likely to be a major boost to the study of individual differences in the normal organisation of writing and spelling systems.

Most crucially, none of the effects discussed in this section undercut the separation between functionally distinct lexical and non-lexical procedures. They merely complicate our understanding of the lexical procedure, which was already by no means simple! In addition, these complications do not affect the distinction between the central and the peripheral sub-types of agraphia or its functional relevance. Both these contrasts fit reasonably with the normal literature, and both suggest the existence of subsystems within the overall writing system, which can be independently impaired. If, then, one considers the agraphias as a whole, the research programme of cognitive neuropsychology is strongly supported. Impairment to a complex functional domain – that of writing – produces a set of complementary disorders that appear to reflect damage to the same underlying structure that one would postulate from an analysis of the normal writing process.

33. Differential ability to use and retain information in a visual short-term store could also be invoked to explain the difference in pattern of performance between the graphemic buffer patients FV and LB$_2$ (see section 6.8).

7 Language Operations: Are Input and Output Processes Separate?

7.1 Separate or Common Input and Output Processes: Are the Two Empirically Distinguishable?

The last three chapters have been concerned with the application of the cognitive neuropsychology method to whole domains, not just with the isolation of individual subsystems. Yet if some form of modularity framework is assumed as a general design principle for cognition, the conclusion that the orthographic, phonological, and semantic analyses of words should be conducted by functionally distinct subsystems is not too surprising. The sights, sounds, and meanings of words are phenomenologically very different. If one were to design a system to categorise words orthographically from the output of earlier visual processing, another to categorise them phonologically from the output of earlier auditory processing, and a third to specify them semantically from the outputs of the orthographic and phonological analyses, then the computational requirements of the three processes would be sufficiently distinct to make a modular 'solution' plausible.[1]

In this chapter, an issue will be addressed for which general design principles and phenomenology do not provide any obvious answer. What is the relation between the sets of conclusions reached in chapters 5 and 6? To put it more generally, are the central representations and processes used by output systems the same as those used by input systems? On the claims being made for the cognitive neuropsychology method, this is just the sort of question that the approach should be suited to answer. The problem is whether pairs of subsystems are the same or different and not how they operate.

The issue is one with a long history, and in both the past and the present the answer has often been that common central systems are used for input and for output. So in his pioneering work on the alexias in the last decade of the nineteenth century, Dejerine (1892) assumed that the orthographic processes involved in reading and writing were one and the same. The motor theory of speech perception makes an equivalent assumption for the phonological processes used in speech perception and production (Liberman, 1957). It certainly seems an economical way to

1. The issue of whether the relation among these processes is better represented in terms of a 'cascade' framework (e.g. McClelland & Rumelhart, 1981) rather than a modular one will be considered in chapter 11.

organise the cognitive system. If one needs to map in different directions between one code – or what might appear to be one code – say, a phonological one, and another, say, a semantic one, why duplicate the representations?

Yet have conclusions based on theoretical economy and simplicity proved so fruitful in psychology's past? What could be simpler than having one type of component, from which to build all cognitive processes, as assumed in stimulus-response theory? What could be more economical than having one type of store, into which all types of information can be placed, or one limited-capacity system, which could be used in any type of task? None of these notions has, however, been particularly successful.

At first glance, the neuropsychological evidence appears to support both sides of the input–output argument! A surprising and relevant phenomenon is that found in RG, the original – very pure – lexical agraphic patient described in chapter 6, who writes by relying on the non-lexical phonological route alone and so can write non-words but not irregular words (Beauvois & Derouesné, 1981). This syndrome was explained as a result of the loss of the orthographic representations of words in spelling. Yet RG was also the first phonological alexic patient to be analysed (see chapter 5). Phonological alexia is a syndrome in which orthographic processing of words must be intact because irregular words can be read, even though this is not the case for non-words. Thus the one kind of material RG cannot read is the only kind he can write correctly, and the type he cannot write is what he can read! This counterintuitive dissociation has also been observed in certain children with reading difficulties (Frith, 1980).

This contrast between the properties of RG's reading and writing impairment cannot be put down to any relative difference in difficulty in the reading and writing of irregular words and non-words. Thus unlike RG, phonological and deep agraphic patients can show non-lexical reading at a much higher level than non-lexical writing. PR (Shallice, 1981a) read 72% of non-words, only 18% of which he could write. In JC (Bub & Kertesz, 1982b), the effect was even stronger; he read 85% of non-words, only 5% of which he could write. RG, then, is a patient who has a strikingly different pattern of performance at input and at output. It is most simply explained by assuming that the input and output systems are distinct.

Some patients, though, show the same characteristics in their reading and writing, which seems to fit the common input/output (I/O) store position. For instance, deep dyslexics whose writing to dictation has characteristics similar to their reading aloud have been described; thus GR (Newcombe & Marshall, 1980b) makes somewhat similar types of error in the two cases (see Table 7.1; Nolan & Caramazza 1982, 1983). In fact, no deep dyslexic has been described, to my knowledge, who can write – an important proviso – and who is not also a deep dysgraphic. However, the converse does not hold. Deep dysgraphics have been described who are not dyslexic (e.g. Bub & Kertesz, 1982b; Baxter & Warrington, 1986), and others who are at least partly surface dyslexic (Newcombe & Marshall, 1984; Goldblum, 1985).

The patients in the recent neuropsychological literature who contrast more sharply

Table 7.1. *GR's responses on two different tasks using the same set of 60 stimuli*

	Oral reading	Writing to dictation
Correct	39	17
No response	2	9
Semantic	4	11
Derivational	0	2
Structural	2	21
Multiple-word semantic	13	0

From Newcombe and Marshall (1980b)

Table 7.2. *JS's performance on matched tests with auditory and visual stimuli*

	Auditory	Visual
Picture–word matching[a]	26/150	127/150
Lexical decision	47/80	73/80

[a]The Peabody Picture-Vocabulary test (Dunn, 1965)
From Caramazza, Berndt, and Basili (1983)

with RG as regards inferences about a common I/O subsystem are the patient JS of Caramazza, Berndt, and Basili (1983) and related patients of Levine, Calvanio, and Popovics (1982) and Denes, Ballellio, Volterra, and Pellegrini (1986). As a result of a stroke, JS had a large left hemisphere lesion, including damage to the posterior superior temporal lobe and the neighbouring parts of the parietal lobe. In their interpretation of JS, Caramazza and his colleagues attempted to explain a wide set of similar deficits related to the phonological aspects of word processing in terms of damage to a single subsystem. The most striking aspect of JS's performance is that he was far superior on visual–verbal than on auditory–verbal tasks (Table 7.2). His problem in comprehension of words presented auditorily was only one of a number of difficulties he had in the phonological domain. In addition, there were:

1. A chance performance on discrimination of stop consonants.
2. A near-chance performance on matching a written pseudohomophone with a picture (e.g. picture of a leaf with *leef, luaf,* or *leab*).
3. The inability to detect whether visually presented words rhyme.

4. The presence of a large number of phonemic paraphasias in reading aloud and object naming.
5. No effect of phonemic distractors on short-term memory performance with visual presentation, unlike normal subjects (Martin & Caramazza, 1982).[2]
6. Fluent paraphasic spontaneous speech.

Thus the patient has many deficits – some input and some output – all of which have a phonological aspect. If a single phonological system existed, damage to it would produce a pattern of this form.

These two patients, RG and JS – one with a disorder in the orthographic domain and the other, in the phonological – have a very different pattern of deficits as regards the relation between input and output. I will use them as an illustrative contrast.

How is one to account for these different patterns of input–output relation?[3] Two main types of explanation have been advanced (see Allport & Funnell, 1981). Both can be applied to either the phonological or the orthographic domain. For convenience, though, consider the phonological domain. The economical position is to assume that only a single morphemic-level processor, a single word-form system, exists within each domain. This I will call the common I/O position, illustrated in Figure 7.1 (I), derived from Allport and Funnell's analysis.[4] Thus Caramazza et al. (1983) explain the various impairments of JP as arising from a single malfunctioning mechanism, the result being a central phonological deficit. On the common I/O position, if the patient shows the same characteristics at input and output, then this is due to damage to the processing system itself. But if different characteristics are observed, they can be attributed to impairment to input or output pathways. To give an example from orthographic processing, RG would have the route from the orthographic to semantic subsystem intact, but not the one in the reverse direction.

The alternative position is that different processors exist for input and output – the separate I/O position (e.g. Morton & Patterson, 1980). Similarity in input and output characteristics can be explained as resulting from a non-functional anatomical association.[5] Such an explanation would be implausible if the different deficits

2. This paper provides converging evidence with that described in chapter 3 for the existence of a visual STS independent of auditory–verbal STS.
3. I am ignoring the fact that one example is chosen from the orthographic domain and the other from the phonological. I assume that this not to be a relevant factor, but see Monsell (1985) for possible differences between the two domains in these respects.
4. Unfortunately, Allport and Funnell (1981) phrase the theoretical alternatives in terms of the relation between 'codes'. It is not, however, clear under what conditions different processes produce the same code. In this book, processing subsystems that transform information are depicted by boxes, as are stores that hold it; lines should merely represent flow of information. The 'code' just reflects the function of the processing system that has produced it. It should be noted that in the account of JS given by Caramazza, Berndt, and Basili (1983), his deficit is not only lexical; other aspects of phonological processing are also involved.
5. In special cases, other explanations are possible. For an example, see the discussion of surface dyslexia and surface dysgraphia in chapter 4.

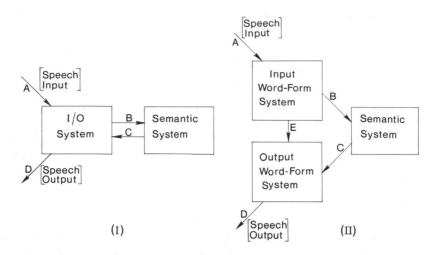

Figure 7.1. The common I/O (input/output) system position (I) and the separate I/O system position (II).

actually had parallel *quantitative* characteristics, as was shown, for instance, for word and non-word writing errors in the graphemic-buffer patients FV and LB$_2$ in chapter 6. For JS, however, no such evidence was presented. Moreover, in the acquisition of language, there must be considerable communication between the phonological aspects of comprehension and of production, so it would presumably be functionally adaptive if subsystems that eventually become functionally distinct are anatomically close. Thus the 'associated deficit' explanation for patients like JS is quite plausible. It is of the nature of neuropsychological evidence that an explanation of a similar pattern of impairments in two domains in terms of associated deficits is hard to refute. No attempt at refutation has been made in the cases under discussion. Instead, the principal arguments for preferring a common I/O position have been the dubious ones of plausibility and economy.

Starting from the opposite perspective, one can ask whether the common I/O position could potentially be refuted by the discovery of certain types of dissociation. The position has been expressed in two different forms. The stronger version is that taken by Caramazza et al. (1983) that a unitary phonological-processing system exists. On this hypothesis, dissociations within the phonological realm are difficult to explain. Yet in chapter 3, it was argued that an impairment of auditory–verbal short-term storage – a phonological input buffer – could coexist with intact phonological processing in speech production. I will therefore primarily consider the main version of the position to be where commonality of processing is restricted to the lexical domain (e.g. Allport & Funnell, 1981). On this theory, a single word-form system exists that is common to speech perception and production. How does this more restricted hypothesis fare?

The most serious problem for this theory would seem to be observation of a

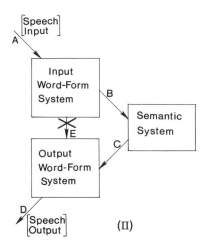

Figure 7.2. The one locus of impairment within the separate I/O position (to route E), which has no correspondence within the common I/O position.

patient who had lost the use of a word-form system at input but not at output or vice versa. In practice, though, on the common I/O subsystem position, it would be possible to reinterpret any such finding in terms of a disconnection of an intact common I/O subsystem from either input or output (e.g., damage to route A or route D in Figure 7.1[1]). On psychological evidence alone, it would be extremely difficult to differentiate between the effects of damage to a system and of the transmission routes into it.

One seems to have arrived at an impasse. It would appear that without a detailed mechanistic theory of the system and of the effects of impairments to it, which I have argued should be avoided in first-pass neuropsychology, any deficit interpretable within a separate I/O subsystem position could be reinterpreted within a common I/O subsystem account, substituting an impairment to a transmission route for an impairment to a processor. There is, however, one exception to this isomorphism between the rival explanations. This is the effect of a lesion to any transmission route, which on the separate I/O subsystem position, carries information from the input to the output system without the involvement of the semantic system (see Figure 7.2). This transmission route is involved in the 'reproduction' of a heard word into its spoken form. If the model is correct, then a specific impairment to this process should be possible.

In contrast, consider the common I/O position. There is no way that this model, as represented in Figure 7.1(I), can be damaged to give rise to such a syndrome. If the common I/O subsystem is itself damaged, one should have a syndrome similar to that exhibited by JS. If a common I/O subsystem exists and the input to it and the output from it are intact, then the patient should be able to repeat (or copy) information normally. Therefore, the main source of evidence that might produce difficulties for the common I/Os position lies in specific disorders of the process of reproducing heard words into a spoken form by non-semantic means. It is therefore these theoretically critical disorders that will now be considered.

7.2 Classical Conduction Aphasia

A specific difficulty in repeating or reproducing a heard utterance into a spoken form is the cardinal feature of conduction aphasia. In chapter 3, two versions of this disorder were distinguished. In a repetition disorder, the patient has a difficulty in a span task involving a set of short high-frequency stimulus words, but individual words can be repeated perfectly. The process stressed is auditory–verbal short-term memory. In a reproduction disorder, the problem is that of echoing back a single item. This latter situation is relevant here.

Historically, specific disorders of reproduction have been viewed within two main conceptual frameworks. Originally, they were analysed in terms of the classic Wernicke–Lichtheim theory, which was basically a separate I/O system position, if a rather complex version of it.[6] Much more recently, they have been analysed by analogy with modern acquired dyslexic syndromes. Thus the first reproduction disorder that is relevant to the separability of input and output word-form systems was thought of as the auditory analogue to deep dyslexia (Morton, 1980b). Morton's main example was patient R (Michel, 1979; Michel & Andreewsky, 1983). A second patient, MK, who appears to be functionally similar to R, has been described by Howard and Franklin (1987).[7] The two patients differed in aetiology; R had had a head injury and MK, a stroke affecting the left posterior parietal lobe. They both appeared intellectually intact; indeed, R had a performance IQ of 107. However, they differed in their spontaneous speech; R made numerous phonemic paraphasic errors, while MK made very few such errors and had fluent, if rather empty, speech with occasional literal paraphasias.

The most striking aspect of the performance of both patients was that they made semantic errors in reproducing single words. Clinically, it was clear that they were trying to repeat and not to give associations. Both, too, showed a set of dissociations analogous to that found in deep dyslexia – a marked effect of imageability on word reproduction and an inability to reproduce non-words (Table 7.3). MK also made phonologically related errors in word reproduction – for example, '*missile*' → '*whistle*'. These errors, however, involved real-word responses in nearly all cases. Of R, it was stated that 'when the patient tries to repeat the word exactly, he

6. See chapter 1. The input system is required for both comprehension and production.
7. Given the criticisms that were made of the concept of deep dyslexia in chapter 5, the assumption of functional similarity can be only tentative. The two patients, however, present similar problems for the common I/O position. Morton (1980b) also discussed a second patient originally described by Cruse (see Morton, 1980b) and Goldblum (1980) has reported two further cases. However, no baseline information is available on these patients. A more appropriate analogue for the repetition of Cruse's patients would appear to be semantic access dyslexia, which will be discussed in chapter 12. The theoretical inferences drawn from the reproduction performance of R and MK are similar but not identical to those drawn by Howard and Franklin (1987) from MK's results.

Table 7.3. *Percentage of words of different imageability
levels and of pronounceable non-words correctly reproduced
by R and MK*

	Words		
	High I	Low I	Non-words
R[a]	60	6	0
MK[b]	60	29	0

[a] Michel and Andreewsky (1983)
[b] Howard and Franklin (1987)

is so burdened by phonemic inaccuracies that he prefers to write the word. By contrast semantic errors are usually given at once and, interestingly enough, in a correct phonemic form' (Michel & Andreewsky, 1983, p. 219). Phonologically related errors generally consisted of non-words. Both patients also made semantic errors in writing to dictation.

Empirically, then, the syndrome is analogous in the repetition domain to deep dyslexia in the reading one. It is natural, therefore, to attempt to explain it in a parallel fashion. There are many different competing explanations of deep dyslexia. However, one characteristic that the accounts have in common is that the phonological route (or routes) cannot be used. The visual word-form system is disconnected from the phonological output word-form one (see, e.g., Figure 5.5). Reading has to be carried out by the semantic system. An analogous explanation for the present syndrome would require the adoption of the separate I/O system position, with the auditory input word-form system being disconnected from the phonological output one. Words would be reproducible only by means of the semantic system; this provides the opportunity for semantic errors to occur and for *semantic* word-class effects to operate (see Figure 7.2).

Perhaps, though, this argument buys the analogy with reading too readily. If the syndrome is to be used as a refutation of the common I/O position, a more detailed examination is required of whether it could be explained on the basis of that model. At face value, on the common I/O position, word reproduction need not involve the semantic system at all. So there seems little reason why semantic errors should occur in that situation or why semantic variables should affect the ease with which words can be echoed back. There do, however, seem to be ways by which one could attempt to defend the common I/O position.

Morton (1970) some time ago made the suggestion that a weaker level of activation of a word-form unit than that required to support an explicit output may be sufficient to allow some information to be transmitted to the semantic system.[8] If

---

8. At the present stage of the argument, an assumption of this type is completely ad hoc. Neuropsychological support for it will be given in chapter 12.

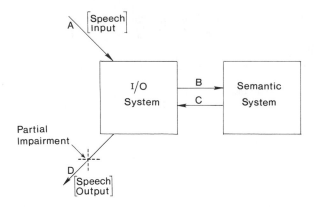

Figure 7.3. The output-blockage explanation for the impairments of R and MK on the common I/O position. A functionally equivalent version is an impairment in the I/O system that affects only outputs via route D.

this suggestion were valid, could partial damage to the common I/O system lead to its producing sufficient activation for some semantic representation to be achieved, but an insufficient amount to support an immediate response?

There are a number of reasons why this tortuous explanation is an implausible explanation for R and MK. The low level of performance on particular semantic classes of words – abstract words – means that correct reproduction must virtually always involve looping through the semantic system. So the phonological word-form system must be severely impaired. Why, then, can it perform so well when information is transmitted top-down from the semantic system, as in, say, naming pictures (82% correct in MK)? How can it provide a sufficiently strong signal for the semantic system that MK, in particular, can do very reasonably on the Peabody picture–word matching test? He scored 113/150, equivalent to an IQ of 104. To make this explanation credible, detailed answers to such questions must be provided.

A second alternative is the possibility considered, although rejected, by Morton (1980b). Could one explain the syndrome on a common I/O position, assuming some blockage on the output of the common system – in route D or at its entrance – with the system working normally otherwise (Figure 7.3)? Might this not explain the impairment in R's spontaneous speech and at the same time be the source of his reproduction problem? If the appropriate word cannot be produced, then an associated word would be substituted. This argument, however, contains a host of holes. If it were valid, why did R appear to be unaware that he was not reproducing words correctly when he made semantic errors? Why was MK better at naming pictures than at reproducing high-imageability words (82% vs. 50%)? Why was he so much better at reading high-imageability words, even if they were irregular (67%), than in reproducing them (33%)? Any blockage in entering route D should affect all these processes equally. Another objection to the account comes from the types of words that could in fact be reproduced. What characteristics would one expect of words that could be successfully reproduced if there was a partial blockage in entering route D? High-frequency words, short words, or phonologically simple ones might be expected to have an advantage. In fact, if anything, long words were reproduced better than short ones (MK: one syllable, 73%; three syllables, 90%). Moreover, the variable that dramatically influences performance is imageability, which affects processes that are functionally quite distinct from the suggested source of the difficulty. At the very least, then, a blockage involving route D could be only part of an explanation of the syndrome in terms of a common I/O system.

One possibility is that in addition, imageable words are retained better, so that they allow – consciously or unconsciously – the possibility for a number of attempts to be made to pass the 'blockage'. Imageable words would indeed be retained better at a semantic level, but do the patients not have auditory–verbal short-term storage available to hold the presented word, whatever its meaning? The retention of one word does not greatly strain auditory–verbal STS capacity (see, e.g., Murdock, 1961). In fact, both patients have a span of only one digit, so the explanation begins to appear more credible. If they had severe auditory–verbal STS impairments, then they would need to fall back on a semantic trace to have more than one try to produce the word. There is, though, a hidden flaw in this argument. Their single-word reproduction impairment makes span an inappropriate means of assessing STS capacity. Using a matching span procedure, MK performed over 90% correct with sets of four digits where the 'different' items involved only a small change in order – for example, 5739→5379. Intuitively, an auditory–verbal STS that will sustain a matching span of four items seems more than adequate to hold one word for repeated attempts at reproduction. The 'response blockage' explanation does not work, even in this extended form.

A second neuropsychological argument can be obtained from two patients with a related syndrome – the classical form of conduction aphasia (chapters 1 and 3) – who were studied by McCarthy and Warrington (1984). One, ORF, was left-handed and had sustained a right parietal stroke; the other, RAN, however, was right-handed and had the standard lesion for conduction aphasia – a left parietal one. The spontaneous speech of both patients contained some paraphasic errors, and in single-word reproduction, frequent phonemic paraphasias occurred, particularly on longer low-frequency words. Table 7.4 gives their scores on age-scaled WAIS subtests. It shows quantitatively how selective the difficulty is; performance on one verbal subtest – Digit Span – is far inferior to performance on the others, at least in ORF. The selectivity of the deficit makes them especially appropriate for single-case analysis because theoretical inferences are less likely to be confounded by associated deficits.

The superior performance of ORF on the Vocabulary subtest suggests that he had no single-word auditory comprehension problems. On the Peabody picture–word matching test, RAN obtained a score of 102/150, equivalent to an IQ of 91, a comparable level to his Performance IQ. He, too, would seem to have relatively

Table 7.4. *Scaled scores on WAIS subtests for ORF and RAN*

	ORF	RAN
Arithmetic	10	4
Similarities	11	7
Digit Span	1	1
Vocabulary	15	6
Picture Completion	10	9
Block Design	7	7
Picture Arrangement	6	10

From McCarthy and Warrington (1984)

intact single-word comprehension. It is reasonable, therefore, to view the patients as having grossly impaired word-reproduction performance in the context of intact auditory–word perception – the classical combination for conduction aphasia.

The critical experiment concerned whether increasing the degree of semantic processing would facilitate word reproduction; this would be expected on the separate I/O store position, according to which the semantic system which is required for reproduction in such patients. The task employed involved the comparison between reproduction of an *individual* low-frequency word with reproduction of the same word when it was the last word in a sentence. This latter condition was used to increase semantic processing of the word, and the need to analyse it semantically was further reinforced because the patients had the additional task of deciding whether or not the sentence made sense; this they indicated by nodding their head after attempting to reproduce the last word. Both patients improved by a small but significant amount from the isolated word to the sentence condition – 47 to 65% for ORF, and 50 to 66% for RAN – and the result was replicated on both patients. The small size of the effect is perhaps misleading. The condition on which they did better seems potentially much the more difficult. In that condition, there is a loss of the attentional advantage for memory of dealing with an isolated word (Kohler & Von Restorff, 1935), and two tasks have to be performed, not just one. These results again then are far easier to explain on the separate I/O position than on the common I/O one. Reproduction is easier in the sentence condition because processing the sentence encourages the use of the less impaired route BCD instead of route E (see Figure 7.2).[9]

What can one conclude after these somewhat lengthy arguments? It cannot be

9. It might be possible to produce an additional memory problem version of the common I/O store explanation analogous to that considered for R and MK. However, the load on auditory–verbal STS of the word in context condition seems likely to be considerably greater than for the single-word condition. It does not therefore seem a likely candidate explanation.

said that the common I/O system position has been refuted. However, since its modern popularity within the neuropsychological literature dates from only 1981, there has been little time for theoretical analysis to be carried out on the relevant disorders. It is already looking fairly sickly. Any defence of the common I/O system needs to be tortuous and ad hoc.[10] The separate I/O position is much the more plausible on the neuropsychological evidence.

7.3 A Comparison with Normal Subjects

Dissociation methodology points fairly strongly to separate input and output phonological word-form systems. Does a consideration of the normal literature lead to the same conclusion? In fact, an increasing amount of research has been devoted to the issue in the recent past.

The most favoured paradigm has been so-called priming. A stimulus is presented, and a certain time later – say 15 min or so – another stimulus, identical to the first or in a related form, is presented. Under certain specific conditions, presentation of the first stimulus facilitates processing of the second. An analysis of these conditions made by Morton (1979a), which was analogous to that used for neuropsychological dissociations, supported a separate I/O model.[11] However, more recent research, reviewed by Monsell (1985), suggests that priming is too complex a phenomenon to be a good vehicle for comparison with the neuropsychological literature.

Can one attempt to obtain an experimental paradigm that would provide a clearer analogue of the dissociation situation in neuropsychology in order to offer a more direct test of whether parallel inferences can be obtained from normal and neurolog-

10. This conclusion may need to be qualified somewhat after the consideration of the possibility of relateralisation of function, to be discussed in chapter 10. The arguments given there for protecting inferences about normal function against this possibility do not apply in the present case. Another line of argument is that on the single I/O system position, it is necessary for a control mechanism to exist to determine how the system is to be utilised on any particular occasion. One does not echo every word one hears! Norris (personal communication) has therefore argued that the reproduction deficit could lie in the control mechanism rather than in the processing mechanism; maybe the system would not be able to enter reproduction mode, but could operate in perception or production mode. However, the typical error made by ORF and RAN in word reproduction is a literal paraphasia. The system appears to be in the correct mode, but just not working too well.

11. Initially, it was found that presenting a word in a particular modality facilitates later recognition of it in the same modality (e.g. Murrell & Morton, 1974; Scarborough, Cortese, & Scarborough, 1977; Kempley & Morton, 1982). Yet reading aloud a written word or saying the name of a visually presented object does not facilitate subsequent auditory recognition (Ellis, 1982b; Gipson, 1986). Morton (1979a) argued that priming was occurring at the word-form (or input lexicon) level. Therefore, one must have separate word-form (or lexicon) systems at input and at output. However, research to be discussed in chapter 14 suggests that one needs to view the phenomena within a specifically memory framework and not just in terms of the architecture of processing systems.

ical evidence?[12] One possibility is to use a so-called dual-task procedure. It has been shown by various workers that in some situations, two fairly demanding, if routine, tasks can be carried out simultaneously, with little increase in the rate of errors (e.g. Allport, Antonis, & Reynolds, 1972; Spelke, Hirst, & Neisser, 1976; McLeod, 1977). It is plausible that a prerequisite for being able to combine two routine, but demanding, tasks is that they utilise separate functional subsystems. Such tasks that can combine should therefore dissociate in neurological patients.

As an example of the correspondence between dual-task performance and neurological dissociations, consider the case of music and speech. Allport et al. (1972) demonstrated that music students can sight-read fairly difficult pieces of music and at the same time echo back, or 'shadow', an unknown text, making very few errors. Neuropsychological evidence supports that conclusion. Double dissociations exist between impairments to music and speech processing. Basso and Capitani (1985) presented a case study of a conductor who, as a result of a large left middle cerebral artery stroke, became severely globally aphasic, as shown by his performance on many language tests.[13] Yet his ability to play piano pieces up to a difficult level was good, although not perfect. Even more impressively, deliberate errors of rhythm and pitch in Mussorgsky's *Pictures at an Exhibition* and errors of a harmonic nature in Beethoven's Piano Sonata no. 2 were all detected, and he conducted correctly from memory the intermezzo of Act 3 of *Carmen,* including the appropriate entry point of all instruments. He even conducted a number of concerts, after one of which the music critic of the Italian newspaper *Republica* wrote that 'his extraordinary gifts remain untarnished'. The complementary syndrome – amusia with intact language processing – also exists (see, e.g., McFarland & Fortin, 1982).

The dual-task procedure together with the structural-separation assumption have been used to address the theoretical issue of whether separate or common I/O systems exist (Shallice, McLeod, & Lewis, 1985). The relevant empirical question is how well two tasks can be combined if one of them stresses the input part of the I/O system and the other, the output part. The phonological output word-form system was occupied by having subjects read random words at close to the maximum rate – roughly 400 msec per word. Subjects also had to *listen* to a stream of random

12. Other types of argument have been concerned with this issue, using approaches somewhat more distant from neuropsychology. For instance, Fay and Cutler (1977) developed an argument from the existence of malapropisms, a class of speech errors in which words are uttered that are close in sound but different in meaning from the intended one. These authors consider the operation of a purely output lexicon, which they conceive of as a list of mappings between semantic and phonological features. They argue that there would be no reason to assume that it would be organised on the basis of phonological similarity. Therefore, if an output lexicon separate from the input one were to exist, malapropisms would not be expected in spontaneous speech. The problem disappears if one replaces Fay and Cutler's concept of an output lexicon by the one used in this and previous chapters, which stores the phonological specification of words for output and can be addressed not only from the semantic and syntactic subsystems, but also from (input) phonological and orthographic word-form systems. As the subsystem can be addressed by many sorts of inputs but produces only one sort of output, it is entirely plausible that near neighbours in the store are related in terms of the output they produce.

13. He showed some sparing of individual word comprehension.

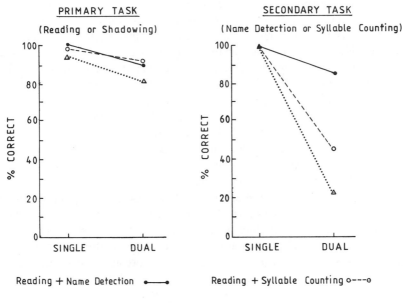

Figure 7.4. Performance on three dual-task combinations: reading aloud and name detection; reading aloud and syllable counting; shadowing and name detection. Reprinted from Shallice, McLeod, and Lewis (1985); *Quarterly Journal of Experimental Psychology 37A:520*; © The Experimental Psychology Society.

words presented at approximately the same speed and attempt to detect any given name. Subjects could combine the tasks with only a 10% decrement. By contrast, when pairs of tasks that used the same part of a separate I/O subsystem were combined, the decrement was much greater (Figure 7.4). For instance, detecting a name and shadowing, both of which use the auditory input lexicon, could not be combined. Thus where the separate I/O approach would predict interference, it is found; where lack of interference would be predicted, it is also found.[14] The common I/O approach has no explanation for the overall pattern of performance. The dual-task procedure therefore provides a result with normal subjects that parallels the dissociation finding in patients, just as it does for the much broader distinction between speech and music processing.

7.4 Multiple Syntactic-Processing Systems

The question of whether the systems involved in perception and production are separable or common can be posed of any class of actions. However, it is for

14. The dual-task decrement for the basic pair of tasks was, however, greater than for, say, shadowing and a visuo-spatial task. This suggests that separability may not be all-or-none (see chapter 11).

complex and specific skills like language or music that the common subsystem approach seems most plausible. For such complex skills, the question can in turn be asked about many different subsystems. In language, for instance, it arises for the perception and production of individual phonemes, semantic representations, and syntactic processing as well as in the selection of individual word-forms.

Neuropsychologically, dissociations between perception and production can occur. Thus in an impressive paper on one phonetic dimension, Blumstein, Cooper, Zurif, and Caramazza (1977) found a double dissociation between perception and production. In the production of voiceless stop consonants, such as /t/, there is a brief delay between release of the noise burst and the onset of glottal pulsing, which is not present in a voiced stop with the same place of articulation, such as /d/. Normal subjects reliably produce a voice-onset time (VOT) with a certain range – say, 50 to 75 msec – when uttering /t/ and can also in perception reliably use this brief delay as a cue to discriminate between the voiceless and the voiced phonemes. Blumstein et al. described three aphasic patients who showed a quantitatively normal VOT discrimination function in their speech perception, but in whom the distribution of VOTs failed to cluster in the appropriate range in their spontaneous speech. They also described one patient who showed the complementary dissociation. It might be possible to explain these results in terms of different types of disconnection of a single centre responsible for phonetic processing. However, because there appears to be little correlation over aphasic subjects in how well they perform the perception and production tasks, it is more natural to assume that separate subsystems are involved.

There is more to language than individual sounds and the phonological forms of words. Can neuropsychology be used to examine the input–output organisation of the higher level aspects of language? In particular, one can ask if there is neuropsychological evidence relevant to whether the syntactic operations involved in speech comprehension are separately organised from those used in speech production.[15] The attempt to answer this question leads into the thickets of one of the most tangled and complex areas of cognitive neuropsychology – the study of agrammatism.

Apart from the occasional reference to function words, syntax has not so far been discussed in this book. In chapter 1, I introduced the classical nineteenth-century account of Broca's aphasia as an impairment in the motor aspects of speech. However, as the field developed, it rapidly became apparent that prototypic cases had a difficulty that did not involve merely 'motor images'. There was a selective problem in using certain vocabulary items, especially function words. Consider this characteristic protocol of a patient describing the scene in a widely used clinical

---

15. In general, the first part of this book has been concerned with relatively restricted issues about which a convergence of evidence can be obtained from normal human experimental psychology. This does not apply to the rest of this chapter. It is, however, natural to consider at this point the issue of whether other input and output language processes have a common or separate functional base. For wider reviews of agrammatism than the one presented here, see Berndt and Caramazza (1980), Saffran (1982), and Howard (1985b).

test, the 'cookie jar' picture of Goodglass and Kaplan (1972), which shows a minor domestic disaster:

Well . . . see . . . girl eating no . . . cookie . . . no . . . ah . . . school no . . . stool . . . ah . . . tip over . . . and ah . . . cookie jar . . . ah . . . lid . . . no . . . see . . . I don't know, but . . . and . . . let's see . . . water all over . . . spilled over . . . yuck . . . Mother . . . daydreaming. (Helm-Estabrooks, Fitzpatrick, & Barresi, 1981, p. 425)

As Howard (1985b) points out, no articles are used and no auxiliary verbs or pronouns, except expressions that are probably stereotypic, such as 'I don't know'. In addition, some verb inflections are omitted. There is also a tendency for verbs to be used in the gerund form.

The dissociation between the use of these expressions and nouns does not arise just because these items are in some general sense more difficult, perhaps more 'abstract'. In the complementary types of difficulty, the fluent aphasias – anomia or Wernicke's aphasia – the speech can be syntactically well formed, but may contain pauses where there should be content words or be full of indefinite terms such as *thing, stuff,* or *guy* or pronouns such as *it* (e.g. Saffran, Schwartz, & Marin, 1976; Buckingham, 1979). Indeed, a patient, WLP, has been described whose content words were eventually reduced almost to one word 'shopping centre', which she used whenever a content word was required in an utterance. Earlier, when her stock of content words had been somewhat more intact, the patient had described the different reactions of one of her two daughters to her language problem as

Oh yeah, *she's* real nice. She, you know . . . she tells me something and I say 'oh, oh, oh' and she says, 'Hon, why don't you say that?', and I say 'well, ah . . .' Then, when she says it, I say 'Oh yeah!' But, oh Lord, my other . . . ah . . . girl, you know, my girl that I have, she says 'Mom, now you tell me something!' (feigning anger) and I say 'Oh, I can't tell you anything!'[16] (Schwartz, Marin, & Saffran, 1979, p. 280).

When the agrammatic characteristics of the Broca's aphasic difficulty began to receive attention, a common explanation was that the omission of function words is a compensatory strategy designed to maximise the information content when speech production mechanisms are impaired (e.g. Isserlin, 1922). In the simplest version of this hypothesis, the underlying deficit is in phonological production (see, e.g., Lenneberg, 1973). However, patients with difficulties in the production of phonemes do not necessarily have agrammatic speech. Thus in the so-called phonetic disintegration syndrome, speech can be phonetically extremely poor, with, for instance, consonant clusters frequently reduced to a single consonant. Yet in such patients, spontaneous speech is not necessarily agrammatic (see, e.g., Lecours & Lhermitte, 1976). As agrammatism became more widely studied, the strategy explanation receded in popularity and an explanation of the agrammatic aspects of

---

16. Other aspects of this patient's language are discussed in chapter 12. Whether in a patient like WLP, content words are selectively lost or whether the preservation of function words, say, can be attributed to their high frequency has not been determined. (See also chapters 5 and 6.)

Broca's aphasic speech in terms of specifically linguistic disorders – particularly, syntactic ones – became increasingly common (e.g. Jakobson, 1956; Luria, 1970b).[17]

The increasing tendency to view agrammatic speech as due to an impairment in some linguistic faculty has run parallel with a great increase in the linguistic sophistication of empirical investigations of the syndrome stimulated by the Chomskyian revolution in linguistics. Indeed, many of the major early modern contributions to the study of agrammatism were actually made in the Boston area by Goodglass, Zurif, Caramazza, and their co-workers. During the late 1970s, one theory came to dominate the field. Agrammatism was seen as resulting from an impairment to a central syntactic-processing mechanism used in both comprehension and production (e.g. Von Stockert, 1972; Zurif, Caramazza, & Myerson, 1972; Kremin & Goldblum, 1975; Caramazza & Zurif, 1976; Berndt & Caramazza, 1980).

Unlike the analogous approach at the word-form level, this theory did not result from considerations of theoretical economy alone. The classical view of Broca's aphasia was that speech comprehension was spared, or at least relatively so, and this had remained the dominant position until the early 1970s (e.g. Geschwind, 1970). The origin of the central syntactic-processing theory lay in the development of a new type of group-study procedure in the 1960s by Goodglass and his colleagues.

7.5   The Modern Aphasia Group-Study Method

In the early 1960s, the general consensus was that interesting sub-types of aphasia could not be discriminated by quantitative means and, in particular, that the classical syndromes of the diagram-makers had no quantitative basis (see, e.g., Bay, 1962; Schuell, Jenkins, & Carroll, 1962). However, it was demonstrated by Goodglass, Quadfasel, and Timberlake (1964) that if more refined measures were taken, a fair percentage of aphasics could be separated into two fairly clear subgroups. The primary measure that Goodglass and his colleagues used was what they called 'phrase-length ratio', derived from transcriptions of the spontaneous speech of the patients. The length of the number of words between neighbouring pauses was measured, and the ratio of groups of five or more words to groups of one and two words was calculated. The results are shown in Figure 7.5.

Shortly afterwards, Benson (1967) took this measure and a number of others of spontaneous speech, including rate, prosody, phonetic intelligibility, effortfulness, word choice, and the amount of perseveration and paraphasia. Using a combined fluency scale, he again found a clustering of patients into two different ranges. In addition, he was able to use a primitive localising technique – radioisotopic brain scans – to give rough localisations of the lesion sites in 61 of 100 patients. There was a strong tendency for the 'non-fluent' patients to have a more anterior lesion

---

17. Strategic explanations of agrammatism have not been completely rejected. Indeed, in recent years, they have been having a minor revival (see chapter 10 for one aspect of the debate).

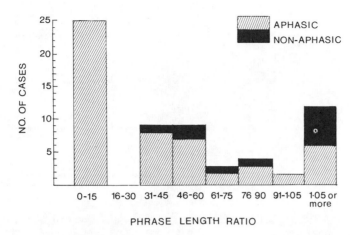

Figure 7.5. The distribution of the phrase-length ratio across a group of aphasic patients and a group of controls. It can be seen that the aphasics fall into two clusters, one of which has a similar distribution to that of the controls. Reprinted from Goodglass, Quadfasel, and Timberlake (1964) by permission of Masson Italia.

site than the 'fluent' ones. So the approach developed of dividing aphasic patients into two main types: 'fluent' versus 'non-fluent' or 'posterior' versus 'anterior'.

More subtly, the work of Goodglass and his colleagues (1964) legitimised the use of two major sub-groups of aphasics. They attempted to relate these sub-groups to the classical aphasia types – Broca's and Wernicke's – as defined by clinical criteria. The use of conventional clinical criteria was not, however, a straightforward matter, as indicated by the following problem:

A set of six characteristic symptoms for each of the . . . diagnostic categories (Broca's, Wernicke's, amnesic [i.e. with naming difficulties only] and mixed aphasia) was agreed on by the three authors. They then independently assigned each patient to one of the categories after having listened to the tape recorded Conversational and Expository Speech and inspected the auditory comprehension subtest scores. The method was abandoned when only 6 cases of agreement among the three raters were found in the first 28 cases classified. (pp. 139–140)

They adopted instead the use of profiles, the relative performance on a set of quantitative, if somewhat narrow, spontaneous-speech, comprehension, and naming tests (Figure 7.6). For instance, Broca's aphasics were held to have no more than the median aphasic comprehension impairment. They found that their sub-groups, defined by phrase length, now fitted fairly well with a differentiation into Broca's and Wernicke's types. However, because length of uninterrupted word group is one of the dimensions used in the profiles, there is an element of circularity in the reasonable fit of the phrase-length-ratio measure with a division of the patients using classical categories. The conceptual basis for the use of classical categories was by

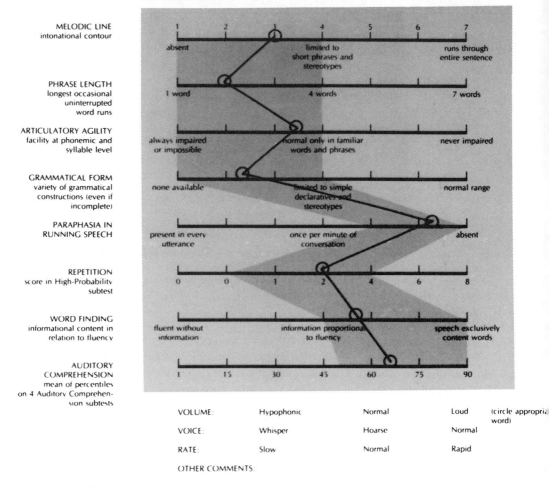

Figure 7.6. The appropriate profile for a Broca's aphasic patient in the most recent version of the Boston Aphasia Battery. The rating scales used in Goodglass, Quadfasel, and Timberlake (1964) were more primitive, but otherwise closely related. Reprinted from Goodglass and Kaplan (1983) by permission of Lea & Febiger.

no means as secure as it appeared. However, the existence of clearly quantitatively differentiable subgroups of aphasics with different characteristics could no longer be denied.

The comprehension tests used by Goodglass et al. (1964) in their methodologically important study were not theoretically based. When more linguistically motivated tests were given to groups of patients who had been selected as Broca's aphasics in terms of their aphasia profiles, a surprising result was obtained. The comprehension of the Broca's aphasics, like their speech production, was asyntactic. Such a group performs poorly when comprehension depends on grammatical morphemes or on word order. So a sentence such as *The cat that the dog is chasing is black* gives trouble if it has to be matched to the correct picture from a set of four possibilities that factorially vary in terms of which of the chased and the chaser is white or black and which is a cat or a dog. Irreversible sentences of equivalent *syntactic* complexity, such as *The apple that the boy is eating is red,* do not give a problem (e.g. Caramazza & Zurif, 1976; Goodglass et al., 1979; Schwartz, Saffran, & Marin, 1980b). Indeed, it had already been discovered that when contrasted with Wernicke's aphasic patients, the Broca group performed more poorly on those comprehension tests that require processing of syntactic structure (Von Stockert, 1972; Kremin & Goldblum, 1975; Von Stockert & Bader, 1976). The conclusion drawn was that the Broca's aphasic suffers from an impairment to a common I/O syntactic system.

Almost as soon as the central syntactic-processing theory began to be widely accepted, attempts to specify it further were made. A commonly held position was that there was a specific difficulty with function words. One well-known version was that of Kean (1977), who argued that the impairment could be characterised as an inability to process a particular class of words. Kean's theory was that the Broca's aphasic tends to reduce the structure of a sentence to the minimum string of elements that can be lexically construed as 'phonological words' in the language. A 'phonological word' is a concept developed by Kean. It refers to those lexical items in a sentence that influence the determination of stress. So Kean argued that the omission of inflections and function words in the speech of a Broca's aphasic follows from the way that such words do not normally carry stress and do not affect which other words in the sentence are stressed.

A variety of criticisms of this theory have been put forward (see Kolk, 1978; Berndt & Caramazza, 1980). Perhaps the most convincing is that of Saffran, Schwartz, and Marin (1980a). They asked five agrammatic aphasics to describe pictures in which a sentence about the participants could potentially be reversible, as in one showing a boy running to his mother. Normal subjects gave the expected active-construction word order on 99% of occasions. The agrammatic patient made over 30% 'errors' in the order in which they produced the two substantives. Yet if the loss of those sentence elements that are not phonological words is the key problem for a Broca's aphasic, the order of substantives should be correct.[18] In addition, as discussed in chapter 5, when patients have difficulty with function words, it is not that they do not attend to them or neglect them, since they can process them semantically (see also Goodglass, Gleason, & Hyde, 1970). Therefore, agrammatic production does not seem to be reducible to just a difficulty – at any level – in the production of 'phonological words'.

The major alternative proposed was that agrammatism represents an impairment in the carrying out of algorithms utilised by a central I/O syntactic parser (Zurif & Caramazza, 1976; Berndt & Caramazza, 1980). Within the broad class of theories

---

18. A similar word-order deficit occurs in the comprehension of these patients (Schwartz, Saffran, & Marin, 1980b).

of this type, some alternatives are now being articulated in an impressively detailed and linguistically sophisticated form (e.g. Lapointe, 1985). Indeed, if one compares these modern theories with earlier versions within the same broad class, such as the position of Caramazza and Zurif (1976), one has the impression of a field advancing in power and technical sophistication. There are, however, a few anomalies for this common I/O position. It is beginning to appear that these anomalies may be more problematic than was originally thought.

7.6   The Central Syntactic-Processing Mechanism: Problems

The first problem is far from being a direct refutation of the common I/O position. Instead, it is an odd paradox discovered by Linebarger, Schwartz, and Saffran (1983), which makes the common I/O position a somewhat less natural explanation. Linebarger et al. did not study just the inability of agrammatic patients to comprehend syntactically complex sentences by techniques such as picture–sentence matching. In addition, they looked in considerable detail at the performance of their patients on grammaticality judgements about sentences. They found that their patients, especially the ubiquitous VS, who has already appeared in chapter 5, could perform these judgements very well. VS, for instance, was able to make near-perfect discriminations between grammatical and ungrammatical sentences of a whole range of types. Thus *I want you to go to the store now* and *I hope you will go to the store now* were accepted as grammatically correct, but not *I want you will go to the store now* and *I hope you to go to the store now*. Yet VS was agrammatic in spontaneous speech and was poor, although not at chance, in picture–sentence matching tests that stressed syntactic processing.[19]

Linebarger et al. suggested that the problem for agrammatic listeners is not in actually constructing syntactic representations, as held by earlier theorists, but in providing the syntactic representations with a semantic interpretation. This does not have a direct implication for the issue of whether the impaired system is common to both input and output, as a related explanation could be applied to agrammatic production, too (e.g. Saffran et al., 1980a). Yet it must certainly be premature to argue that a mechanism is used for both input and output, if there is no agreement on the function it carries out in either input or output.

There is, however, an even more fundamental problem. Is the disorder being discussed – agrammatic aphasia, non-fluent aphasia, Broca's aphasia, anterior aphasia, or what have you – a unitary functional disorder that has properties well captured by the standard aphasia group study? It has been cogently argued by Schwartz (1984), Badecker and Caramazza (1985), and Howard (1985b) that this belief is misplaced. Badecker and Caramazza go further. They argue that the aphasia group-study approach in which, say, Broca's and Wernicke's aphasics are contrasted, is inherently faulty.[20] Indeed, the historical process that gave rise to the adoption of

19. A similar dissociation was discussed for short-term memory patients in chapter 3.
20. Badecker and Caramazza (1985) also claim that linguistically sophisticated theories of 'agrammatism' are now being developed, with some theorists using idealised data of a type that would never occur in practice!

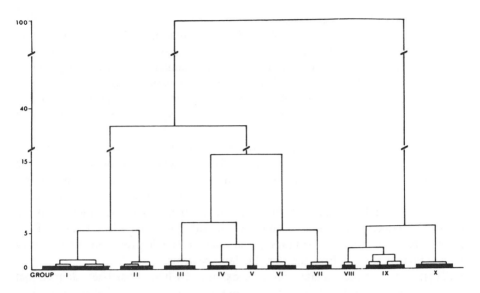

Figure 7.7. Hierarchical 'dendogram' for aphasia using a cluster analysis. Globals are in groups I and III; Broca's, in II, III, and IV; isolation of the speech area, in III and IV; transcorticals, in IV and X; conductions, in VI and VIII; Wernicke's, in VII; and anomics, in IX and X. Reprinted from Kertesz and Phipps (1977) by permission of Academic Press.

the methodology militates against its effectiveness as a research tool. The origin of the approach and, indeed, its rational basis lie in the critical investigation of Good-glass et al. (1964) discussed earlier. They showed that contrary to the dominant belief at the time, it is possible to subdivide aphasic patients into sub-groups with broadly similar symptoms. These sub-groups have been used to form the basis of a classification system widely employed for clinical purposes. Yet a clinical instru-ment like the Boston Aphasia Battery of Goodglass and Kaplan (1972) is concerned with dividing the space of aphasic disorders into a number of sub-groups for diag-nostic efficiency. There is no simple principled way to decide what 'grain' the classification should have, whether it should be broad or fine. There are no a priori reasons why a clinical procedure useful for, say, lesion localisation should be an effective research tool.

More recently, the approach of grouping patients with similar symptoms has been applied more systematically by the use of a cluster analysis. Kertesz and Phipps (1977) applied this procedure to the scores of 142 aphasics with infarcts[21] on a test battery derived from that developed by Goodglass and Kaplan (1972). Far more than two groups emerged. The authors derived 10 clusters of patients (Figure 7.7), and these clusters cut across the classical categories.[22] So cluster 2, for instance,

---

21. A lesion arising from an embolus lodging in an artery.
22. In fact, the difficult conceptual problem of what level of grain should be used to determine the clusters is not confronted in this paper either.

contains 57% of the Broca's aphasics; cluster 3 has 13%; cluster 4 has another 30% and these clusters also contain 'global aphasic', 'isolation of the speech area', and 'transcortical motor aphasic' patients. Thus more systematic use of measures of the similarity among patients does not reinforce the standard group-study presuppositions. In any case, the similarity of symptoms across patients whom one is investigating – the basis of the methodology – may represent merely a similarity of lesion sites across patients rather than a functionally unitary impairment (see chapter 2; Poeck, 1983).[23]

A group of Broca's aphasic patients, then, could well be functionally heterogeneous, with the overlap of symptoms arising because a group of subsystems that are anatomically close together have been damaged. Moreover, the operational definition used in standard screening tests allows patients with known comprehension deficits to be included, even though these impairments must be milder than the patients' production problems. Therefore, the difficulty that at least some of the patients have on comprehension tasks that stress syntactic processing could easily be functionally distinct from their production problems.

This, then, is a second situation to be examined where it has been claimed that there are dangers in basing a functional inference on an association observed in a group study. The first was the discussion of amnesia in chapter 2. Can, though, the argument that there is such a danger be made more concrete? Is, for instance, the greater variety of aphasic syndromes that is suggested by the results of the cluster analysis borne out if the impairments of those patients who have difficulty in producing syntactically correct utterances are examined in detail? It is increasingly accepted that functional differences among such patients do exist. In 1973, Tissot, Mounin, and Lhermitte suggested that such patients may differ according to whether their difficulty lies at the level of syntactic organisation – 'syntactically impaired' – or at the level of the utilisation of function words – 'morphologically impaired'. A related position was taken by Saffran, Schwartz, and Marin (1980b).

Strong support for this view was provided by two Italian patients studied by Miceli, Mazzucchi, Menn, and Goodglass (1983); both patients had 'agrammatic' disorders. Their difficulties of speech production were pure. On a wide variety of neuropsychological tests, both patients scored within normal limits, and the content words in their speech were generally correctly produced. Statistical analyses of spontaneous speech showed, however, great differences between the two patients. If one considers the omission of function words and the substitution of the infinitive for an inflected form, then case II is clearly the more severely impaired (Table 7.5). But if one ignores the omission of function words, case I has a median string length of 2 items; he is a fairly typical slow, effortful Broca's aphasic. Case II, by contrast, has a median string length of 7.5 items – very significantly more – and has a wide

23. The idea that the Broca's aphasia 'syndrome' may be a semiartefact of the anatomy of the vascular system (Berndt & Caramazza, 1980; Poeck, 1983) is indirectly supported by anatomical studies. Long-standing classical Broca's aphasia typically arises from large lesions in the territory of the upper division of the left middle cerebral artery (Mohr et al., 1978). They can therefore be expected to damage a number of processing systems.

Table 7.5. *Percentage of occurrence of certain types of syntactic errors in the speech of two agrammatic aphasics studied by Miceli et al. (1983) by comparison with the number of times used correctly*

	Case I	Case II
Substitution of infinitive for inflected form	19	47
Omission of clitic (or weak) pronouns	13	100
Omission of auxiliary verbs	0	73

spread of string lengths in speech, as does a normal subject; indeed, the patient spoke at normal rate. It was argued by Miceli et al. that case II has a morphological deficit, not a syntactic one; he has primarily lost the ability to produce function words. Case I, though, is held to have a syntactic disorder. This contrast supports the position advocated by Tissot et al. (1973). Agrammatic disorders in production therefore appear not to be functionally unitary. Further quantitative evidence supporting this view has been put forward by Berndt (1987) and Parisi (1987).[24]

This finding does not refute the theory of a syntactic-processing mechanism common to input and output, but it makes the evidence on which it was based – associations between comprehension and production impairments in groups of 'agrammatic' patients – seem much less secure, since not all Broca's aphasic patients seem to have damage to such a mechanism. There is another aspect of the results of the study of Miceli et al. (1983) that causes more direct problems. Despite the very different pattern of spontaneous speech in these two patients, they have one major characteristic in common. Both appear to have normal comprehension of syntax. Case I, in particular, performed normally on the shortened version of the De Renzi and Vignolo (1962) Token Test, on the type of centre-embedded sentences that Caramazza and Zurif (1976) found gave great difficulty for agrammatic patients, and on a number of other tests of syntactic comprehension. In case II, syntactic comprehension was not adequately tested in a quantitative fashion. However, two patients with a similar pattern have recently been reported by Kolk, Van Grunsven, and Keyser (1985) and by Nespoulous et al. (in press). The second of these patients, despite a severe problem in producing function words – although having a mean phrase length of six words – made no errors at all on a wide range of tasks that stress the comprehension of syntax.[25]

What then, can one conclude about the possibility of a common input/output system being utilised for syntactic processing? The theory is far from being refuted. One could argue that case II of Miceli et al. and the two similar cases who have a

---

24. The possibility has not been ruled out that this difference is a strategic one, but this seems implausible (see also chapter 10).
25. Howard (1985b) has recently pointed out that similar dissociations occur in the reading and writing domains.

morphological difficulty do not represent 'true' central agrammatism. Case I clearly presents more problems for the theory, but it would be possible to argue that the common I/O syntactic-processing system was disconnected from other subsystems involved in speech production. There is, though, a more basic point. It is increasingly clear that there is no adequate justification for drawing theoretical inferences from associations between deficits in studies involving groups of Broca's, or non-fluent, aphasics. The positive support for the common I/O syntactic-processing theory must, therefore, be highly suspect. Moreover, the application of the modern single-case approach to the study of agrammatism is very recent. It has, however, produced some interesting results, and in chapter 12, we will see that other aspects of the disorder are coming to light that also do not fit easily into the common syntactic-processing position – in particular, concerning the Broca's aphasics' use of verbs. This approach has not yet led to a coherent overall theory of syntactic production disorders, but it has certainly shaken existing theoretical conceptions severely.

In this chapter, we have seen how related issues concerning whether the systems involved in input and output processing are or are not distinct have been tackled using different methodologies. The analysis of impairments at the word-form lexical level has used single-case studies. The work is very much in its infancy by comparison with, say, the study of the alexias and the agraphics. However, a promising convergence of normal and neuropsychological evidence has been obtained, pointing to the existence of separate input and output systems at this level. Much more work has been carried out on investigating syntactic-processing systems. Here, though, the dominant theory since the mid-1970s – that a system common to input and output exists – is looking increasing sickly. Moreover, a major cause of the difficulty seems to be the basic methodology that has been widely used – the aphasic group-study approach, by which the groups are defined in terms of categories that are partly operational and partly based on classical syndromes. Overall, the balance sheet seems to be strongly in favour of the use of single-case studies.

8   The Generality of the Approach: The Case of Visual Perception

8.1 Introduction

The last few chapters have shown the cognitive neuropsychology approach to be applicable to a number of different topics. Yet the areas treated have actually covered a fairly narrow range by comparison with those that are conventionally included in, say, either clinical neuropsychology or cognitive psychology. The topics discussed so far have all been aspects of language. In later chapters, the approach will be applied much more widely by considering areas where the method provides fascinating glimpses into relatively unexplored terrain. In general, though, these areas are not too helpful for an overall assessment of the solidity of the cognitive neuropsychology methodology.[1] One area outside language – visual perception – does contain a set of interesting and solid neuropsychological studies, and the inferences drawn from these investigations can be compared with those derived from completely different disciplines.

This area is important to consider for another reason. So far, it has been argued that the only effective methodology in cognitive neuropsychology is the single-case study. Group studies, it has been suggested, particularly in chapter 7, are not an effective source of evidence. This view is too extreme. Indeed, some of the more interesting studies on disorders of visual perception have been group studies, although of a type somewhat different from those discussed in chapter 7.[2] These will be discussed in conjunction with the individual case studies because contrary to much opinion in cognitive neuropsychology, under certain conditions the inferences that can be drawn from the two types of study are not substantively different.

The neuropsychology of visual perception is a large topic with a more extensive literature than that of almost all the areas discussed so far. The treatment will therefore be more selective and less detailed than that of earlier chapters.[3] What is critical for the overall argument being developed is whether parallel inferences about nor-

1. In certain aspects of other areas considered – in particular, attention and episodic memory – some convergence of inferences from cognitive neuropsychology and other disciplines does exist.
2. In this chapter, group composition is determined by lesion site and not by a gross psychological characterisation of the disorder. Moreover, theoretical inferences are based primarily on dissociations. Relevant methodological issues are discussed in chapter 9.
3. For reviews of the overall topic, see Hécaen and Albert (1978), De Renzi (1982), Ratcliff and Newcombe (1982), Warrington (1985), and Bauer and Rubens (1985).

183

mal function can be drawn from the neuropsychological findings to those reached from other disciplines. Visual perception also makes an interesting contrast with the earlier topics covered, in that the conceptual links are with neurophysiology and artificial intelligence rather than with cognitive psychology. Thus the efficacy of the neuropsychological approach can be assessed more broadly.

8.2   Dissociations Between Disorders of Sensation

In chapter 1, I alluded to the 'craft' knowledge that 100 years of clinical neurology has produced. One excellent example is the great variety of disorders of visual sensation that has been discovered (see, e.g., Hécaen & Albert, 1978). For instance, at the most basic level of visual sensation, it is known that cortical injury can produce specific deficits – all independent of acuity – in the perception of colour, shape, and movement and in the visual information necessary for the accurate guiding of actions.

Well established are the achromatopsias, in which the visual world appears drained of colour to such an extent that in extreme cases, only black, white, and shades of grey may be discriminable (for a review, Meadows, 1974). Such patients can perform very poorly in standard tests of colour vision (see, e.g., Critchley, 1965). But other visual functions can be intact. For instance, on quantitative tests, case II of Damasio, Yamada, Damasio, Corbett, and McKee (1980) had normal acuity, could read normally, discriminated visual forms normally, and judged line orientations correctly. However, the world appeared to her in shades of grey, with occasional black and white, and she had a defective performance on the Ishihara test of colour vision, colour matching, and colour naming.[4] Moreover, in one such patient, it was clearly established that the three types of cone in the retina were operating normally (Mollon, Newcombe, Polden, & Ratcliff, 1980), showing that one is dealing with a central colour disorder.

There have been only rare reports of isolated disorders of the primitive perception of shape. Efron (1968) described a patient, S, who could make fine discriminations in hue and had an acuity that, although not normal, was described as 'adequate'. Yet he was unable to discriminate squares from rectangles, being barely above chance at very simple contrasts of this type. Efron's finding was replicated by Warrington (1986) in two patients. One, JAF, performed so poorly that she obtained less than 70% correct in discriminating a square from a 65×40 ratio rectangle. Normal subjects, of course, perform at 100% level for far more difficult discriminations.[5] In spite of a gross difficulty in perceiving shape, acuity was nor-

---

4. This patient also had a prosopagnosia, a difficulty recognising faces (see section 8.3 and chapter 16). Damasio, Yamada, Damasio, Corbett, and McKee (1980) also report a case in which achromatopsia is limited to one visual field.

5. A priori, one possibility is that the disorder can be explained in terms of the loss of particular spatial frequencies. Warrington and Weiskrantz (personal communication) have assessed the spatial-frequency sensitivity curve of JAF. It appears that the impairment of shape perception in this patient cannot be reduced to a loss of particular spatial frequencies.

Table 8.1. *Reaction time (in msec) to carry out three different discriminations by LM and a control subject*

	LM	Control S
Red versus *green*	315	285
Diamond versus *circle*	306	296
Moving versus *stationary*	999	275

From Zihl, Von Cramon, and Mai (1983)

mal in both patients. JAF could also read fine small print, which adds yet one further dissociation! Both patients were, however, extremely poor at tests of object and face perception. Warrington argued that the basic analysis of shape precedes these two types of perceptual process. Letter perception can be preserved, though, because letters are so highly distinctive in shape, and *quantitative* determination of their internal dimensions is not critical in their identification.

Selective disturbances in the perception of movement have been even more rarely observed. A well-documented case was reported by Zihl, Von Cramon, and Mai (1983). After suffering a stroke, the patient, LM, complained of loss of movement vision in all three dimensions. When she poured tea or coffee into a cup, the fluid appeared frozen, 'like a glacier' (p. 315). With perception of people or cars, they 'were suddenly here or there but I had not seen them moving' (p. 315). Many experiments were performed that showed defective perception or detection of movement (Table 8.1). In peripheral vision, discrimination of direction of movement was only marginally better than chance, and rapid motion could not be perceived in central vision. By contrast, her visual field, acuity, binocular vision, colour discrimination, and object and word recognition were all normal.

Isolated disorders of the ability of a patient to localise a visually presented object have been known since the first decades of the twentieth century and, in particular, the classic work of Holmes (1918). Holmes described six soldiers with parieto-occipital gunshot or shrapnel wounds who were unable to take hold of an object presented to them or reach out to touch it accurately. They would at times project their arms in quite the wrong direction. The difficulty, which can be very gross, was present whichever hand they used and whichever visual field was stimulated. Holmes showed that it did not result from a specifically motor problem, for when he asked a patient to touch a part of his body, the task could be carried out satisfactorily. In addition, the patient can be impaired in describing the position of an object (Holmes, 1918).

'Visual disorientation' is classically described as affecting not only reaching, but also the eye movements necessary to fixate an object and the judgement of distance or size (see, e.g., Riddoch, 1917). It can even lead to the patients giving the appearance of being blind. Yet if by chance, fixation happens to be satisfactory, the patient can report tachistoscopically presented material (see Godwin-Austen, 1965). Fixation can even be specific to a half-field and occur whichever hand is used for

Left eye
Left hand

Right eye
Left hand

Left eye
Left hand

Right eye
Left hand

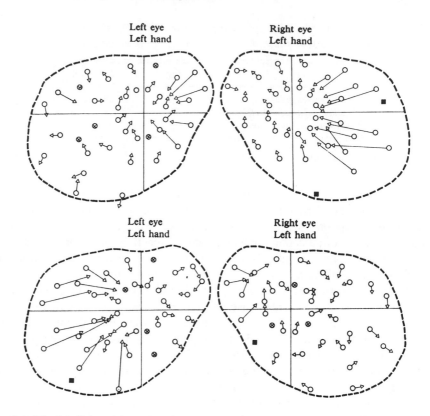

Figure 8.1. The localising ability of patients with a left hemisphere lesion (above) and a right hemisphere lesion (below). A cross indicates accurate performance. It can be seen that the impairment is confined to a half-field. From Ratcliff and Davies-Jones (1972); *Brain 95:*54; by permission of Oxford University Press.

reaching (Cole, Schutta, & Warrington, 1962; Ratcliff & Davies-Jones, 1972) (Figure 8.1).[6] This further supports the idea that the reaching process is not the critical factor. Indeed, it was even observed in one case to be limited to an otherwise intact

---

6. More complex combinations of the visual field and the hand that are affected can occur (see Rondot, de Recondo, & Ribedeau Dumas, 1977); it is presumed that these have a functional origin 'later' in the information-processing system. Visual disorientation has sometimes been treated as related to another syndrome, 'neglect', to be discussed in more detail in chapters 13 and 16. In 'neglect', the patient tends not to respond to stimuli in one part of the world, particularly the left in the case of lesions to the right hemisphere (for discussion, see De Renzi, 1982). The two syndromes – visual disorientation and neglect – were both present in a famous early case of Balint (1909). As Holmes (1918) originally pointed out, patients with visual disorientation can claim to see the object but to be unaware of where it is. This is phenomenologically very different from neglect, where the patient appears to be unaware of the stimulus. Therefore, it seems more plausible that visual disorientation and neglect stem from damage to separate functional systems.

quadrant of the visual field (Ross Russell & Bharucha, 1984). This suggests that the organisation of the damaged function is retinotopic.[7]

Are these impairments in fact distinct? Warrington (1986) investigated this issue for all dimensions other than movement, by considering five patients who had sensory disorders resulting from bilateral occipital lobe lesions. All were assessed quantitatively for their ability to perceive location, colour, and shape; in addition, their acuity was tested. Combining these five patients with Godwin-Austen's (1965) case, every possible pair-wise combination of intact and impaired dimensions is obtained. All four aspects of visual sensation dissociate. For instance, two of the patients, BRA and THR, produced quantitative evidence supporting Holmes's (1918) observations of intact experience of a stimulus that the patient is unable to localise. BRA, for instance, was 20 times worse at visual localisation than two of the other patients. Yet she correctly identified all the primary colours and made only very occasional errors when the full range of hues was tested. A later patient with visual disorientation performed normally on colour identification (Warrington, personal communication).

These findings, of course, fit well with ideas on the parallel modular organisation of the analysis of sensory input familiar from sensory neurophysiology, (e.g. Van Essen, 1979; Zeki, 1980), physiological psychology (e.g. Cowey, 1982), and information-processing psychology (e.g. Treisman, 1986). The dissociation method has therefore suggested the existence of distinct subsystems in an area where, given our knowledge of other fields, it should do so. Moreover, one cannot say that this is just a post hoc discovery. The isolation of the selective deficits of location and colour far predated the corresponding findings in other sciences.

8.3 The Distinction Between Apperceptive and Associative Agnosia

It is hardly surprising that when one moves to higher levels of visual perception, the picture becomes more complex. The perceptions of space, of faces, of objects, of places, of words, and of colours all probably dissociate and so may those of less frequently discussed classes of things, such as buildings (see Hécaen & Albert, 1978; Warrington, 1982b). However, the situation is not completely clear. Take, for instance, prosopagnosia, the inability to identify faces.[8] This is normally accepted as being dissociable from an impairment of colour or object perception (Bodamer, 1947; Hécaen & Albert, 1978). It has been claimed, however, that the dif-

---

7. Visual disorientation has also been considered in the context of the 'syndrome' of simultanagnosia, discussed in chapter 4. The relation between the two syndromes is not clear, especially given the argument presented in chapter 4 that simultanagnosia is not a unitary functional entity! Godwin-Austen (1965) has argued, however, that the two syndromes dissociate, since at a short exposure duration, his patient was as likely to report two letters as one. Unfortunately, his results were not presented in a way that enables this claim to be properly assessed. For a visual function to be retinotopic, it must be spatially organised in a corresponding fashion to the retina.

8. It should be noted that two dissociable types of prosopagnosia probably exist: one concerned with the perception of faces, and the other with their identification.

ferentiation between classes of visual stimuli that contain many similar exemplars may also be impaired in such patients. For instance, a prosopagnosic ornithologist lost the ability to differentiate similar birds (Bornstein, 1963).

In the rest of this chapter, I will concentrate on one area only – the perception of objects. Disorders of object perception are of special importance for three reasons. They have been quite extensively analysed from a cognitive neuropsychology perspective, and are of importance for the discussion of disorders of knowledge representations in chapter 12. In addition, they have had a considerable influence in a somewhat unexpected direction. They were a major stimulus in the development of Marr's (1982) computational theory of visual perception.

In chapter 1, I discussed the distinction drawn by Lissauer (1890) between apperceptive and associative agnosia. According to Lissauer, the construction of a conscious percept from sense data constituted the apperceptive process; the accessing of semantic information required the associative process as well. In both types of disorder, the sensory processes that have just been discussed need to be normal. In the case of the apperceptive agnosic, however, the correct three-dimensional, appropriately oriented conscious percept of an object cannot be constructed. For the associative agnosic, the percept has been constructed but, to use Lissauer's ideas, it is stripped of meaning.

The distinction drawn by Lissauer was put onto a more solid quantitative basis by two studies (De Renzi, Scotti, & Spinnler, 1969; Warrington & Taylor, 1978) that used the methodology of testing a consecutive series of patients with localised cortical lesions restricted to one hemisphere and then grouping them for analysis according to site of lesion. In both studies, it was found that processes that would be thought of as 'apperceptive' are more impaired by posterior right hemisphere lesions, whereas visual 'associative' processes are more affected by posterior left hemisphere lesions.

A number of earlier studies had shown greater deficits in patients with right posterior lesions than left posterior ones on tests of pre-semantic visual processing of objects (e.g. Milner, 1958; De Renzi & Spinnler, 1966; Warrington & James, 1967). Of particular interest, because of its links with the computational approach, is the study of Warrington and Taylor (1973), which was concerned with how patients perceive objects in so-called unconventional views (Figure 8.2). Patients with unilateral lesions were subdivided into three groups per hemisphere: If their lesions involved the frontal lobe, they were classed as anterior; if it was confined to the temporal lobe, they were placed in the temporal group; and the rest were placed in the posterior group. The patients were given 20 pictures of objects taken from an unconventional view and afterwards the same 20 objects from a more conventional direction. On each occasion, they were required to identify the object, either by name or by a description.

With the unconventional-view pictures, each of the three left hemisphere groups made between 1.5 and 1.7 errors out of 20 identifications. The right anterior and the right temporal groups made just a little more. However, the right posterior group made, on average, 4.8 errors, roughly three times as many as the other groups.

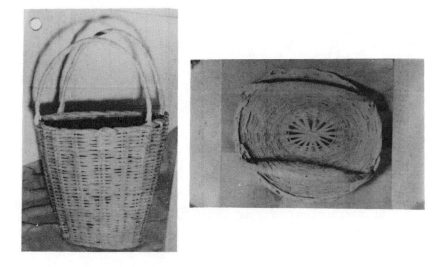

Figure 8.2. An example of one conventional and one un-conventional view used by Warrington and Taylor (1973).

With the conventional view pictures, error scores were very low in all groups, with no significant differences among the lesion groups. Thus the problem on the unconventional-view test cannot arise at the semantic level. On more basic discriminations, including shape discrimination, however, the right posterior group behaved in a similar fashion to the left posterior one (see Taylor & Warrington, 1973). Thus the disorder cannot be explained by a deficit at the visual-sensation level. The errors made by the right posterior group are of interest, for the patients do not necessarily see only a jumble of lines. Instead, they quite often see something incorrect. For instance, a common right posterior response to the unconventional version of Figure 8.2 is a mat.

Specific deficits of aspects of object perception in groups of patients with posterior left hemisphere lesions have been less widely reported. The initial study in which a double dissociation between posterior right hemisphere and posterior left hemisphere perceptual deficits was found was that of De Renzi et al. (1969). They obtained a contrast between performance on the Ghent Overlapping Figures Test (Figure 8.3) and on an object–figure matching test. On the Ghent Overlapping Figures Test, the group with posterior right hemisphere lesions[9] was significantly worse than all other groups. On the object–figure matching test, the patient was required to match each of 10 coloured photographs – one at a time – to each of 10 objects laid out on a desk. The correct match in each case was the same type of

9. Technically, this group was defined by the presence of both a right hemisphere lesion and a left-visual-field defect.

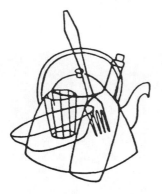

Figure 8.3. An example of an Overlapping Figures Test. The subject must identify all the figures.

object as that shown in the photograph, but was physically very different – say, two physically quite different dolls. The test therefore required that the two be matched conceptually. Two different series of 10 items were used. The left hemisphere group performed significantly worse, making roughly 50% more errors than the right hemisphere group.

Warrington and Taylor (1978), in their study, contrasted performance on a slightly different version of their 1973 unconventional-view test with that on a test somewhat like a simpler version of the matching test used by De Renzi et al. To circumvent naming difficulties, they used a two-alternative forced-choice procedure for both tests. Again, on the unconventional-view test, the right posterior group performed significantly worse than the left posterior group, which, in turn, was not significantly different from the controls.[10] But on a test of matching the *functions* of objects (Figure 8.4), which requires comprehension of the function the object has and contains distractors that are conceptually very similar, both left and right posterior patients were significantly impaired, and there was no sizeable difference between the two posterior groups.

In the control group – patients without cerebral lesions – there was a relation between the scores that individual patients obtained on the two tasks. This is natural because one would expect the two processes critical for the two tests to be in series. If a regression line is obtained from the scores of the control group, then the scores of the right hemisphere group fall squarely on the regression line, indicating that the function-matching score can be predicted from the different view-matching score. The left hemisphere group is different. Their function-matching scores are significantly worse than one would expect, given their reasonable unconventional-view scores (Figure 8.5). This suggests that the deficit on the function-matching task of the left posterior group has a different origin from that of the right posterior group.

On the basis of these two experiments, Warrington and Taylor (1978) developed

10. In this study, the posterior and temporal groups of their earlier study were combined.

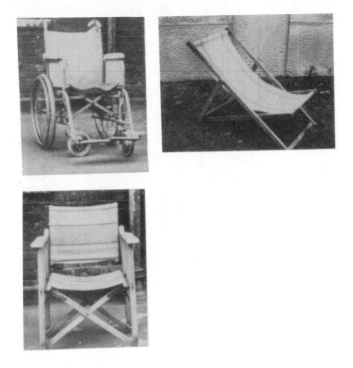

Figure 8.4. The function-matching test of Warrington and Taylor (1978). The subject must match one of the pair of items (above) to the single one (below). Reprinted by permission of Pion.

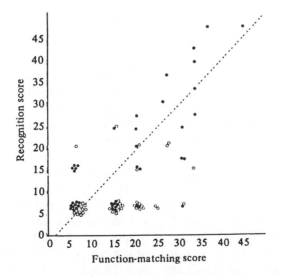

Figure 8.5. The results of the function-matching test study. The open circles represent the left hemisphere patients; the filled circles are the right hemisphere patients; and the dotted line is the regression line obtained from normal controls. Reprinted from Warrington and Taylor (1978) by permission of Pion.

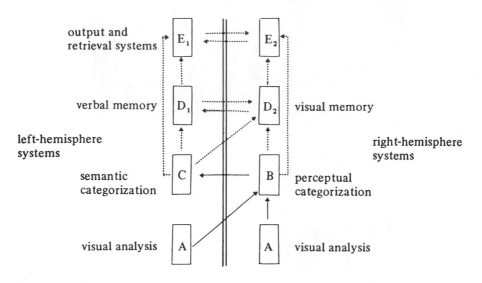

Figure 8.6. Warrington and Taylor's (1978) model of the stages in perceptual processing. Reprinted from Warrington and Taylor (1978) by permission of Pion.

a three-stage theory of object perception (Figure 8.6). Initial analysis of the stimulus is held to be of different sensory characteristics – including shape – in parallel, with both visual fields being separately represented in their corresponding hemispheres. Evidence was discussed earlier that the perception of colour and location is indeed retinotopically organised. Damage at this level that impairs object perception is held to be a 'pseudo-agnosia'. They then followed Lissauer (1890) and argued that there are two postsensory categorical systems in object perception in an analogous fashion to word-form and semantic systems in word recognition, as discussed in chapters 4 to 7. Apperceptive agnosia would arise from an impairment of the first of the subsystems, which they called 'perceptual classification' and held to be localised predominately in the posterior part of the right hemisphere. Associative agnosia would be the consequence of the impairment of the second subsystem, their 'semantic categorisation' one, which would be localised predominantly in the posterior part of the left hemisphere.

One possible difficulty with this explanation is that the left hemisphere impairment might be arising from errors in implicit naming by the left hemisphere group. In the study of De Renzi et al. (1969), this seems to be a major problem. Faced with having to select from an array of 10 objects in the matching task, it would seem natural for the patient to adopt a strategy of naming the presented photograph when scanning the objects. De Renzi et al. pointed out that of their 18 left hemisphere patients who performed worse than any control, 8 were not aphasic on the basis of the Token Test.[11] However, the Token Test is a test of comprehension, not

11. This test was discussed in chapter 3.

naming, so that this is not a solid refutation. In Warrington and Taylor's (1978) study, there was a low but significant correlation (0.43) between a naming score and the function-matching score. However, where only two alternatives are available for the forced choice, it seems less likely that errors in implicit naming are the cause of the left hemisphere function-matching difficulty.

8.4 Converging Proposals from Other Fields

A related conceptual distinction to the one drawn by Warrington and Taylor (1978) on neuropsychological grounds had been suggested within cognitive psychology by Seymour (1973, 1979). He argued that corresponding to a pre-semantic 'logogen', or lexicon unit, for words there is a 'pictogen' unit for pictures or objects. A more surprising connection with the neuropsychological findings on object perception was that made by Marr and Nishihara (1978) in the development of the more central stages of Marr's (1982) computational theory of visual object recognition. On Marr's overall model, recognition of an object depends on information being processed through a series of four stages.

1. In the first stage – the primal sketch – a scene is represented in terms of edges, bars, and blobs that have attributes of orientation, contrast, length, width, and position, and that can also be grouped.
2. Cues to the depth of surfaces, such as stereopsis, surface texture, and contour occlusion, are added in the second stage – the 2½ dimension (2½D) sketch.
3. The third stage is the attaining of a 3D structural description of the object in object-centred space and its classification using a catalogue of stored structural descriptions.
4. In the fourth and final stage, a semantic interpretation is achieved.

The connection between the neuropsychological findings and Marr's theory is not just that a functional separation is made between attaining an appropriate structural description of an object and making a semantic interpretation. The process suggested by Marr and Nishihara for the derivation of the structural description of an object from the 2½D sketch was also stimulated by neuropsychological observations. Marr and Nishihara argued that the first move in obtaining a structural description from the 2½D sketch is the assignment of a principal axis for the represented object.[12] It follows that if the principal axis cannot be directly obtained from the 2½D sketch, additional and more complex processing operations would be required. Marr noted that a characteristic of some of Warrington and Taylor's (1973) unconventional-view stimuli that gave difficulty to right posterior patients was that the principal axis of the object is not represented as such in the photograph (see Figure 8.2). He analysed the 20 unconventional-view stimuli used by Warrington and Taylor and considered that for nearly all the stimuli, it was indeed difficult to obtain the principal axis directly from the 2½D sketch (Warrington, personal communication). He therefore viewed the difficulty of extracting the real principal

---

12. For further arguments for the importance of principal axes, see Hinton (1979).

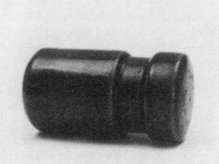

Figure 8.7. An example of the minimal-distinctive-feature condition. Reprinted from Humphreys and Riddoch (1984); *Quarterly Journal of Experimental Psychology* 36A:401; © The Experimental Psychology Society.

axis from the photograph as the source of the errors made by the right posterior patients. This supported his theory of the way in which structural descriptions are obtained from the 2½D sketch.

There seems to be a rather tight correspondence between neuropsychologically derived theory and computational models. It should, though, be noted that the interpretation of Warrington and Taylor's results made by the experimenters themselves and the one made by Marr and Nishihara (1978) are subtly different. Warrington and Taylor (1978) followed Sutherland (1973) in arguing that object perception depends on the accessing of a stored abstract structural description of the object. This is entirely compatible with the third stage of Marr and Nishihara's computational model. However, Warrington (1982b) argued that perceptual classification would fail if either the stored abstract description were damaged or access to it were impaired. It might seem that if the stored description itself were damaged, then the object would not be perceived in its conventional view either. This would, however, not necessarily follow if partial damage to the structural description had occurred, leaving sufficient cues for identification under perfect conditions. For Marr and Nishihara, however, it is only the more complex processing required when the principal axes of the object and its representation do not correspond that needs to be selectively impaired.

The first direct attempt to test Marr and Nishihara's (1978) account of the unconventional-view deficit was made by Humphreys and Riddoch (1984), who contrasted two different ways of rotating an object. In one, it was rotated so that its principal axis was foreshortened, in much the same way as shown in Figure 8.2. In the other, it was rotated so that its primary distinctive feature was less salient, but it was not foreshortened (Figure 8.7). In their experiment, subjects also had two two-alternative forced-choice tests, one for each type of transformation. The authors report findings on five patients: one (HJA) with bilateral parieto-occipital le-

Table 8.2. *Number correct (out of 26) in two three-alternative forced-choice picture–picture matching tasks that stress the perceptual process in different ways*

	Manipulation	
	Foreshortening	Minimising distinctive features
RH 1	12	23
RH 2	11	22
RH 3	11	22
RH 4	11	22
HJA	24	20
Controls	22.6	24

From Humphreys and Riddoch (1984)

sions, and four with right hemisphere lesions. The results are shown in Table 8.2.[13] The four right hemisphere patients performed at a significantly different level on the two tests, but HJA did not.

Humphreys and Riddoch suggested that two different procedures exist for obtaining the structural description of an object (in their terms, achieving 'object constancy'). One is basically the procedure discussed by Marr (1982), in which the structural description of the object is determined relative to its principal axis. This route, they argued, is impaired in the right hemisphere patients. The other, following Sutherland (1968), is held to involve 'processing the local, distinctive features of objects in isolation from volumetric properties of shape' (Humphreys & Riddoch, 1984, pp. 412–413).

The primary argument given for the presence of two routes is the existence of a double dissociation between the right hemisphere patients and HJA. In fact, for reasons to be discussed in chapter 10, to make a secure inference to normal function, it is necessary that a double dissociation be of a cross-over form between patients. HJA did not perform significantly worse than any of the right hemisphere patients on the reduced-distinctive-feature condition.[14] Even if the double dissocia-

13. The control data are, however, suspect because the age of the controls was on average 82, 17 years older than the patients.
14. Even using the criterion that Humphreys and Riddoch (1984) adopted – significant differences between the two conditions in different directions for the two types of patient – their claim does not hold. HJA was initially said to perform at a significantly different level, but in the opposite direction. However, this was based on an analysis that was statistically invalid (see Humphreys & Riddoch, 1985). The authors, somewhat surprisingly, continue to claim that a double dissociation exists, despite the absence of a significant difference between HJA's performance in the two conditions.

tion claimed by Humphreys and Riddoch had been adequately established empirically, their argument for the existence of two routes would still be shaky. As will be shown in chapter 10, a double dissociation where one patient is not normal on either condition – a non-classical dissociation – can occur from lesions that are in series, and this is plausible in the present case.[15]

The interpretation of the performance of the right hemisphere patients as a difficulty in obtaining a structural description when the principal axis is not evident in the picture is not, however, dependent on the adequacy of HJA as a complementary patient. Humphreys and Riddoch found that adding extrinsic depth cues somewhat improved the performance of the right hemisphere patients on the foreshortened condition; moreover, the foreshortened condition itself, on which they were more impaired, was rated as having more salient features than the reduced-distinctive-feature condition. The results are entirely compatible with Marr's (1982) idea that obtaining an appropriate principal axis can be a major hurdle in perception for right posterior patients. However, they also fit the wider Warrington and Taylor (1978) position of an impairment in the perceptual-classification process.

Warrington and Taylor's position can also explain a number of other specific deficits that patients with right posterior lesions show. There are the right posterior deficits obtained by De Renzi et al. (1969) on identifying one of a group of overlapping figures that were discussed in chapter 1. Warrington and James (1967) and Warrington and Taylor (1973) found a deficit in right posterior patients on the Gollin figures test, in which an outline figure has much of its contour deleted, making it difficult to recognise. The finding most related to the unconventional-view one is that of Warrington and Ackroyd (see Warrington, 1982b), who obtained a significant right posterior deficit by changing the lighting conditions in a conventional view. None of these results seems to be interpretable simply in terms of an impairment to processes required when the principal axis is not directly realisable from the 2½D sketch.

For the narrower Marr and Nishihara–type theory to be supported, patients who showed the foreshortening deficit would have to perform normally on these other right posterior tests. To my knowledge, a deficit among right hemisphere perceptual tests specific to foreshortening has not yet been obtained. Moreover, a recent group study by Warrington and James (1986) makes the prospect of finding one seem rather less plausible than more so.

Instead of using photographs, as in their earlier studies, Warrington and James used real objects. The objects were placed in an apparatus that projected three-dimensional shadows of the object to form a single stereoscopic shadow image lying in the space in front of a ground perspex screen. An object was then slowly rotated

---

15. No clinical neuropsychological evidence was presented on HJA. However, since he was poor at naming objects, even in prototypic view, he was held to have an associative agnosia. In fact, he had field defects in both visual fields, suggesting that he had bilateral lesions. In addition, he had major deficits in matching the location of a gap in two circles and in size discrimination. It therefore seems plausible that he also had a pseudo-agnosia, a disorder of the pre-categorical sensory processes, discussed earlier in this chapter, and the authors now appear to hold a related view.

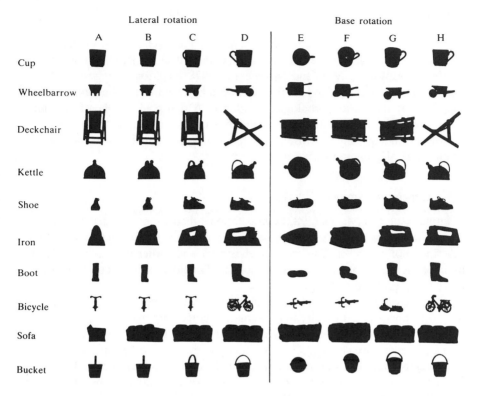

Figure 8.8. The two types of rotation, A–D and E–H, studied by Warrington and James (1986). A and E are the two initial positions; D and H, the two easiest versions used. The stimuli were rotated continuously from the most difficult to the easiest version. B and C, and F and G illustrate intermediate positions. Reprinted from Warrington and James (1986) by permission of Pion.

around its vertical axis or the main horizontal axis through its base so that it became progressively easier to see (Figure 8.8). The task of the subject was to identify the object at the smallest possible angle of rotation. Two groups of subjects were used: patients with right hemisphere lesions and normal controls. As expected, the right hemisphere patients were impaired on the task. If right hemisphere patients have a specific difficulty with foreshortening, then they should do worse if the principal axis is not initially available than if it is. In fact, their median performance summed over objects was 9.7° worse than controls in the first case and 9.8° worse in the second. There was no detectable effect of not having the principal axis directly available initially. Warrington and James argue that the right hemisphere perceptual-classification system contains representations of objects as a hierarchy of sets of distinctive features and presumably some representation of the spatial relations among the parts of the object they represent. On this view, the two procedures claimed by Humphreys and Riddoch (1984) to be separate routes to object recognition become different aspects of the same 'route', and both are impaired by right posterior lesions.

It can therefore be concluded that there is neuropsychological evidence for a subsystem specifically concerned with the attainment of the structural descriptions of objects. However, Marr and Nishihara's (1978) additional suggestion that the extraction of the principal axis of the object is a key subprocess is no longer so well supported by the neuropsychological evidence. A rich potential therefore remains for a relation between computational theories of visual perception and neuropsychological findings, but as close a link has not been obtained as seemed possible when Marr's theorising first became known.

8.5   Associative Agnosia

A further aspect of Marr's (1982) computational theorising on visual perception is that visual semantic processes are separated from the attainment of a structural description of an object. The group studies reviewed earlier provide strong neuropsychological evidence for the validity of this functional separation. They are not, however, entirely convincing.

There have also been single-case studies of associative agnosia, the syndrome that corresponds to a difficulty in the semantic processing that is specifically visual – the understanding of the visually presented object. The study of associative agnosia, however, faces certain difficulties not present in that of apperceptive agnosia. Apperceptive agnosia is fairly common in patients with posterior right hemisphere lesions, at least in a mild form. However, putative associative agnosic patients are rare. Hécaen and Angelergues (1963) considered that only 4 out of a series of 415 patients with localised lesions had this disorder, and in 3 patients, it occurred in conjunction with other severe cognitive impairments. De Renzi and Spinnler (1966) similarly identified only 1 associative agnosic patient in the 124 patients in their series. Second, an associative agnosia can be effectively studied only if the patient has neither a pseudo-agnosia nor an apperceptive agnosia. Good tests for apperceptive agnosia became available only in the 1970s. Earlier methods of establishing that an apperceptive agnosia was not present used procedures such as the ability to copy a drawing; these may well eliminate only the possibility of a pseudo-agnosia and not an impairment in attaining the structural description of an object.[16]

A fair number of case studies of associative visual agnosia exist in the neuropsychological literature. However, in some of these, the interpretation of this aspect of the patient's overall impairments is made difficult by the presence of additional cognitive disorders (e.g. the reports of Taylor & Warrington, 1971; Lhermitte, Chedru, & Chain, 1973; Warrington, 1975; Mack & Boller, 1978; Pillon, Signoret, & Lher-

---

16. Associative agnosia also needs to be distinguished from another syndrome that has not yet been discussed – optic aphasia, which is both complex and not well understood. The distinction between associative agnosia and optic aphasia will not be considered in this chapter. The issues involved are complicated and relate to the structure of semantic systems; the matter will be discussed in chapter 12.

mitte, 1981). In other cases, the presence of extensive bilateral lesions suggests that apperceptive agnosia or pseudo-agnosia problems might well have been present, and psychological testing did not convincingly exclude this possibility (e.g. the reports of Benson, Segarra, & Albert, 1974; Newcombe & Ratcliff, 1974; Davidoff & Wilson, 1985).

Two patients have been reported who have relatively restricted unilateral lesions, which involve primarily the left occipital lobe, and no confounding aphasic or other cognitive disorder. These are DEL of Hécaen, Goldblum, Masure and Ramier (1974) and FRA of McCarthy and Warrington (1986b). Both patients had normal spontaneous speech and performed normally on most quantitative language tests that do not involve visual input, including verbal WAIS IQ (DEL: 107; FRA: 111). Deficits were present on writing (DEL) and on naming from auditory description (some difficulty in FRA, 9/15 only). DEL was also impaired in calculating. Both patients had a hemianopia, but visual sensory functions in their intact fields were satisfactory. Thus FRA had normal acuity and performed in the normal range in distinguishing squares from rectangles, in detecting shapes, and in discriminating dot position. Both patients were given the overlapping figures test (see Figure 8.3), which presents difficulties for patients with apperceptive agnosic problems of right posterior origin. DEL scored well on the Ghent test and correctly differentiated the five objects of one of the more difficult Poppelreuter tests, which use the same principle. FRA was given three of the Poppelreuter tests and, although unable to identify any of the items, easily coloured in all the objects correctly. Without an adequate structural description of each object, it would not seem possible to correctly segregate the areas appropriately in the colouring task. DEL also performed within the normal range (22/24) in pointing out differences between two otherwise identical complex pictures, and FRA performed as well on visually complex scenes as on simple ones. It seems unlikely that either patient had any special difficulty in attaining structural descriptions.

In contrast to their intact language, cognitive, and apperceptive visual perceptual skills, both patients were impaired in all tasks requiring the identification of objects or pictures, DEL fairly mildly so and FRA severely. Thus DEL made 22% errors when naming objects and 46% errors when naming pictures; by contrast, familiar noises were well named. Similarly, FRA made 47% errors when naming pictures, but only 1% when naming the same items from a verbal description. Thus both had an identification difficulty specific to visual presentation. Moreover, this difficulty also appeared when naming was not required. For instance, in a test of saying which of nine items presented one at a time were in the same semantic category as a target stimulus, DEF made 20% errors, while control subjects made at most 4%. FRA had to select which of five items presented at the same time was semantically the same as a visually dissimilar target item, the two having not only the same function, but also the same name; for example, one type of razor had to be matched with another. He made 43% errors, even though there was no time pressure, and in another similar test, 28% errors.

Their problems also occurred in everyday life situations. Thus according to his wife, DEL poured water into a spoon instead of a glass, put ash into a sugar-bowl instead of an ashtray, and asked for a sugar-bowl when it was in front of him. FRA frequently became muddled when performing tasks such as setting the table, which require simple object recognition.[17]

Associative visual agnosia, since it was first described by Lissauer (1890), has been a controversial syndrome that has almost always had its critics as a functional entity. Ironically, the increasing sophistication of neuropsychological investigations of the topic have nearly been matched by the growth in complexity of the alternatives from which the syndrome has had to be pruned away. However, it now seems that impairments to visual semantic processes can be dissociated from those involved in attaining a structural description.

The establishment of three stages of processing in the course of identifying objects, to which both single-case studies and group studies speak, is an important conclusion that fits well with ideas derived from other disciplines. However, it, in turn, gives rise to other questions. As far as the semantic aspect of the processing is concerned, one can ask about the specificity of the semantic-processing subsystems that are involved. Can the deficits be specific to individual modalities? If so, can there be disorders of the visual-to-verbal transmission of information at the semantic system? These complex issues will be discussed in chapter 12.

Overall, neuropsychological studies of visual perception dovetail well with investigations from other disciplines. Together with the alexias, the agraphias, and short-term memory disorders, they provide a solid block of empirical evidence that suggests that the cognitive neuropsychology approach works. That the conclusions derived from cognitive neuropsychology fit those obtained from other fields is reassuring, but it is not conclusive evidence that the methodologies used are valid. In the next three chapters, I will look in more detail at the methods used.

17. Optic aphasic patients do not make such errors in real-life situations. Moreover, their errors, to be discussed in chapter 12, are qualitatively different from those of FRA, at least.

Part III

Inferences from Neuropsychological Findings

9   On Method: A Rejection of Ultra-Cognitive Neuropsychology

9.1   Introduction

Cognitive neuropsychology is too young a field to have an accepted set of methods, let alone a training or apprenticeship procedure common to different centres of research. So those who come to work or study in the field tend to continue using the principles of the disciplines from which they arrived, and these are many and varied! However, two main approaches can be distinguished.

For the majority – those arriving from the neurosciences and some branches of psychology, particularly traditional human experimental psychology and those areas of clinical neuropsychology where test batteries are widely used – cognitive neuropsychology as represented in the earlier chapters in the book must at first seem to be a field fixed in a nineteenth-century mould. There tends to be little equipment, hard neuroscience evidence on patients tends to be ignored, and in its concentration on the individual case it uses methods that seem highly idiosyncratic if not positively dubious. For readers of this persuasion, it will be obvious that one needs to justify theoretical inferences based on single cases and the lack of discussion of hard neuroscience evidence, such as lesion localisation.

There is, however, an increasing minority who have arrived from other parts of cognitive psychology and the speech sciences. For some of them, the emphasis on the individual case, a rejection of the group study, and a lack of concern with the neurological basis of behaviour are becoming almost elements of a creed. There is also a tendency to reject as irrelevant the clinical aspects of a case. This general cluster of positions I will call ultra-cognitive neuropsychology.

With respect to group studies, consider the indirect message in the instructions to authors discussed in the first issue of the journal *Cognitive Neuropsychology* (1984):

In reports of group studies, criteria for selecting and for grouping patients must be detailed and explicit, and related to the particular hypotheses being tested. . . . A set of patients classified as Broca's aphasics can be extremely heterogeneous, and any conclusions reached in such a study may, in fact, be true for only a few of the patients in this group. One way round the problem is to treat each patient as an individual. . . . Another is to provide explicit evidence of homogeneity of the group in a group study. (p. 118)[1]

Standard group studies, the journal is implicitly claiming, do not provide appropriate evidence in cognitive neuropsychology. This view has recently been made much more explicit by Caramazza (1986) in a lengthy analysis of the logic of cognitive neuropsychology. He rejects group studies entirely as having no relevance for understanding normal function.

On the irrelevance of the neurological bases of a patient's behaviour, consider Morton's (1984) view of the use of information on localisation of the lesion for answering questions on function. He says, with little discussion of the evidence, 'It is likely that this approach does not and cannot help to answer the questions being asked by some people who study the brain and behavior' (p. 59) – namely, those concerned with the functional organisation of cognition. He continued simplifying history: 'The diagram makers failed because they, and their critics, could not separate out the different questions' (p. 61).

These two aspects of ultra-cognitive neuropsychology are primarily concerned with rejecting certain types of evidence as not relevant for theorising. They are held for well-articulated reasons and will be separately considered. The third aspect – the neglect of the clinical aspects of a case – has not been defended in print, to my knowledge. It will be considered further in section 9.5.

The position to be presented in this and the next two chapters is that cognitive neuropsychology practice not only must steer very well clear of the Scylla of sole reliance on a standard reductionist approach that relies solely on group studies, but also would do better to avoid the Charybdis of ultra-cognitive neuropsychology. The single case should be the preferred method, but not the only method. One should not anticipate that knowledge of localisation will produce great pay-offs, but it should not be ignored. Implicit in these claims is the assumption that the procedures advocated in chapter 2 and used in chapters 3 to 8 are at present the most appropriate ones for carrying out cognitive neuropsychology. One way of testing this is to see whether the method works in practice. However, such are the variety of approaches competing in the field and of implicit assumptions of those interested in the findings that direct consideration of the methodologies available must also help to distinguish the more from the less useful.

I am therefore going to discuss in more detail than in chapter 2 the methods available for making inferences about normal function from impaired performance. Chapter 10 concerns the practical pitfalls that occur in making inferences to normal function from neuropsychological findings. It is devoted primarily to single-case studies. Chapter 11 deals with what theoretically one can infer as far as the organisation of the normal cognitive system is concerned. Most of the examples needed

1. All sorts of questions may be posed of these instructions. Why should the procedure for grouping patients be related to the hypothesis being tested? Is this not a dangerously circular procedure? And why does one need to provide explicit evidence of homogeneity of a group when, say, a classical dissociation has been established? However, the main relevance of the instruction is, in fact, ideological not methodological.

to give the discussion concrete content are drawn from the previous six chapters. This chapter considers the procedures that were formerly standard. It is addressed primarily to the adherents of ultra-cognitive neuropsychology who reject such approaches.

9.2 Inferences from Group Studies: Are They Ones of Principle?

Within ultra-cognitive neuropsychology, it is held that group studies generally provide misleading or uninterpretable information as far as inference to normal function is concerned. The argument has been presented by Caramazza (1986) in an elegant and rigorous fashion, but it is essentially simple.

Caramazza argues that to explain the impaired behaviour of a single patient in any domain formally, one basic assumption must be made about the way that neurological damage affects cognitive processes, and two types of information are then needed. The simplest basic assumption, which is the one most frequently used – often without its being stated – is that impaired behaviour is explicable in terms of the same model as normal behaviour, except that certain parameters of the model are changed; for instance, in an absolute pure deficit, one and only one parameter would be set to zero, the rest would be unaltered. This is the subtraction assumption, introduced in chapter 4, which is in practice a much more slippery entity than its simple formulation might lead one to expect. The problems in applying it are, though, practical rather than conceptual; they will be discussed in chapter 10.[2] The two types of information needed are, first, the specification of the model of normal function and, second, a characterisation of the effect that the lesion has created – that is, the alterations to be made to the parameters of the normal model.

A key conceptual problem for theoretical inferences in cognitive neuropsychology is that this second type of information – how the parameters are altered as a result of the lesion – cannot in practice be known independently of the patient's behaviour. Does this mean that inferences from cognitive neuropsychology findings have no theoretical power? This is not the case. The results obtained with a particular patient may not be compatible with *any* plausible alterations that can be made to the parameters of a particular model of normal function in a given domain. The patient's behaviour could therefore be incompatible with a theory of normal function. This means that standard procedures for scientific-theory testing can operate for theories of normal function, with neuropsychological results used as data. An example of the application of this type of logic, if not in a formally specified way, was the discussion of the common I/O system theory of speech perception and production (chapter 7).

Can this type of theory-testing inference also be used with 'facts' that are the average performance of groups of patients? Caramazza (1986) shows formally that it cannot. In essence, the argument is that if the group is not functionally homogeneous, then the individual patterns of data of the homogeneous sub-groups, not the

---

2. More complex 'link' assumptions are possible in principle. These would correspond to the strategies specific to particular patients discussed in chapter 10.

average over the whole group, would be relevant for theorising. The average would be at best irrelevant, but also potentially misleading. Moreover, the only way to know that the group is functionally homogeneous is to perform a series of individual-case studies, which reduces the group study to case studies. He therefore claims that the only valid form of neuropsychological data is that from single-case studies.

The argument presented by Caramazza seems simple and powerful. Yet it proves both too much and too little. It proves too much because it can be extended to show that formally, one cannot even reliably refute theories of normal function using group data from normal subjects. Indeed an analogous argument was presented by Audley and Jonckheere (1956) that the use of results averaged across normal subjects should not be used to test mathematical theories of normal function. Suppose, for instance, that on a theory of reaction time for some task in which the difficulty of a discrimination can be measured in terms of some objective variable x, the following relation should hold:

$$RT = a + x^b \ (b \neq 0 \text{ or } 1)$$

where a and b are personal constants that differ across individuals. Then, averaged group data would not in general obey the same function.[3] Audley and Jonckheere conclude that

if we attempt to estimate the parameters for the group as a whole the only practical assumption would seem to be that all display the same stochastic processes with the same parameter values. Such an assumption is so improbable that in general it seems better to estimate the parameters separately for each individual. (p. 91)

The fact that in normal experimental psychology, the average performance of groups is, in general, an unreliable datum for testing the predictions made from complex quantitative models for individual subjects has not prevented the group study from being the standard effective means of testing theories of normal function in human experimental psychology. The critical point is that psychological data frequently consist in the direction of a difference between two conditions or the absence of such a difference. Averaging artefacts are much less likely to be a problem when simple predictions of this type are being assessed than when a precise mathematical function is being tested.

As has been amply illustrated in earlier chapters, neuropsychological data, too, normally consist in relatively crudely specified effects. This, therefore suggests that the formal argument of Caramazza (1986) proves too little. It demonstrates that averaging effect fallacies can in principle occur. It does not show that they do in fact occur for all types of neuropsychological group data.

---

3. Audley and Jonckheere (1956) pointed out that there are many mathematical functions for which the average of a set of functions that differ only in the value given to one or more of the parameters is not a function of the same type. Technically, the function is not closed under addition. For instance, the average of a set of functions $y = ax$, where a varies, is indeed of the form $y = \bar{a}x$, where $\bar{a}$ is a constant. The same does not apply, say, for $y = a^x$. Of course, it would be possible to consider what possible functions the theory would predict could occur for averaged data, but this would normally produce a highly complex and much less powerful empirical test. In any case, the same procedure could be employed for group data in neuropsychology.

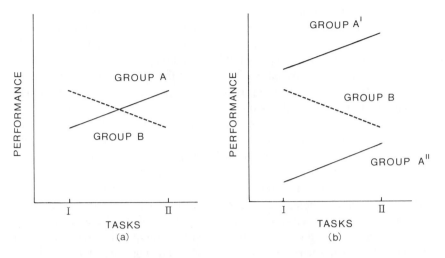

Figure 9.1. An example that illustrates that when a double dissociation exists between groups, one does not necessarily exist between any pair of individuals, selected one from each group. Group A in (a) is split into two subgroups, A' and A," in (b).

How do neuropsychological group studies fare if one restricts concern to the type of basic findings treated as primary in earlier chapters – associations and dissociation between deficits? To argue from the existence of an association between two deficits shown by a group of patients that the overall pattern arises from damage to a common system would be unwarranted. One deficit might well be occurring in entirely different patients in the group from those suffering the other deficit. However, the situation is completely analogous to the inference from associated deficits observed in a single patient. As pointed out in chapter 2, one disorder might arise from damage to an entirely different functional system from the other, within the individual subject. It is the logic of inference from associated deficits that is faulty, not necessarily the use of group data.

If one turns to dissociations, it appears at first that the general thrust of Caramazza's argument is valid. A double dissociation may be observed between the performance of two groups without *any* pair of individuals, one selected from each group, showing the effect! An example is shown in Figure 9.1. Assume that all members of group B perform in exactly the same way, but that group A is composed of two equal subgroups, A' and A", in each of which all members behave identically. Then under the conditions illustrated in Figure 9.1, there will be a double dissociation between the two groups as a whole, but not between any individual members of group A and group B.[4]

4. It might be argued that the individuals illustrated in Figure 9.1(b) show a double dissociation, since group A is better on task II than task I, and group B shows the opposite pattern. It will, however, be argued in chapter 10 that what is critical for a double dissociation is that on task I, group A performs significantly better than group B, and on task II, the significant difference is reversed.

This example is highly artificial, though. It depends on the distribution of group A's scores on *both* tasks being completely bimodally distributed *and* having a much larger variance than the distribution of group B's performance. On any reasonable distribution of group A's scores, there would be some members of groups A and B who would show a double dissociation. This means that in normal circumstances, a double dissociation obtained from group data incorporates a double dissociation between individual members of the two groups.

In fact, there is at least one sort of double dissociation to which this type of artificial counter-example cannot apply – where both dissociations are what I will term *classical,* in which each group performs its better task at a normal level. In the example illustrated in Figure 9.1, at least one dissociation cannot be classical; group A is not normal on either task. The inference to separable processes appears no more suspect, even in principle, for a classical double dissociation based on group data than for one based on two single cases. In practice, classical double dissociations are not frequent with group data! However, the example illustrates the point that inferences from certain patterns of group data are not subject to averaging artefacts. General critiques of the potentially misleading nature of neuropsychological group data will therefore not suffice. The patterns of data that occur in practice need to be specifically discussed; this will be done in chapter 10.

A second point needs to be made about this example. Consider the cross-over interaction illustrated in Figure 9.1(a) but assume that it is derived from two individual patients, each performing significantly better on one task than on the other, but with neither patient performing normally on either task. Then, as we will see in chapter 10, the inference to normal function is subject to a potential individual-difference artefact. This artefact is much less likely to cause trouble when group data are used. Therefore, by 'monster-barring'[5] group data as, in principle, inappropriate for functional inferences while supporting single-case data, Caramazza (1986) has ignored the specificity of patterns of data that can occur and has overemphasised one type of artefact over others. The argument does, though, draw attention to the way that the *principles* of inference from group data are best considered in the light of principles that apply to single-case data. This will be done in chapter 10. However, the main problems with the use of group data lie elsewhere.

9.3   Pragmatic Difficulties in Conducting Group Studies

The real problem with using neuropsychological group studies to make inferences to normal function lies in the variety of practical difficulties for obtaining findings that are both valid and interesting. The difficulties are of three main types. The first is, indeed, related to Caramazza's (1986) principled criticism. It is difficult to avoid

---

5. Lakatos (1963–64) has shown that in the history of mathematics, apparent refutations of theorems were quite often ruled out of consideration at the time they were developed as using examples too bizarre to be taken seriously. The theorems were later found to be invalid! This process of ruling out apparent evidence by fiat, he termed 'monster-barring'.

potentially interesting findings being masked by the noisy nature of group data; it is only too easy to obtain negative results. Then there are the problems of the necessary rigidity of the group study and of selection artefacts.

In practice, it inevitably takes a long time to collect enough patients to form a *series*. The time depends on the problem under study and the patient population that is available to the clinician or research worker. However, one or two years would probably be a normal duration for a specifically planned study.[6] The slowness with which the series is assembled generally means that it is necessary to set very wide criteria for the patients to be included. Very heterogeneous groups with large variance become impossible to avoid. Given the wide variety of cognitive disorders that exist, only a few patients in a group may show a theoretically relevant impairment, so a finding of potential theoretical interest is liable to be lost in the noise of inter-subject heterogeneity.

The length of time it takes to obtain enough patients has another effect on group studies. As the parameters of the investigation have to remain fixed while the study is being carried out, all flexibility is lost, and, of course, all possibly relevant control conditions need to be considered and included in advance, a difficult task that can lead to a costly error. In a small, fast-moving case study, by contrast, a phenomenon can be observed clinically one day, some experiments planned the same evening, and the experiments constructed and carried out in the following few days![7]

The rigidity of the group study has a more dangerous side. There is a strong temptation to attempt to interpret the averaged results of previously obtained clinical test findings for functional purposes, when the single measure studied may be an unsuitable one for theoretical inferences. An example is the attempt to make inferences from the relation between laterality of lesion and the difference score WAIS Verbal IQ–Performance IQ. On the average, patients with left hemisphere lesions have a lower score on the measure than do patients with right hemisphere lesions. McGlone (1977, 1980) extrapolated from this empirical finding to argue from the smaller effects of laterality of lesion on this measure in women than in men that women's brains are less lateralised.[8] Yet a host of processes contribute to the measure, so that to attempt to relate differences to a single underlying cause seems foolhardy (see Walsh, 1978). There are, for example, *male left* hemisphere cases who, for valid functional reasons, show quite the opposite effect from the average patient – large Performance IQ deficits relative to their Verbal IQ. Examples would include some associative agnosic and optic aphasic patients, a syndrome to be discussed in chapter 12 (e.g. ML of Shallice & Saffran, 1986), and

6. Post hoc analyses of the results of patients tested at the time for clinical reasons can even range over 10 to 20 years of testing (e.g. Basso, Capitani, Laiacona, & Luzzatti, 1980; Warrington, James, & Maciejewski, 1986). Such investigations suffer even more from the second of the problems – that of the rigidity of the study.

7. Most single-case studies, especially larger and more theoretical ones, in fact have a considerably slower pace than this. Some can take years.

8. Actually, a very large study, involving over 600 patients, has failed to replicate the effect (Warrington et al., 1986). The result is therefore empirically doubtful, as well as conceptually irrelevant.

some left frontal patients (e.g., these described in Lhermitte, Derouesné, & Signoret, 1972; Derouesné, personal communication, to be considered in chapter 13). In addition, there may well be different strategies by which particular tests, such as Block Design can be carried out. All sorts of confoundings of gender with aetiology and so with syndrome and between gender and strategy are possible.

There is yet a third problem with the use of group studies in neuropsychology. When carrying out a group study, strict criteria should be set for the patients to be included. Yet the clinical and administrative reasons for the particular patients being in the hospital or hospitals where the series is being carried out are many and complex. Also, each patient who is included in the series must be clinically capable of being tested and willing to be so, and it has to be possible to arrange testing to avoid more important claims on the patients' time, such as clinical examinations. The variables under study may interact with any of these practical issues.

The possibility exists that one or more of these stages in determining which patients are included in a study might produce a selection artefact. That this needs to be taken seriously can be shown in a simple way. The age distribution of patients in many group studies is not what one would expect on a priori grounds. Assuming that all patients over 70 years of age are excluded from consideration – which is preferable, given that after that age, mean performance tends to decline much more steeply than before – the mode of the incidence distribution for both vascular disease and tumours lies in the 60s. Some studies give frequency distributions of the age of patients in the study that do show a very rapid rise in numbers from about age 40, with the peak in the 60s decade. One example is the very large series of Basso, Capitani, Laiacona, and Luzzatti (1980); in their study, when patients over 70 are excluded, the mean age of the sample is roughly 53. Yet many studies have a mean age for their patients of 45 or so. The most likely explanation is that the number of patients in the 60s in such studies is much lower than would be expected on grounds of the incidence rate of the disease. The other patients in their 60s have presumably been lost somewhere along the selection process, probably more frequently for women than for men.

Two examples where anomalous results appear to have arisen from the way in which patients were selected for a series are known. There was much discussion in the 1960s about whether the comparison between the effects of left and right hemisphere lesions was confounded by the lesions of patients in the right hemisphere group being on average larger (see, e.g. Arrigoni & De Renzi, 1964; Benton, 1965; De Renzi, Scotti, & Spinnler, 1969). One argument was that patients with left sided lesions are more easily detected at an early stage of a slowly developing disease process than are patients with right sided lesions; the left sided lesions tend to give rise to more obvious symptoms, such as aphasia. A second possibility is that patients with very severe left sided lesions tend to be excluded from an experimental investigation because they do not understand the instructions.

De Renzi (1982) reviewed studies that compared the percentage of patients with left and right hemisphere lesions showing constructional apraxia, a deficit in the execution of tasks where individual elements must be arranged in a given spatial relationship to form a unitary structure, under the guidance of a visual or mental model; an example of such a task would be drawing. De Renzi noted that in seven studies on the topic in the literature, the incidence of constructional apraxia among patients with right hemisphere lesions remained remarkably constant; in all papers, the value lay between 32 and 38%. However, for left hemisphere lesions, the picture was quite different. In the first three studies, carried out in the early 1960s, only 14 to 18% of left hemisphere cases were reported as showing constructional apraxia. In the last three, carried out in the 1970s, the incidence in left hemisphere patients lay between 31 and 37%. The hemisphere difference had disappeared! De Renzi pointed out that some of the conflicting results had been obtained by the same authors using a similar patient population! He therefore concluded that the earlier studies had been subject to a selection artefact.

A second controversy where the explanation of discrepant results is assumed by both sides to lie in a selection artefact is that concerning the effect of gender on the incidence of aphasia. In 1977, McGlone published a dramatic paper that appeared technically to be of high quality. She argued that aphasia is far more frequent in men than in women. In her sample of 52 patients with left hemisphere lesions, 48% of the males were aphasic but only 13% of the women were on formal testing. She also referred to a report that men are greatly over-represented in aphasia rehabilitation clinics (Messerli, Tissot, & Rodriguez, 1976). From her study, she made the major functional claim that language processing is less lateralised in women than in men, with the result that a unilateral lesion is less likely to result in aphasia.

This finding did not fit with the general impression held by clinicians. Moreover, it fairly soon became apparent that it was difficult to replicate. Two studies with a much larger number of patients – one of 850 stroke cases (Brust, Shafer, Richter, & Bruun, 1976), and the other of 390 left hemisphere lesions (Miceli et al., 1981) – found no sex differences in incidence of aphasia. Moreover, Kertesz and Sheppard (1981) quote neurological estimates of the percentage of men among stroke victims as a whole as lying between 55 and 61%, and in three studies much larger than McGlone's, the proportion of aphasics with vascular aetiology who were male was 61% (Basso et al., 1980), 59% (Kertesz & Sheppard, 1981), and 54% (De Renzi, Faglioni, & Ferrari, 1980). This means that given that a patient has had a stroke, the chance of it leading to aphasia does not depend on gender.

McGlone's vascular patients were tested a long time after their stroke, so there would be ample opportunity for biases to influence the selection process.[9] By comparison, in some of the other studies (e.g. Brust et al., 1976), patients were tested on initial admission to hospital normally only hours after the stroke, so that selection artefacts are much less likely. The conclusion drawn by Kertesz and Sheppard (1981) and by De Renzi et al. (1980) is that McGlone's study is subject to a selec-

---

9. There is, in fact, some evidence for a more rapid recovery from aphasia in women than in men. Basso, Capitani, and Moraschini (1982) found a greater recovery in verbal expression in women than in men, but no difference in the rate of recovery in comprehension. By itself, though, this factor is not quantitatively sufficient to explain the discrepancy between McGlone's (1977, 1980) study and the others.

tion artefact. McGlone has retorted that it is their studies that are subject to selection artefacts! Both sides at least agree that selection artefacts are a problem; they differ on whose studies are subject to them.[10]

Even though group studies are subject to these three types of problem, it should not be concluded that anatomically based group studies produce essentially non-replicable results.[11] Many examples of direct or indirect replications exist, such as the perceptual studies discussed in chapter 8 and the later studies on constructional apraxia (see De Renzi, 1982). It is, moreover, noteworthy that the discussion of second-order potential confoundings is a real part of this literature (e.g. De Renzi, 1982).[12]

Group studies require a great outlay in time and effort, but they should not be rejected as a methodology. Reliable results can be obtained. Moreover, the organisation of some functional systems cannot easily be studied by the single-case approach. It may be difficult to generate enough equivalent stimuli to obtain sufficient quantitative data for statistical analysis within the individual case; not all domains have stimuli that are as numerous and well understood as words! There are also situations in which subjects learn. If they do, qualitatively different results over different testing periods or even different trials would occur, so that static performance necessary for quantitative statistical analysis of the individual case would not be obtained.[13] In these situations, the group approach may well be preferable.

10. Another possible confounding factor is that in a series having a mixture of aetiologies, patients with different types of aetiology may be differentially represented in different groups if the groups are defined by location of lesion. This is unlikely to be a problem in the comparison between hemispheres but is potentially one for the comparisons between anterior and posterior groups to be discussed in chapter 13.

11. One unsolved problem in the methodology is what cortical boundaries should be used in allocating patients to groups. A division between right and left hemisphere groups is obviously appropriate. However, it is less clear what within-hemisphere subdivisions should be used. The most frequent course is to use the different lobes, but lesions are more likely than not to involve two or more lobes. An anterior–posterior division is also widely adopted. In either case, one needs to make an additional decision about whether to allocate lesions that cross a boundary to the area that they maximally involve or to both regions, or to exclude such patients. The latter is in principle preferable and was just about possible before CT scans indicated that lesions tend to be larger than they had previously appeared. Now the first of the three alternatives seems in practice preferable, except in special cases, such as the methodology used in the studies of Milner and her collaborators with the Montreal epileptic patients (see, e.g., Milner 1971).

12. The selection procedure involved in studies where the criterion for inclusion in a group depends on the functional deficit seems less secure, as the discussion of amnesia group studies in chapter 2 indicated. For instance, the selection processes involved in studies that contrast fluent and non-fluent aphasias, discussed in chapter 7, are rather obscure, and potential confounding factors are now widely recognised. Thus patients with fluent aphasias tend to be older than those with non-fluent aphasias and to be more frequent with vascular aetiology than with tumours (Obler, Albert, Goodglass, & Benson, 1978; Basso et al., 1980; Miceli et al., 1981). Yet lesion size tends to be larger in non-fluent aphasia (Basso et al., 1980).

13. Examples in which these two types of constraint operate are (1) a topic such as right–left disorientation, which has a vocabulary so limited in number (two items) that it can hardly be studied by statistical means in the individual case (and in which there seem to be pronounced premorbid individual differences), or the study of complex perceptual transformations of real objects where many

9.4 The Relevance of Localisation

Most cognitive neuropsychologists are little concerned about the site of the lesion in the patients they are studying. Why should this be so? Modern techniques, such as CT scans, PET scans, and so on, provide only a rough and erratic measure of the functional lesion. Yet even if a reliable and accurate technique were developed, what would it tell us? In practice, many of the patients whose impairments have been satisfactorily analysed from a functional perspective have proved to have large lesions. How, then, does one determine what the effective lesion site is for the functional syndrome under study?

A common method that has been frequently used is to attempt to establish the effective lesion site by superimposing the positions of the lesions of all patients considered to have a deficit and looking for a 'hot spot', where they all overlap. Yet this procedure is subject to a whole host of problems. Particular diseases can damage different parts of the brain with incidence rates that differ greatly. Thus the application of a simple 'hot-spot' approach is liable to be confounded by statistical artefacts; the more frequently damaged areas will be especially liable to be included in the 'hot spot'. A second problem is that a lesion in area X may be strongly correlated with a lesion in area Y because they have, say, a common blood supply or because X contains a neural or chemical pathway that provides non-specific input necessary for the functioning of Y.

If one puts on one side these practical difficulties, the method will work – even in principle – only if isolable systems are not only functionally modular, but also anatomically so. As Morton (1984) points out, this additional assumption might be unjustified, at least for higher mental functions, so it would be dangerous to place too great a reliance on it unless there is a clear pay-off.[14]

Assume, however, in line with most assumptions on modularity, that the local-isation-of-function principle is at least roughly correct for many processes. A major advantage of localising syndromes for understanding function would exist if 'bridge laws' can be developed to link functional theories with ones on a more microscopic level, the multi-level theory being potentially stronger than any of its component parts. This is a possible means of advance in areas like perception or attention, where animal analogues of the processes being studied clearly occur. Indeed, part of the beauty and power of a theory like Marr's (1982) is that the computational model makes linked predictions on both the psychological and the physiological levels. However, most of the areas in which cognitive neuropsychology has made major advances concern processes that are either unique to humans (e.g. all aspects of language) or much better understood in humans (e.g. semantic memory; see

comparable stimuli may be difficult to obtain (e.g. the stimuli of Warrington & Taylor (1973) or of Warrington & James (1986); see chapter 8); and (2) an inference test, such as the alternation test of Chorover and Cole (1966), on which subjects have to infer that a sequence obeys, say, a single alternation.

14. An example of functional separability in the absence of a gross anatomical difference between the loci of the two processes is given in chapter 11.

chapter 12). For ethical reasons, the experimental neurological manipulations and detailed cellular-level observations of human cortical function within such fields must lag far behind the procedures used in neurophysiological and physiological psychology research on animals. At present, therefore, for most of the issues discussed in the earlier chapters, information about localisation is not, in practice, of great value for understanding function.[15]

There are exceptions to this general position. The most obvious is that group studies of the type in which the groups are determined anatomically clearly require information on lesion location. Even in single-case studies, there are a variety of ways in which anatomical information can be useful. The first is pragmatic and clinical. When working with a patient who exhibits a potentially novel syndrome, one needs to consider many different types of explanation for the patient's behaviour. Neurological information can provide useful cues. As a simple example, if the patient's lesion involves frontal lobe structures, one must be especially sensitive to the possibility of a disorder of control processes; if the corpus callosum is affected, one needs to be particularly careful to check for different syndromes being exhibited by the two hands; if thalamic structures are affected, then disturbances of attention would be a priority, and so on. In other words, localisation information may play an implicit part in the discovery process for new syndromes.

A second example from single-case studies is that in certain syndromes, functional and anatomical arguments are interleaved, as in consideration of the right hemisphere theory of deep dyslexia. Also, the bridge laws can at times be very simple, as whether a syndrome results from a lesion to a system itself or from a disconnection. An obvious example is letter-by-letter reading (chapter 4), which has classically been viewed as resulting from a disconnection (e.g. Dejerine, 1892; Benson & Geschwind, 1969), but on another theoretical position, it arises from damage to a subsystem – the word-form system (Warrington & Shallice, 1980). If the word-form system was assumed to be *entirely* within the left hemisphere and the lesion was anatomically completely restricted to fibre tracts, this would support, *for that patient,* an explanation in terms of a transmission deficit at the functional level. Such a patient has indeed been observed (Saffran, personal communication).[16]

To reject anatomical considerations as irrelevant, in principle, for functional theorising is therefore as misguided as to reject group studies as a method. Despite coming to this conclusion on the level of principle, in one major way, Morton's (1984) warning related to the fate of the diagram-makers is valid. To hope for an advance in theories of the functional organisation of cognition by paying special attention to issues of localisation is not, at present, a promising strategy.

9.5   Conclusion

In the last two sections, I have argued that the use of group studies is not likely to lead to rapid theoretical advance and that, in general, information about the local-

15. These arguments are a development of those given in Caplan (1981).
16. Another example concerning episodic memory will be given in chapter 15.

isation of lesions is not vital for cognitive neuropsychology. However, this is not to argue that group studies and information on lesion localisation should be excluded from cognitive neuropsychology. The rather negative assessment made of group studies and localisation information is not one of principle, but a pragmatic one specific to the methods available at present. With, say, advances in neurological measurement techniques, the situation might very well change. The existence of effective non-invasive techniques for studying localisation of function in the normal brain during task performance would undoubtedly offer many opportunities for links with cognitive neuropsychology, and their development seems increasingly likely. Historically, it may prove that cognitive neuropsychology will be an almost entirely psychological field for only a limited period of time.

The adoption of the ultra-cognitive neuropsychology approach may, then, narrow the empirical armoury of the investigation. This is not, however, its principal danger. The elements of the approach do not occur together for any logical reason. They have, instead, a common social origin. Modern cognitive neuropsychology is a much more purely academic pursuit than was the type of clinical neuropsychology that preceded it. The neurological and general clinical aspects of a patient's impairment are frequently not part of the day-to-day reality of the work situation of cognitive neuropsychologists. It is a standard part of the clinician's assessment of a patient to compare the patient's behaviour with that of controls and of patients who may have similar lesions. The undertaking of group studies to establish norms and the obtaining of anatomical correlates are part of the clinician's routine practice. The daily use of this sort of information is foreign to ultra-cognitive neuropsychology, and this is a major problem.

This tendency to be relatively insensitive to the general clinical aspects of a patient's impairment is evident in the way that standard quantitative clinical baseline information on single-case study patients is not given by many cognitive neuropsychology authors. This has much more serious consequences than the ignoring of group studies and of localisation information. The single-case method is a tightrope. It is easy to select a patient with a mixed syndrome – a 'multi-component' disorder – and to generalise from some particular quirk in the patient's behaviour, some consequence of the interaction of multiple deficits, to some invalid abstract conclusion.[17] The possibility of making such an error is much reduced if good clinical neuropsychological and neurological information exists on the patient; potential anomalies in the misleading analysis are then much easier for the reader to observe.

The most negative possible scenario for cognitive neuropsychology would be for an anti-clinical anti-reductionist, ultra-cognitive variant to lead to the publication of a rash of studies that seem technically highly sophisticated but are made at best irrelevant and at worst positively misleading by being subject to clinical errors. Such errors would be especially difficult to spot for two reasons. The information

---

17. For instance, if one draws inferences from an agnosia without giving information on high-level visual sensory processing or from an acquired dyslexia providing no results on the patient's aphasic difficulties.

that would enable critics to appreciate the error would not be available. In addition, the increasing technical sophistication of papers written by those trained as research cognitive psychologists could greatly reduce the clinical readership, who would be more liable to spot a hidden clinical error. If this were to happen, the use of case studies – good as well as bad – might fall into disrepute. Thus the practice of the case study requires detailed attention. It is the topic of the next chapter.

10   On Method: Single-Case Studies

10.1   Introduction

In chapter 9, it was shown that the use of neuropsychological group studies is not likely to lead to rapid advance in our understanding of normal function. Earlier, it was argued that, by contrast, the single-case study approach is an effective source of evidence. The argument was, however, a pragmatic one. The method leads to conclusions that are internally consistent and that mirror those arrived at by other means. Yet the theoretical structures used to interpret the different types of evidence may, as Rosenthal (1984) has pointed out, seem satisfactory as much for the ease and simplicity with which we can use them as for their empirical adequacy in modelling reality. If one examines the theoretical inferences made from single-case studies in earlier chapters, it becomes clear that they are delicately balanced on a set of implicit supporting assumptions.[1] The inference procedures therefore need to be examined directly to assess whether they can bear the theoretical weight placed on them. In fact, those who have adopted the single-case approach have only rarely attempted to justify their leap from findings on a single patient to a general conclusion.

The most rigorous treatment of the inference procedure is that of Caramazza (1986). He argues for a four-component explanation of neuropsychological findings:

1. A hypothesis (plus subsidiary hypotheses, initial conditions, and so on) of how the task is carried out by a normal subject (essentially his 'M', for model).
2. A hypothesis about how this normal model is modified in this particular case by brain damage (his 'L', for locus of damage).
3. An assumption that behaviour *directly* reflects the operation of M subject to L — the transparency assumption (also known as the subtraction assumption).[2]
4. The assumption that all cognitive systems are basically identical — the principle of universality.

From this four-component position on how to account for neurological data in terms of models of normal function, Caramazza draws a number of conclusions

---

1. For discussions see Kinsbourne (1971), Shallice (1979b), Badecker and Caramazza (1985), Caramazza (1986), and Sartori (1988).
2. Systematic discussion of this assumption derives from Klein (1977) (see also Caplan, 1981).

about the way such data should be used to test theories of normal function. He argues that:

1. Each case should be treated as an independent test of theory; generalisation should not be made over patients pre-theoretically.
2. The use of an association among symptoms as a theoretically relevant result has been unduly maligned. What is critical is having a sufficiently detailed model of the cognitive system to be able to explain the patterns of associations and dissociations occurring over patients in a domain.
3. A double dissociation observed in a second patient has no greater inferential importance than any other type of theoretically relevant observation.
4. Group studies do not provide a valid data-base for generalising to normal function.
5. The direct replication of a finding is impossible in neuropsychology.

I consider that for what Caramazza was trying to do – provide a solid base for inferences from neuropsychological findings to theories of normal functioning – his overall approach was innovative and appropriate. In my view, though, his specific conclusions are a dubious guide to neuropsychological practice.

Part of the problem lies in the way he treats his assumptions as givens, which are not assessed. More critically, inferences from neuropsychological findings are subject to a host of potential artefacts. His argument stresses certain dangers (e.g. averaging artefacts) but ignores others, either by hiding them as unquestioned assumptions (e.g. individual differences) or by employing a limited set of basic assumptions that does not allow him to deal with them fruitfully (e.g. differences in task difficulty).

Overall, he is concerned principally with the logic of theory testing – that is, selecting among well-articulated theories by using existing observations on a set of extensively studied patients. However, what is at least as critical for neuropsychology is how to select patients and make observations on patients to produce the best chance of developing valid theories and avoiding invalid ones. Caramazza's approach offers no guidance in this respect.

In order to make the methodology adopted in chapters 3 to 8 more rigorous, it is necessary to employ a more complex set of initial assumptions than Caramazza used. The bulk of this chapter will be concerned with the plausibility of the assumptions and the conditions under which they are likely to be satisfied. Throughout, the issue being considered is the same as that tackled by Caramazza: what can one infer about normal function from the particular patterns of performance shown by individual patients? It will, however, be assumed in this chapter that the normal system under consideration is modular. In chapter 11, the question of whether non-modular systems are compatible with neuropsychological findings will be addressed. The assumptions themselves fall into three groups.

The type of models to be considered

1. The cognitive system being investigated contains a large set of isolable processing subsystems.
2. This modularity operates on a number of levels. As far as neuropsychology is

concerned, however, there is a limit to the fineness of the grain of the modularity.[3]

3. Following Marr (1982), isolable processing subsystems may be viewed as having functions carried out by algorithms implemented by particular mechanisms.

From the model to performance

4. Cognitive systems are qualitatively similar across individuals for tasks that are routinely performed in a culture.
5. Task performance requires the use of a 'procedure' – a temporary activating or inhibiting of sets of inter-subsystem transmission routes.[4]
6. Tasks may at times be carried out by more than one procedure – that is, more than one combination of subsystems. However, if the procedure for carrying out each task is specified, the *overall pattern of performance* – namely, the gross pattern of associations and dissociations shown by the patient – depends on the *amount of resource* available in each subsystem required.

The effect of lesions

7. Lesions vary greatly in the modules they affect, and in any particular case, the identity and the number of subsystems that are impaired is not ascertainable independently of the behaviour of the patient.
8. The effect of a lesion on task performance is equivalent to
   (a) a pattern of quantitative loss of resources across the normal set of subsystems, *with*
   (b) a procedure determinable by the investigation; possibilities would be the procedure that normal subjects use or the one that optimises performance, given the impairment, by making use of intact subsystems in an appropriate fashion.
9. Individual differences among normal subjects in the amount of resource available in the relevant subsystems is relatively small by comparison with the destruction in resource that neurological disease can produce.

The assumptions serve different functions in the overall argument. A first group – assumptions 1, 3, 5, and 6 – are the core of what is required to show that individual models can produce predictions about the conditions under which a certain overall pattern of performance will be observed across tasks. Assumption 8 allows predictions to be made about the effects of lesions. Assumptions 4 and 9 are required for model testing to be in principle based on the results of individual subjects. Assumptions 2 and 7 allow this approach to be possible for all types of isolable subsystem, down to a certain grain of modularity.

In general, the assumptions are self-explanatory. The exception is assumption 6,

3. In some cases, this may be a conceptual limit. For instance, a system that is macroscopically modular may operate by mass action at a somewhat more microscopic level (see, e.g., Allport, 1985). Alternatively, the limit may be set by neurological factors. If the physical size of lower level subsystems is smaller than those of higher level ones, then the physical grain of lesion boundaries may not be sufficiently sharp to allow the isolation of subsystems of below a certain level in the rough hierarchy of modular organisation. The physical distance in which effective presence of function switches to relative absence of function may therefore determine the potential functional discriminability of the approach.

4. This is a simplification of the relation used in later chapters between procedures and modules. The issue is discussed in chapter 13.

which introduces two concepts: the *overall pattern of performance* and *amount of resource*. The presupposition is that the effectiveness of the operation of each sub-system can, to a first approximation, be measured by a single variable – the re-source. This means that each procedure requiring a subsystem makes qualitatively equivalent demands on its resources, so that if the subsystem functions in an im-paired fashion for one task, it does so for all those that require its resources to the same degree. It presupposes that the demands that different tasks make on the sub-system can be ordered on a continuum.

It would not be reasonable to assume that the effects of different types of damage to a subsystem can be placed on a continuum for the detailed aspects of its behav-iour, such as its speed of operation or the proportion of different types of error made. However, the grosser the measure of the subsystem's behaviour, the more adequate the assumption is likely to be. The assumption is therefore restricted to the effect of whether or not damage to a subsystem produces impaired performance on the tasks that require it.[5]

It would appear logical to discuss the validity of the assumptions before consid-ering their implications for methodology. However, whether the assumptions are valid depends in part on the approach taken by the investigator and on empirical issues. Thus a major part of the methodological suggestions to be made concern how to improve the likelihood of the assumptions being valid. Such a discussion is more concrete if the implications of the assumptions are assessed first.[6] This is carried out in the next two sections. After this, individual critical assumptions are considered.

10.2   Neuropsychological Evidence and Theory Development

An empirical finding in science may be important because it confirms in a quanti-tatively precise fashion specific predictions of the theory – corroboration. The find-ing may also be of value because it focuses attention on a theory previously con-sidered implausible or even one not previously conceived – discovery. By contrast, the finding may be useful because it disconfirms some established theory without necessarily favouring any other alternative – falsification. The different types of finding that occur within neuropsychology can be considered in the light of these three functions of scientific data.

In chapter 2, it was argued that neuropsychological data are not likely to fulfil the first of these functions, that of corroborating precise quantitative predictions. This is well borne out by the empirical evidence considered in chapters 3 to 8. Only twice have fairly precise quantitative data been used, when arguments for function-ally related associated deficits were given in chapter 6. They involved a special

---

5. A type of model in which this does not hold will be discussed in chapter 11.
6. The purpose of the next section is to present more formal arguments for the theoretical importance of the dissociation by comparison with the other forms that neuropsychological data can take. The argument is more abstract than that in much of the book, and if its conclusions are accepted, the section may be skipped.

case, to be discussed later, and were not concerned with precise corroboration of theoretical predictions. Neuropsychological evidence, then, seems unlikely to fulfil the first of the three functions of scientific evidence at all frequently.

How does neuropsychological evidence fare with respect to the two remaining inferential functions of scientific results? First, under what conditions can the over-all performance of a patient most effectively guide one towards a theory that is not currently accepted? How, in other words, can one maximise the efficacy of the case-study approach as a heuristic procedure for theory development? Second, how can this type of evidence be used to falsify invalid theories? For both issues, I will first consider the overall pattern of performance of a patient across a variety of tasks. For the present, I will consider only tasks that involve a single flow of information through the system – a single procedure; by analogy with pure cases, they can be called 'pure tasks' (Sartori, 1988). Moreover, to avoid the complexities required by assumption 6, I will initially assume that all tasks 'stress' the individual subcomponents they require in an all-or-none manner.[7] Impairment of a subcomponent therefore means damage sufficient to lead to impaired task performance on all tasks that require it.

It turns out that these two different scientific goals are best achieved by similar means. The most basic point is that patients who exhibit a set of dissociations are especially important. This may seem obvious, but it needs emphasising because there have recently been influential critiques of the dissociation–fractionation approach. Thus one of Caramazza's (1986) conclusions was that there is no essential distinction between the inferential power of associations and dissociations. Ellis (1987), in a discussion of the methodology of cognitive neuropsychology, did not even mention dissociations at all; in addition, he attacked the syndrome–pure case approach, to which they can be linked.

As far as the theory-development function is concerned, it has frequently been assumed since Lichtheim's (1885) classic paper that pure cases are critical. On the present approach, the concept of a pure case or a single-component syndrome can be obtained from assumptions 1 and 6; it corresponds to the effect of damage to only a single subsystem. Nearly all the theories of normal function that have their origin in neuropsychological findings have been based on the assumption that the syndrome that led to the theory was indeed a single-component one. This applies as much to theories rejected in earlier chapters as it does to those accepted. Thus to give examples from chapter 5, it applies to the theory of the inherent instability of the semantic system or the idea that reading aloud an abstract word requires the use of the phonological route as much as to the claim that non-semantic morphemic spelling-to-sound correspondences exist. The argument against the first two ex-amples hinged directly on the patients' having additional deficits that were relevant to the theoretical issue.

Ellis (1987) has made an important objection to the aim of studying patients who have pure syndromes. He argued that if it is adopted, 'the cognitive neuropsychol-

---

7. Whether these assumptions can be relaxed is considered in later sections of the chapter.

ogist will pass over 999 patients to find the one thousandth who comes close to being a pure case of ''word meaning deafness'' or whatever' (p. 402). He also held that 'we would be deluding ourselves if we thought that any *actual* set of modules we were to propose today might bear anything more than a passing resemblance to the ultimate ''true'' set (assuming they are discoverable)' (p. 401).

For the theory-discovery function of neuropsychological evidence, these objections appear to pose a major problem. There are two means of responding. The first is based on the way that the concept of a pure case – like that of an 'ideal gas' in physics – is useful, even if it is not realised in any real patient. Any dissociation observed in a multi-component syndrome also occurs in a pure syndrome. Consider, for the present, a prototypic dissociation in which normal performance is obtained on one task (I) and grossly impaired performance on another task (II) of roughly comparable difficulty. Then the result follows very simply. Given the assumption of all-or-none operation of subcomponents, the impaired performance on task II entails that at least one subcomponent necessary for performance of the task is damaged. The dissociation can be produced by damage to any one of these subcomponents alone, since it cannot be involved in task I, given the satisfactory performance on that task. Therefore, in a dissociation, even when observed in a mixed syndrome, both the intact performance and the impaired performance will 'coexist' in at least one pure syndrome. An analogous argument applies to the situation that is more important in practice – namely, a set of dissociations, or a group of tasks in which only one is impaired.

The argument does not apply for an observed association. If the impairment on task I arises from damage to subsystems that are not involved in task II, then the association of deficits on the two tasks will be observed only in the mixed syndrome; it does not occur in any pure syndrome. Therefore, sets of dissociations are heuristically important. They are safer than associated deficits in that they necessarily mimic what happens in a pure syndrome. Moreover, they occur reasonably frequently in neuropsychological practice. So they make the pure syndrome approach a viable one.

The second response to Ellis's (1987) criticisms relates to his fear that 'recognised syndromes will inevitably be prone to multiply and change at an alarming rate' (p. 401). If we are to be alarmed at this prospect, presumably the set of syndromes that are multiplying and changing are doing so in a chaotic fashion, and so they do not provide any solid leads to the organization of the underlying structure. Change could, however, be progressive if a procedure for determining the relative purity of a syndrome existed independently of the specific explanatory theories available. Does such a procedure exist?

Fractionation, of which examples were given in earlier chapters, has been considered to be a procedure that enables purer syndromes to be obtained (e.g. Shallice, 1979b). Fractionation occurs when two patients show the same set of impairments, except that one shows intact performance on a task or tasks where the other is impaired; the *more* selective disorder is chosen over the less selective one as a

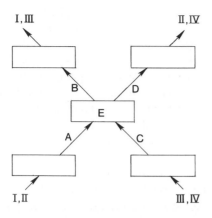

Figure 10.1. An example that illustrates that fractionation does not necessarily result in purer syndromes. *A,B,C,* and *D* are connections; *E,* is a subsystem. I to IV correspond to the routes used by pure tasks.

candidate single-component syndrome. Does continual application of this procedure lead to the set of theoretically relevant syndromes becoming more and more refined?

Unfortunately, the process of fractionation applied as suggested does refine the data-base, but at the cost of eliminating potential pure syndromes. As pointed out by Sartori (1988), a syndrome that fractionates into more selective ones may itself be a single-component one. Thus in the simple example model (Figure 10.1), the syndrome corresponding to an impairment to subsystem E – a single-component one – has the same properties as an impairment to a combination of A and C and to a combination of B and D. Therefore, a single-component syndrome fractionates into two combinations of other single-component ones. This is hardly surprising, since the syndromes into which the initial one fractionates represent deficits to the two inputs and the two outputs of subsystem E.[8]

At least, it might be argued, can one not conclude that if a syndrome fractionates, and if the 'parent' syndrome is a pure one, its more selective progeny will be pure? This claim does not hold either! Thus in the model example, the mixed syndrome corresponding to impairments to connections A and D is more selective than the pure syndrome corresponding to an impairment to subsystem E. Performance of one task (III) is intact in the former case but not in the latter. There seems to be no way, other than through a satisfactory model of the whole system, to know that the 'parent' syndrome is a single-component one, but that a syndrome that combines, say, impairments to connections A and D is mixed.

It is not, however, necessary for fractionation to be a logically certain procedure

8. A more concrete example is that a memory-retrieval difficulty will produce a more selective impairment than the storage deficit that corresponds to it; both would, however, be equally pure.

for obtaining purer syndromes in every case in which it is applied for it to be a useful heuristic for generally obtaining theoretically more appropriate cases. For any given system, as the number of subsystems damaged increases, the average number of tasks that cannot be satisfactorily carried out will also increase. Thus the adoption of a fractionation approach – selecting selective impairments for study – will lead on the whole to the analysing of purer and therefore more heuristically valuable syndromes. As a heuristic procedure, though, it should not be rigidly applied; the possibility needs to be considered that the more general parent and more selective progeny syndromes arise from a situation similar to that of damage to subsystems E and A in Figure 10.1.

Thus the approach of studying the most selective disorders – fractionation – is justifiable as far as theory discovery is concerned. It gives one the best chance of actually observing single-component disorders. In addition, it necessarily involves the establishment of a set of dissociations, which has inferential power even if the syndrome is, in fact, a mixed one. Thus the 'pure case'–dissociation–fractionation approach seems appropriate as far as theory discovery is concerned.

This section has been concerned with only the overall pattern of performance. What can be said about other qualitative aspects of behaviour and, in particular, the *nature* of the errors produced by patients? At times in the empirical chapters, such data have provided important evidence. Consider, for instance, the role of regularisation errors, discussed in chapter 4 and 5, which provide valuable evidence for a theory of reading by multiple routes, one of which uses spelling-to-sound correspondences. This shows that the nature of errors can be heuristically valuable. In this case, the error occurs through the normal operation of subsystems in parallel with the one that is damaged. Many types of error, though, would seem to result, at least in part, from the output of a damaged subsystem itself. The literal paraphasias that occur in reproduction conduction aphasia would be one example (chapter 3). To explain why such errors occur, one needs a detailed understanding of both how the impaired subsystem should operate and how it has been impaired. Thus this type of error would probably not reflect in any simple fashion the nature of the underlying architecture. This means that not all errors are likely to be of heuristic value.

10.3   Neuropsychological Evidence and Theory Falsification

Sets of dissociations are even more critical where model falsification is concerned. Any multi-component model that is held to account for normal behaviour can explain the simple fact of impaired behaviour across any group of tasks – if it is considered in isolation – and generally it can do so in a variety of ways. If all subsystems were damaged, this behaviour would be observed. However, for pairs of tasks requiring certain combinations of subsystems, impaired performance on one task is incompatible with intact performance on the other. The simplest such situation is when the two tasks are held, on the model, to depend critically on one set of subsystems. For instance, the dissociation in amnesia between the spared

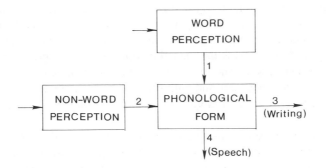

Figure 10.2. An idealised single-route model of writing.

recency in free recall and impaired performance on the earlier part of the serial position curve (see Figure 3.3) is incompatible with the two parts of the curve being derived from one set of component processes. More complex cases also occur when one task requires a subset of the subsystems required by the other.[9]

Model falsification can, of course, depend on the results on more than two tasks, and it normally does. Granted that each task is pure, then each subsystem and interconnection used to perform each task must be intact for normal performance to be obtained. A model is falsified if and only if impaired performance occurs on a task that utilises subsystems and interconnections that are employed in other tasks on which performance is intact. For instance, if performance is normal on tasks I, II, and III – which use subsystems A, B, and C; A, D, E, and F; and G and H, respectively – then any task that uses any combination of subsystems A to H must be performed normally if the model is correct.[10] As an example, consider the simplified logic of the inference from phonological agraphia against a single-route model in which spelling necessarily utilises the phonological form of the stimulus (Figure 10.2). Three tasks are involved. Writing words, which uses routes 1 and 3, and repeating non-words, which involves routes 2 and 4, are both performed well. Thus all routes must be intact. Writing non-words, which requires routes 2 and 3, should also be performed well, but it is grossly impaired. This does not fit the model.

The conclusions obtained in this section depend on the assumption that each task can be satisfactorily carried out by only a single procedure. If this assumption is

9. For example, consider two tasks that can each be performed by a single procedure. If task I requires the operation of both subsystems A and B, then impaired performance necessitates that subsystem A or subsystem B or the connection between them be damaged. Thus task II, which requires all the subsystems – A, B, and C – and the connections AB and BC, should not be performable. These inferences will be modified when varying resource demands of tasks are considered in section 10.5.

10. For simplicity, interconnections among subsystems are ignored in notation statements in the rest of this section. They are entirely equivalent as far as the logic of the inference is concerned. Again, difficulty differences among tasks are ignored. In this example, it is dealt with by double dissociation (see chapter 6 and this chapter section 5).

relaxed, the conclusions change radically. To illustrate this, consider the situation in which each of a group of tasks can be performed by a set of alternative procedures, with each procedure utilising at most one subsystem – which may, however, differ among the procedures. This is the logical complement of the previous case, and here falsification depends on one intact task and a set of impaired ones.[11] In cases where both multiple procedures and multiple subsystems are relevant, falsification clearly requires a complex combination of this type of inference and that discussed above.[12]

The example just considered shows that if falsification is treated purely from a logical perspective, then associated deficits are as relevant as dissociations. Thus Caramazza (1986) is logically correct in considering associations as relevant for falsifying models as dissociations.[13] However, in practice, his position is methodologically dangerous because situations in which there are more subsystems per procedure than there are procedures per task are much the more important in neuropsychology. Any cognitive task necessarily requires the use of multiple subsystems. If in addition, the tasks involved can be carried out by various procedures, any falsification inference would become rococo in its complexity and impossible in practice. There would also be many false leads to negate the heuristic value of any observations of impaired behaviour. Thus pure tasks are critical, as are pure patients. In these situations, dissociations and sets of dissociations are more important than associated deficits.

Parallel arguments can therefore be given with respect to the heuristic and falsification roles played by scientific data. For both types of application, patients exhibiting dissociations and sets of dissociations are more valuable than those exhibiting associations. If one contrasts, say, the history of our understanding of the central dyslexias (chapters 4 and 5) and of the central dysgraphias (chapter 6), the study of the latter has been much more straightforward. In my view, this is because the relatively pure central dysgraphic patients studied initially were selected using

11. For instance, if tasks I, II, and III are impaired *and* task I can be performed correctly if any of subsystems A *or* B *or* C is operating correctly; task II, if any of A *or* D *or* E *or* F is; task III, if G *or* H is, then task IV, which involves the utilising of B *or* D *or* H, must be impaired if the model is valid. Thus normal performance of task IV falsifies the model. In this case, falsification operates more through selective preservation than through selective impairment.

12. That the logic of neuropsychological inference differs for subsystems operating in parallel rather than in series was first discussed, although in a different fashion, by Sartori (1988). He argued that a double dissociation necessarily involves damage to two systems in parallel. This is indeed necessarily true if all tasks other than the two key ones are intact and subsystems are held to operate in all-or-none fashion. However, it is not generally true. Thus damage to connections A and D in the example illustrated in Figure 10.1 – which are not in parallel – produces a double dissociation between tasks I and IV.

13. Caramazza's (1986) argument is based on the way that a pure syndrome can involve associated deficits. The difference between Caramazza's approach and the present one stems from his being concerned with the logical issue of how the domain of alternative models and the domain of data can be related in neuropsychology, each being treated as independently achieved. The present approach is concerned primarily with the more concrete issue of the type of patients best studied at an early stage of theory development.

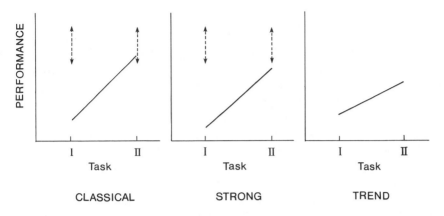

Figure 10.3. Three types of dissociation. The dotted lines indicate the normal range.

sets of dissociations. For the central dyslexias, mixed cases formed the conceptual mould within which later patients were identified.

What can be inferred from aspects of a patient's behaviour other than the overall pattern of performance? It was argued in section 10.2 that the nature of the errors made will at times be heuristically valuable.[14] Other types of information that one can obtain about a patient's performance – the combination of tasks over which performance is impaired, the rough speed of performance, the actual rate of error production, the consistency of performance – may also be useful, but only as a secondary source of evidence that builds on the original dissociations and only when the evidence confronts well-developed theories. As discussed in chapter 2, there are generally too many unknown parameters involved in giving accounts of the detailed aspects of a patient's behaviour.

This conclusion would seem to form a natural end to the chapter. However, the conclusions about the inferential role of dissociations are based on a set of assumptions. One needs to ask about the conditions under which the assumptions are valid. The argument then reverts much more to issues of concrete neuropsychological methodology. Particular assumptions will be considered in turn, with special attention paid to assumptions 3, 4, 6, 8, and 9, although tackled in different order. The most basic assumption, 1, will be treated in chapter 11.

Before considering the assumptions, it is useful to differentiate three types of dissociation according to the levels at which task I and task II are performed (Figure 10.3). In a *classical dissociation*, task II is performed at the same level as before

14. It is unclear whether the existence of an error type can falsify a model. For a model to be falsified by some neuropsychological finding, one would need to know that there are no possible lesions to the model that could produce the observed effects. It is not apparent how a theory of normal function, particularly one at the information-processing level, could specify what errors would be produced for all possible types of lesion.

the onset of the illness, as far as it is possible to tell by the use of appropriate control tests; at the very least, it is performed in the normal range. Performance on task I is, however, much inferior and well below the normal range. In the double disso-ciation between STM patients and amnesics on span and LTM tasks both dissocia-tions are of this type (chapter 3). In a *strong dissociation,* neither task is performed at normal level, but task I is performed very much better than task II. The semantic dyslexic reading of regular and irregular words is of this type (chapters 4 and 5). In relatively pure patients, regular words will be read much better than irregular ones – say, 85% compared with 40% (averaged results of patient HTR; see chapter 5) – but regular-word reading is still not at normal level, which would be close to 100%. If the measure of performance on the two tasks is in terms of the scaled score of normal subjects, then a special form of strong dissociation exists, which I will call a *robust dissociation;* it is less susceptible to resource and individual-differences artefacts. The final form is the *trend dissociation,* in which task I is performed significantly better than task II, but the levels of performance are not qualitatively dissimilar.[15] For instance, in the discussion of surface dyslexia, many of the regu-larity effects reported in Table 4.4 are of this type. Inferences based on trend dis-sociations are susceptible to a number of potential artefacts, and in general are much weaker in inferential power than the other two forms.

10.4   Inferences from Impairments: Task-Demand Artefacts (Validity of Assumption 8b)

Cognitive neuropsychology studies begin from specific impairments on particular tasks. In the last section, it was argued that the more selective the impairment, the more powerful in general are the potential theoretical inferences that can be made. However, even more basic than the selectivity of an impairment is its existence. There has been a tendency so far in this account for two meanings of the word *impairment* to be conflated. One is 'poor' performance on a task, where just how bad 'poor' should be will be discussed in section 10.5. The other is the consequence of damage to one or more cognitive systems. To conflate the two presupposes that poor performance is in fact a sign of cognitive impairment; indeed, in section 10.3, the principal function of assumption 8 is to allow this conflation to be made for the purpose of the analysis that followed. A task was assumed to be carried out by the procedure used by normal subjects or by the most *efficient* use of the subsystems that remain after the illness.

In practice, this conflation may not hold. Patients may perform poorly on a task

---

15. The problem arises of how to distinguish *strong* and *trend* dissociations operationally. For many combinations of tasks, it would be possible to adopt the criterion that for a strong dissociation, performance of task A is more than, say, 2 standard deviations closer to the normal mean than that of task B – that it is *robust.* However, this does not work for tasks on which normal performance is at or near 100%, as in, say, reading aloud from standard word lists. In this situation, the concepts can be applied only fairly loosely; a practical case where the distinction is useful is given in the discussion of individual difference artefacts (section 10.6).

simply because they misinterpret the task requirements. This can result from, say, a comprehension disorder arising from aphasia or dementia. More subtly, though, it can arise because the patient interprets the task demands in a different fashion from a normal subject. This point has been made cogently by Kolk and van Grunsven (1984) in a study of agrammatism.

In the discussion of this topic in chapter 7, I skated over one of the principal techniques used in modern research in the area, that of metalinguistic judgements of sentence structure (see, e.g., Zurif, Caramazza, & Myerson, 1972; Caramazza & Zurif, 1976). The patient is presented with a written sentence, such as *The cat ate a cookie,* and sets of three words from the sentence, such as *the, ate, cat.* The patient's task is to say which of the words in the sentence 'go best together' in that particular sentence. All possible sets of three words are presented, and the results of these triadic comparisons are then subject to a hierarchical cluster analysis technique (e.g. Johnson, 1967), which has the aim of exposing the underlying cognitive organisation used by the subject for the task. Normal subjects typically produce the scaling structure appropriate on linguistic theory, *(the cat) ((ate), (a cookie)).* It was observed that agrammatic aphasics produce anomalous clusters, such as *(the) (cat ate) (a) (cookie).* This was considered to be impaired performance and used as evidence that agrammatic aphasics have difficulties with speech comprehension as well as speech production.

Kolk and van Grunsven (1984) pointed out a major problem. How does one know that agrammatic aphasics interpret the task instructions as requiring *syntactic* judgements? The Dutch research workers investigated the problem by assessing the performance on the test of two patients, M and L, who had only a mild word-finding difficulty. They were not agrammatic in speech production, as indicated by their performance on the Boston Profile of Speech Characteristics – the speech production part of the Boston Aphasia Battery. Both patients performed this at an optimal level, except for some difficulty for one patient on the articulatory-agility scale.[16] In addition, the patients performed well on tests of syntactic comprehension. However, on the triadic comparison test, both patients produced structures characteristic of agrammatic patients. M tended to neglect the first functor in sentences, producing a structure similar to the agrammatic cluster – *(the) (horse kicked) (my son).*

It might be argued that because both patients had recovered from a more severe aphasic disorder, their performance on the triadic comparison test indicates a latent agrammatism, which has manifested itself on what would be presumed to be a more demanding situation. This, however, seems implausible because Kolk and van Grunsven also observed four agrammatic patients, B, H, K, and La (Table 10.1), each of whom produced a normal triadic comparison structure. Kolk and van Grunsven prefer an alternative explanation, that aphasic subjects, unlike normals, do not necessarily treat the instruction to indicate which two of three words go best together as a question relating to syntax. Even when patients have recovered, if they

16. It is widely accepted that articulatory agility can dissociate from agrammatic speech (e.g. Berndt & Caramazza, 1980).

Table 10.1. *Percentage of utterances classed as agrammatic and correct in a story completion task for the six patients in the study of Kolk and van Grunsven (1984)*

	M	L	B	H	K	La
Agrammatic	4	0	50	33	61	68
Correct	82	79	39	50	32	18

have a history of speech comprehension problems, they may approach the task with a semantic set. Yet another possibility is that the patients had frontal lobe difficulties, in which case they may well have produced a more concrete interpretation than the syntactic one.[17] In either case, the 'poor' test performance would not be explicable as a direct consequence of an impairment to the mechanisms that the test was held to be studying.

The problems of dealing with the strategy used by the patient is not specific to agrammatism or to this apparently artificial experimental situation. Again, however, there is a difference between the overall pattern of performance and the specific aspects of the disorder. There is every likelihood that the detailed way in which a patient's impairment is exhibited in terms of the nature of the errors, reaction times, and so on will be influenced by the conscious or unconscious efforts made to try to circumvent the disorder. An excellent example comes from a study undertaken by Butterworth (1979) of jargon aphasia, a form of fluent aphasia in which the patient produces many neologisms. Jargon aphasia has often been thought of as a difficulty in voluntarily inhibiting inappropriate words and words that have become distorted in the production process (e.g. Pick, 1931/1973; Zangwill, 1960; Rochford, 1974). Butterworth, however, in a detailed analysis of the speech of a jargon aphasic patient, KC, showed that 51% of the neologisms were preceded by pauses, as opposed to only 18% of real words. Moreover, a large sub-group of neologisms – 55 out of the total of 96 – shared at least 4 features with the preceding neologism uttered, which was, however, separated from it by other correct words. The end of the chain often differed considerably from the beginning.[18]

Butterworth argued that this characteristic of the patient's speech is not a direct mechanical consequence of an impaired process, but a strategic adaptation to the impairment. He held that if KC failed to find the lexical form of a word that he intended to produce, he ended the pause by generating a 'filler' morpheme – the neologism. For ease of production, each neologism tended to be similar to previous filler morphemes. It follows, if the explanation is accepted, that the nature of these errors made by the patient provides no information about the operation of the normal speech mechanism.

17. Frontal lobe difficulties are discussed in chapter 14.
18. This type of chaining had been noted by Green (1969) and by Buckingham and Kertesz (1976).

This example, however, concerns the specific aspects of a patient's behaviour. The broad pattern of performance is unaffected by the use of this particular strategy. Returning to the interpretation of the overall pattern, what procedures can be used to minimise the possibility that an apparent dissociation arises as a result of an idiosyncratic strategic adaptation to the task by the patient? How can one attempt to ensure that assumption 8 (b) is applicable? It turns out that there are many methods available, so that the danger can be reduced considerably.[19]

Five criteria can be adopted for assessing how likely studies are to suffer from a task-validity artefact.

1. *Performance on baseline tests.* If the patient behaves normally on baseline tests, particularly on WAIS IQ and aphasia tests, then a task artefact is less likely, for an ability to comprehend instructions adequately and co-operate can be inferred.[20] However, as the Kolk and van Grunsven (1984) study illustrates, an artefact cannot necessarily be ruled out.
2. *The use of ecologically valid procedures.* The triadic-comparisons test is an obvious candidate for a task-validity artefact because it is unlikely to relate very directly to anything in the patient's experience. By contrast, a test that relies on, say, only reading words aloud would be much less likely to produce a problem.
3. *Converging operations.* The wider the variety of tests used that require different strategies and yet lead to the same theoretical conclusion, the more robust is the conclusion.[21] The use of converging operations does not entail a reliance on associated deficits. As discussed in section 10.2, a number of different tasks may make demands on the same set of model subcomponents. Inferences from individual patients that are based on only a single test finding are, in my opinion, highly suspect.
4. *The use of strategy-control tests for the critical comparison.* If the patient can be shown to perform normally on a test that requires a closely analogous strategy, then a task-validity artefact is unlikely. For instance, MP, the semantic dyslexic patient of Bub, Cancelliere, and Kertesz (1985), discussed in chapter 5, could not match a written word to a semantically similar word among three distractors (e.g. *table: chair, apple, buy, pen*). Yet immediately before this test, the analogous task was carried out almost perfectly with pictures, so it is highly implausible that MP failed to understand the task.
5. *Instructing or training the patient in the appropriate strategy.* It has been argued by Beauvois and Derouesné (1982) that the most appropriate procedure is to instruct the patient which strategy to use. If this is not possible, then the patient can be trained to use the strategy.[22] If one is attempting to assess whether a particular mechanism is damaged, then this seems an entirely apposite approach because in line with assumption 8 (b), the strategy used is no longer opaque to the experimenter.

19. One rough informal procedure that can be used in assessing a study in which a task-validity artefact seems possible is to see whether the authors of the study discuss the possibility. If they do not, they may well not have considered it.
20. The absence of baseline tests in a study is in certain respects more ominous than poor performance by the patient on such tests, since it suggests an insensitivity to clinical variables on the part of the investigator.
21. An example will be given in the discussion of semantic access dyslexia in chapter 12.
22. An example will be given in the discussion of modality-specific aphasias in chapter 12 (see chapter 12, footnote 28). See also the discussion of phonological alexia in chapter 5.

Given that at least two of these safeguards have been used, one can provisionally assume that assumption 8 (b) has been satisfied.[23]

10.5   Inferences from Dissociations: The Problem of Resource Artefacts (Application of Assumption 6)

According to traditional neuropsychological theory, a dissociation consists of a patient performing task I extremely poorly and task II at normal level or at least very much better than task I. In section 10.2, it was argued that the dissociation allows one to infer that the sets of isolable subsystems used by the two tasks differ. A well-known difficulty for this inference is that the tasks involved may be differentially sensitive to neurological disease. This problem has been avoided in this chapter so far by the provisional assumption that any task that requires the use of a subsystem would make an equal demand on it.

In practice, this assumption is too restrictive. Certain tasks, such as the reading of individual words aloud and the Vocabulary subtest of the WAIS, are relatively insensitive to the effects of generalised neurological disease when compared with, say, the Block Design or Digit Symbol subtests of the WAIS (see Nelson & O'Connell, 1978). It appears that the former pair make fewer demands on the subsystems they employ than the latter ones. More simply, consider a patient who could read frequent words, but not infrequent ones. One would not want to argue that different subsystems were involved in the tasks, but merely that the latter task was the more demanding.

In this section, I will be concerned with whether one can make theoretical inferences from the overall pattern of performance shown by two or more patients, even when tasks may vary in difficulty. The assumption that is critical for dealing with this issue is assumption 6. It is derived from the literature on dual-task performance in normal subjects (e.g. Norman & Bobrow, 1975; Navon & Gopher, 1979) where the idea of one or more resources being shared in some fashion between the two tasks seemed to provide a means of analysing the variations in amount of attention that subjects can pay to either one of the two tasks.[24] In the simpler Norman and Bobrow version, it is assumed that a constant amount of resource is available to the subject to allocate to the two tasks, but how much is given to either one of them is under the strategic control of the subject and is unknown to the experimenter. Performance on each task is describable by a performance/resource curve fixed for the

23. No general rule will be suggested for selecting between the alternative procedures that satisfy assumption 8(b).

24. A former advocate of resource notions within the dual-task literature in the study of normal attention has argued that, in fact, it has been of little use in that field (Navon, 1984). He made three points. He pointed out that in the dual-task situation, a gradual trade-off between performance on one task and on the other is the exception rather than the rule. Performance tends more towards the all-or-none. This is not relevant for the extrapolation to neuropsychology. Second, he argued that the concept becomes much more difficult to apply when one is dealing with multiple resources; this is certainly the case also for neuropsychological applications. Finally, he argued that it is unclear what sort of measure of the operation of a system the concept of 'resource' provides. A neuropsychological perspective can help in this respect.

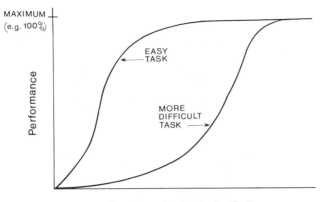

Figure 10.4. Two performance/resource curves. The performance level with maximum resoures need not be 100%; in this case, the curves are said to be 'data-limited'. In most tasks considered in the text, this is not the case.

task, in which performance increases with the amount of resource allocated to it (Figure 10.4).[25]

This approach can be extrapolated to neuropsychology by assuming that neurological disease depletes the amount of each particular resource by an unknown value, which varies with the patient.[26] It can then be applied to determining whether different overall patterns of performance on a set of tasks shown by two or more patients can be explained just by assuming that certain of the tasks are harder than the others. I will initially restrict consideration to the simplest case discussed in section 10.2, in which all tasks under consideration could possibly utilise one and the same subsystem. Even this apparently very simple case produces enough complications!

It would be possible to explain differences among patients in the overall pattern

25. An essential element of the logic is that the performance/resource curves are monotonically increasing, or, more appropriately, monotonically non-decreasing; increasing the amount of the resource available does not decrease performance. It should be noted that the existence of non-decreasing performance/resource curves is subject to a routine check from so-called performance operating curves obtained in the dual-task literature (see Sperling & Melcher, 1978). Accepting that performance/resource curves are non-decreasing eliminates one potential problem for the use of double dissociations – that a double dissociation can arise by comparing patients on two limbs of an inverted-U function (Weiskrantz, 1968).
26. Performance-resource theory has been applied to different neuropsychological issues by Shallice (1979b) and by Friedman and Polson (1981). Friedman and Polson were concerned with hemisphere differences. The rest of the chapter is based on arguments presented in Shallice (1979b). To make the 'resource' concept more concrete, one way of realising it would be in terms of the average proportion of neurons functioning normally in the subsystem necessary to produce a given level of performance when all other neurons in the subsystem are non-functional and all other subsystems involved in the task are unimpaired.

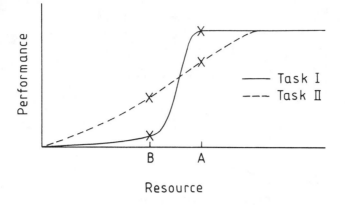

Figure 10.5. Possible performance/resource curves to illustrate how a double dissociation, defined as two complementary dissociations, is not sufficient to eliminate the possibility of a resource artefact. A and B are possible resources of two patients, one of whom does better on task I and the other, on task II.

of performance by variations in task difficulty alone if the pattern of results can be explained by two sets of assumptions: (1) some performance/resource function for each task that is approximately the same for each subject, but may differ from that of other tasks (to satisfy assumptions 4 and 9); *and* (2) a level of loss of resource for each subsystem that is constant over tasks for each patient, but may differ among patients.

Any procedure that ensures that no such pair of assumptions can be satisfied could be used to extend the falsification logic developed in section 10.2 to situations where tasks vary in difficulty. The most obvious procedure is the double dissociation inference (Teuber, 1955; Weiskrantz, 1968; Kinsbourne, 1971), which has become standard in clinical neuropsychology. Double dissociation has, however, been used and expressed in two ways, one valid and one not. It is therefore worth considering in more detail, especially because one theorist has denied that it has any special inferential role (Caramazza, 1986).

One frequent view is that a double dissociation occurs when patient A performs task I significantly better than task II, but for patient B, the situation is reversed (e.g. Coltheart, 1985). However, as shown in Figure 10.5, this pattern of performance is not sufficient grounds for inferring the existence of separate subsystems. One performance/resource curve may merely be steeper than the other, and so one subsystem could be responsible for both tasks. It is theoretically unsound to operationalise a double dissociation merely as two complementary dissociations in two patients, as its dangerously misleading name suggests.[27]

27. It is useful to make a distinction between inferences based on the pattern of performance shown by individual patients, but in which potential resource artefacts are ignored, as in earlier sections of the chapter, and the double dissociation methodology used specifically to counter the possibility of a

The valid formulation of the double dissociation – as far as resource artefacts are concerned – is that on task I, patient A performs significantly better than patient B, but on task II, the situation is reversed. Then, if the two tasks are critically dependent on one subsystem, it would follow from the non-decreasing nature of performance/resource curves that whatever specific form they take,

$R_A > R_B$ for task I (where R_A is the level of resource available to patient A) and $R_B > R_A$ for task II.

These two inequalities are in contradiction. Therefore, performance on the two tasks cannot be explained in terms of the operation of a single subsystem. This form of the classical double dissociation logic is therefore a satisfactory means of falsifying a model where the two tasks are critically dependent on the same subsystem, even when the tasks differ in their degree of difficulty.

Can one make a similar extension to the type of inference procedure introduced in chapter 4 in the isolation of the different acquired dyslexic syndromes – the critical-variable method. If the performance of a certain type of task is affected in one patient (A) by a change in variable X but not by a change in variable Y, and the complementary effect is observed in another patient (B), then is it a legitimate inference that damage to a single subsystem cannot explain the results? This type of pattern can be divided into two sub-types. First, if one of the two interactions obtained between the performance of the two patients – that on variable X, say – is of the cross-over type (Figure 10.6[a]), then by considering the four extreme points, one has a classical double dissociation. If, however, a classical double dissociation is not obtained, the inference is more complex (Figure 10.6[b]). If one considers just variable X, then to explain the pattern of results using only a single subsystem requires the assumption of a performance/resource function for the task that is unaffected by the variable for some, but not all, parts of its resource range (Figure 10.7). To obtain the complementary pattern for another variable would not seem to be possible, given that the two variables operate on the same stimulus set unless one postulates a very bizarre set of performance/resource curves.

By contrast, on the separate subsystem assumption, there are two ways of explaining the pattern (Figure 10.8). Both have been used in earlier chapters. The form in Figure 10.8(a) was the explanation offered for the two forms of phonological alexia differentiated by Derousené and Beauvois (1979) where the variables were graphemic and phonological complexity, respectively (chapter 5). Figure 10.8(b)

resource artefact. In the former case, it is natural and appropriate to base inferences on the dissociation considered as a within-patient effect. In the latter case, however, the double dissociation inference for tackling resource artefacts is not based on two complementary dissociations, but on two complementary inter-subject comparisons. The double dissociation as two complementary dissociations proves useful in another context, that of reorganisation of function (see section 10.7 and footnote 34). It should be noted that the rejection by Caramazza (1986) of the double dissociation as having any special role in neuropsychological inference flows from his divorcing problems of inference from the concrete practice of neuropsychological research (see footnote 13).

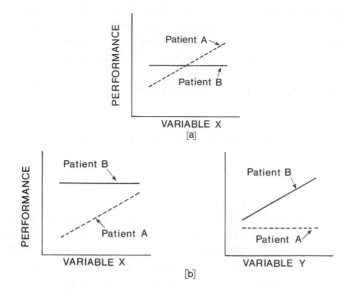

Figure 10.6. Two patterns of results that can be obtained when using the critical-variable methodology: (a) cross-over type, and (b) non-cross-over type.

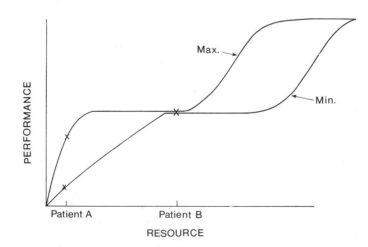

Figure 10.7. Performance/resource curves that could give rise to the pattern shown in Figure 10.6(b) (left), with damage to only a single system (Min. and Max. refer to the minimum and maximum value of variable X used for the two patients).

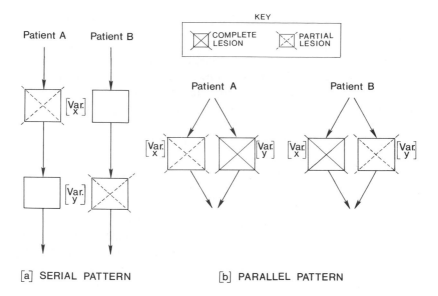

Figure 10.8. Two ways in which the pattern of results shown in Figure 10.6 can be explained using isolable processing systems.

was the form used to explain the contrasting effects of regularity and stimulus concreteness on different types of acquired dyslexic patient (chapters 4 and 5). The orthodox double dissociation thus allows for a serial as well as a parallel relation between the subsystems affected in the two patients.[28] However, the stronger the dissociation, the more likely the parallel version becomes.

The present approach therefore supports traditional neuropsychological practice in confirming that a procedure is available – the double dissociation (given that it is appropriately expressed) – that enables one to deduce that a pattern of performance across patients is not explicable from damage to a single common subsystem, even if the tasks are differentially sensitive to damage. A second procedure – the double critical variable – does not in principle rule out an explanation in terms of a single subsystem, but does so in practice. Thus the classical neuropsychological procedures for guarding against task-difficulty artefacts is justified, given the present set of assumptions.[29]

28. The inferences that can be drawn about the form of the functional architecture from double dissociations were first discussed by Sartori (1988). His conclusions differ somewhat from the ones given here, as do the resource arguments on Figure 10.7 from those given in Shallice (1979b).

29. It should be noted that the argument does not generalise to situations in which resource levels of two different subsystems may vary across patients. Consider two tasks that require the same pair of subsystems, X and Y, and let $x_1 > x_2$ and $y_1 < y_2$, where subscripts 1 and 2 refer to the levels of the two resources for the two patients. Then the two tasks may be carried out by identical subsystems, even if a double dissociation occurs between patients. For instance, let task A require resources

10.6   Inferences from Dissociations: The Problem of Individual Differences (Validation and Application of Assumption 9)

On the dissociation approach, the selection of a patient for study depends on his or her performing selectively poorly on one of a set of tasks. The purpose of selecting such a patient is to be able to differentiate functional components, on the assumption that certain subsystems have been selectively damaged in the patient. The possibility has to be considered, though, that the difference in levels of performance across tasks may not have arisen for this reason. The observed deficit may have been present before the lesion occurred.

Normal subjects differ in their performance across tasks. However, the existence of individual differences in the normal population cannot speak directly to the nature of the functional architecture. Differences in performance across tasks in members of the normal population might reflect just a difference in the degree of development or capacity of particular subsystems across individuals. It could as well reflect differences across individuals in the degree to which a single subsystem is tuned for a particular task. Thus an English and a French person would differ in their performance on reading English and French words; there is no reason to assume different functional architectures.

Might not the use of the single-case procedure, in which individual patients are chosen for investigation because they manifest a dissociation, give rise to a selection artefact? Could the procedure result not just in picking out individuals at the extreme of the discrepancy distribution in the normal population?

No single-case study in which the patient was selected on the basis of a dissociation has, to my knowledge, used any form of statistical justification of the selection procedure. However, it is easy to demonstrate that in particular situations, a selection artefact is unlikely to have occurred. Consider the dissociation between span performance and LTM performance in amnesia, discussed in chapter 3. One long-term memory task that has been extensively used clinically is Warrington's (1984) forced-choice recognition memory test for words. Figure 2.1 illustrated performance on the task for 200 normal subjects and 11 amnesics (Warrington & Weiskrantz, personal communication). On this, the scores of three of the amnesics overlap with those of five of the normal patients. The other amnesics, however, performed well below all normal subjects. By contrast, on the digit span task, the amnesic subjects had a mean of 6.8, with a range of 5 to 9. In other words, they performed in the normal range. For a group of 11 patients, it is obvious from the consistency and magnitude of the effect that the overall dissociation for the group could not

$(x_1 + x_2)/2$ and y_1 for adequate performance, and task B require resources x_2 and $(y_1 + y_2)/2$. Patient I will fail task B only and patient II, task A. It would appear, then, that the double dissociation guards against a task-difficulty artefact only when the two tasks make equal demands on subsystems other than the critical ones. Fortunately, this is a common state of affairs in cognitive neuropsychology; consider the auditory–verbal STM/LTM double dissociation, as manifested in the early and recency parts of the free-recall serial-position curve (chapter 3), *or* that between abstract- and concrete-word reading (chapter 5).

have arisen from a statistical artefact, even though each patient had been included as a result of complex clinical process that cannot be fully analysed. For any individual amnesic who scores below the 200 normals, a selection artefact seems implausible.

Can one as confidently rule out a selection artefact in all investigations where an individual subject is selected for study? In practice, one cannot estimate effectively the number of patients with a similar lesion in whom a dissociation does not occur. Moreover, it is also impossible to determine what percentage of 'normal' subjects would produce scores analogous to those shown by a patient. Consider in the example just discussed the problem of giving a numerical estimate more precise than zero of the percentage of normal subjects who scored, say, 7 or more on digit span and 30 or below on forced-choice recognition memory. The most that can be said is that the proportion of normal subjects who do this must be very low. Also, are the grounds satisfactory for considering a control subject who performed in this way to be 'normal'?

Quantitative statistical arguments therefore will probably not prove a practical procedure to use in order to reject a selection-artefact hypothesis. There are, however, common-sense reasons why the artefactual explanation is generally most implausible. The clinical symptoms displayed by patients are almost always known not to have been present earlier in their lives, and in many patients, there are clear physical signs that a disease process has occurred. Hence, if the test results are consonant with the clinical symptoms, the observed dissociation can hardly be explicable in terms of just a selection artefact. Premorbid differences among patients could influence whether a dissociation does or does not manifest itself clearly. However, the selection artefact is, in general, not a plausible explanation for the dissociations themselves.[30]

In this argument, it is implicitly assumed that the dissociation involved is a classical one. Trend dissociations present a much more severe problem. This issue needs to be considered in the context of the discussion in section 10.5, where a form of the double dissociation procedure was advocated as a means of avoiding resource artefacts. Take the example of the double dissociation that can be obtained for the reading of abstract and concrete words, discussed in chapter 5. Consider two patients, who before their illnesses read either only philosophy (A) or only thrillers (B). Then patient A will have encountered abstract words relatively more frequently than the average person and patient B, relatively less frequently. This means that if words in the abstract and concrete sets are matched for frequency in the population as a whole, they will differ in the personal frequencies for the two patients. An impairment that has the effect of merely making words of low personal frequency unavailable to the patient could result in a cross-over interaction when plotted in terms of frequency for the population as a whole (Figure 10.9)!

30. A supplementary argument can be derived from localisation evidence. If patients with the same functional disorder have similarly placed lesions, then, again, it is implausible to attribute their syndrome just to a selection artefact. For instance, in the short-term memory syndrome, all the patients have posterior left hemisphere lesions (chapter 3).

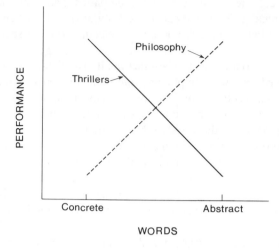

Figure 10.9. Illustration of a possible individual difference artefact.

In practice, if one examines this particular situation, it seems most implausible that the double dissociation between reading abstract words and concrete words can be explained in terms of damage to only a single system. In essence, this is because one of the two dissociations – the concrete-word superiority one – is of the strong variety.[31] It would be very difficult to calculate for any particular pair of tests what spread of performance would be expected to arise in the normal population due to differences in enviornmental history. Clearly, small differences in how pairs of individuals perform across a pair of tests could be easily explained in this way. Thus if both dissociations had been of the trend variety, the interaction obtained might well result from individual differences alone. The overall conclusion is that trend dissociations provide a much less reliable inferential basis than strong or classical ones.

There remains the possibility that, contrary to assumption 4, differences among patients in their functional architecture are not merely quantitative. In this case, the use of group data – either in neuropsychology or in normal experimental psychology – would be very dangerous, since average performance would not correspond to the behaviour of any of the qualitatively different varieties of subjects. Indeed, qualitative differences could probably be discovered only by using a single-case approach!

31. Both PS (Shallice & Coughlan, 1980), who had been a teacher, and PW (Patterson & Marcel, 1977), a former civil servant, showed a large concrete-word advantage, while CAV (Warrington, 1981), who had been a grocer, showed a smaller abstract-word advantage. For the double dissociation to arise from damage to a single system, an AA abstract word for PS (33% correct) would have to be relatively much less frequent for her than a 1–50 per million abstract word was for CAV (44% correct). (On concrete words, PS scored much more highly than CAV.) This is most unlikely.

10.7 Inferences from Dissociations: Reorganisation after the Lesion (Validity of Assumption 8a)

A dissociation may not be attributable to some testing, resource, or individual-difference artefact. Yet it may still not directly reflect the modular structure of the normal cognitive system. After the initial stage of a neurological disease, such as a stroke or encephalitis, or after a neurosurgical operation, such as to remove a non-malignant tumour, patients often recover greatly in both quantitative and qualitative fashion (see, e.g., Newcombe & Ratcliff, 1979). At times, such recovery can occur a remarkably long time after the acute illness. Thus a patient I studied, PR (Shallice, 1981a), was a severe conduction aphasic two years after having suffered a stroke and had a span of two. When his hard-core syndrome of phonological agraphia was studied 18 months later, his conduction aphasia had almost resolved. In addition, the long-term consequences of damage to macroscopically equivalent tissue after operation for a slow-growing tumour, such as a meningioma, and a stroke, where the total damage process occurs rapidly, may well be different. It is known that in animals, multiple-stage and single-stage lesions can produce different effects (e.g. Finger & Stein, 1982).

Little is known about these processes in the human patient (for a review, see Geschwind, 1985). Yet for obvious clinical and practical reasons, observations that are theoretically relevant are normally obtained only a considerable time after the onset of the disease process. Could one be studying a reorganised system whose mode of operation is qualitatively different from the normal? Would this not make inference to normal function invalid? In particular, is it possible that a subsystem might be involved in the operation of two different tasks in the normal subject, but that after a lesion, some substituting system might cope far better with one than the other? Thus any dissociation observed would reflect only the process of compensation, not the original organisation of the cognitive system.

Since we know so little about recovery processes, it might seem almost impossible to refute such a hypothesis. There are, however, at least two relevant lines of argument. First, whether or not the dissociation is a classical one makes an important difference. If reorganisation after a lesion has led to a particular sub-function being carried out by an entirely separate subsystem, which operates on qualitatively different principles from the original one, there are no grounds to assume that *quantitative* measures of the resource available in the original subsystem should remain unchanged. Thus a classical dissociation would not be expected to occur as a result of reorganisation. An essential part of a classical dissociation is that the preserved task is performed at the same level as it was before the lesion and is not at 'ceiling'; this means that the same level of resource is available as before the illness.

This argument can be applied to a frequently postulated form of the reorganisation hypothesis – the possible take-over of a function in a damaged hemisphere by a qualitatively different process in the other one. As an example, take the inference discussed in chapter 3 that the main auditory–verbal STM system is not part of the speech production system. The argument was based on the dissociation between the severe short-term memory impairment of patient JB and her essentially intact speech. Yet JB had had a slowly growing meningioma removed when she was only 24 (see Warrington, Logue, & Pratt, 1971). Moreover, she showed a large right ear suppression effect with dichotic listening on initial testing. An advocate of the right hemisphere relateralisation hypothesis could argue that the speech production process had relateralised, and therefore functional inferences to the normal relation between speech production and short-term memory would be invalid.[32]

The argument is too superficial. If normal left hemisphere speech production involves the principal short-term store used in span, but relateralised right hemisphere speech production does not, then there is a puzzle. The new, qualitatively different, makeshift, speech production process in the right hemisphere gives rise to quantitative measures of error rates and pause patterns that are no different from the normal. The quantitative similarity between the behaviour of the new and the old systems is unexplained. Moreover, if the new system could perform that well with a tiny short-term store, why should a large one normally exist? It is much more plausible to assume that if the speech production process can relateralise – which, it should be emphasised, is very far from having been demonstrated – then before as well as after relateralisation, it does not contain the major auditory–verbal short-term store. Thus the same functional conclusion is reached as when the possibility of relateralisation was not considered.

The double dissociation provides the basis for a second argument against explaining away dissociations in terms of reorganisation of function. From the arguments presented earlier in the chapter, it can be inferred that in a double dissociation of strong or classical types, the different tasks that the two patients perform well are being carried out by different subsystems. Therefore, if the better task for one patient is being carried out by a subsystem that is substituting for the original one, the better task for the other patient must be being carried out by a different subsystem. It seems implausible that when a given subsystem is damaged, two qualitatively different subsystems substitute for it in different patients. There remains the possibility that in one patient, the original subsystem continues to operate in a partially damaged state, but substitution occurs in the second patient. However, to account for the double dissociation, one would then have to explain why the substituting and original systems have opposite characteristics as far as the pair of tasks is concerned.

Take as an example the double dissociation between certain fluent aphasics and certain agrammatic ones in how well they process function and content words, respectively. One might conjecture that the dissociation observed in agrammatism

32. It should be noted that this is a different relateralisation argument from that developed for conduction aphasia in general by Kleist (1916) and Kinsbourne (1972). They argued that relateralisation of *speech perception* processes occurs in conduction aphasia. On this relateralisation hypothesis, the present inference to normal function would be unaffected. In fact, JB was severely aphasic after her operation, so it would be quite ad hoc to assume that speech production returned to normal within its own hemisphere, but speech perception relateralised. Relateralisation hypotheses have the disadvantage that they are beautifully flexible.

– preserved semantic processing but impaired syntactic operations – is a characteristic of a compensatory system in the right hemisphere.[33] It could then be argued that the dissociation observed in agrammatism throws no light on the modularity of the left hemisphere language systems with respect to syntactic and semantic processing. This argument would be powerful if it were not for the existence of the complementary fluent asphasic disorder, in which syntactic processes are relatively intact and yet there is a gross semantic impairment.[34] Fluent aphasia, on this approach, would have to be explained in terms of syntactic processes requiring less of the undifferentiated left hemisphere resource than semantic ones. Thus it has to be assumed that the damaged and compensatory systems are not just qualitatively different, but also qualitatively opposite. To explain a double dissociation in terms of a single-component system that can relateralise requires an additional, rather unlikely assumption. Therefore, the plausibility of the inference to isolable subsystems from a double dissociation is not greatly weakened when the possibility of reorganisation of function is included. This makes the double dissociation an even more critical part of neuropsychological methodology than it was held to be earlier.[35]

10.8 Conclusion

In this chapter, it has been shown that provided one makes certain assumptions about the system that has been damaged, the methodology of using dissociations,

33. The study most frequently cited in support of this possibility is that of Czopf (1972), concerning the injection of sodium amytal into one or another carotid artery in 22 aphasic patients. This technique (Wada & Rasmussen, 1960) was developed to establish the lateralisation of function when this is clinically critical – for instance, when surgery in possible language areas is being considered. The injection is thought to lead to a temporary loss of function in the corresponding hemisphere. For instance, it produces a temporary paralysis of the side of the body contralateral to the side that received the injection. It is unclear what the clinical justification was for the use of such a drastic technique in the group of patients studied by Czopf. He found that in most of the aphasics, right carotid injection affected speech more than left carotid injection, in 10 patients to such an extent that speech was completely abolished. However, in 14 of the right-handed patients, right sided injections were followed by a disturbance of consciousness. Poeck (1983) has argued that this makes the inference to right hemisphere language in the aphasic group 'not very convincing. . . . What was produced in these cases, was . . . a temporary decerebration syndrome, with tetraplegia plus akinetic mutism – a situation far afield from the study of aphasia' (p. 84).
34. This syndrome was briefly mentioned in chapter 7. A patient with these characteristics, WLP, is discussed in more detail in chapter 12.
35. It should be noted that for reorganisation of function discussion, what is critical about the double dissociation is that it involves two complementary dissociations. This differs from the pattern of performance, which is critical for coping with resource artefacts (see section 10.5). The two ways of viewing double dissociations, even though operationally different, are entirely compatible. They coexist in a cross-over interaction. For reasons discussed in the preceding sections, both individual dissociations need to be strong or classical. In future, it may well prove possible to investigate changes in lateralisation of function by neurological methods – for example, by developments in blood flow monitoring. However, the dissociations discussed in the earlier chapters have not yet been investigated using such methods with the occasional exception (see section 5.6).

double dissociations, and sets of dissociations as the primary basis for inference to normal function is valid. The main assumptions are that the system is modular and that the effects of different types of damage to individual subsystems may roughly be considered to lie on a continuum.

In earlier chapters, inferences from the existence of a dissociation to theories of functional architecture were made in a straightforward fashion. Yet from the arguments presented in this chapter, the straightforward inference may seem to rest on a fragile stack of assumptions. This would be an inappropriate conclusion. Instead, one needs to draw a sharp distinction between different types of dissociation. Inferences from trend dissociations, even if significant and even when combined with a complementary trend dissociation, are vulnerable to a set of potential artefacts. By contrast, inferences from classical dissociations and strong dissociations, especially if in complementary pairs, are relatively untouched. Most of the dissociations involved in the inferences made in earlier chapters are of classical or strong form.

The existence of these potential artefacts indicates that one should take care when making theoretical inferences from neuropsychological evidence. Associated deficits, trend dissociations, and single dissociations are liable to lead one astray. Caution, however, does not require the rejection of the approach. In general, the more striking the neuropsychological data, the less are these artefacts likely to be important. Neuropsychology is full of striking data.

11 Functional Specialisation

11.1 Delusions about Dissociations?

The cognitive neuropsychologist shares a conceptual problem with the archaeologist – to infer from a changed system the properties of the original one. Archaeologists have recently begun to consider the inference problem from the other perspective (for a review, see Hodder, 1982). What physical legacy, they have asked, would a society of the type being studied in fact leave? As an illustration of the dangers of making too direct an inference from the data, consider what could be inferred in future about recent Eskimo settlements from the tool remains that would be likely to be left. One would, for instance, find it very difficult to deduce the existence of some of the tools most valuable to the society. The use of other easily made or frequently broken artefacts would be simple to observe, but tools such as bone spears are highly 'curated': carried round, cared for, and reused, and if they are lost or discarded, this normally occurs away from the home site (Binford, 1976). Other things would be left behind, but probably not bone spears! Thus there would be real dangers of theorising inappropriately about the society from what was left. To lessen this danger, there has developed a new field intermediate between archaeology and anthropology – ethnoarchaeology – which studies what traces existing societies would or would not leave.

That neuropsychology might be subject to an analogous danger is illustrated by the development of ideas on dissociations. As has been repeatedly argued, dissociations are the most widespread and strikingly counterintuitive type of data that neuropsychology provides. It has been natural to choose theoretical accounts of normal function that allow them to be explained simply. So, for instance, one has the discrete 'centres' of the diagram-makers, discussed in chapter 1, the functional systems of Luria (1966), and the isolable subsystems and 'modules', discussed in earlier chapters, which are frequently encountered in modern cognitive neuropsychology theorising.

There have long been critics of this type of leap from dissociation to isolable subsystems. Thus when Freud (1891), in his foray into neuropsychology, wrote the first major critique of the diagram-makers and their concept of anatomically and functionally specific centres, he suggested that 'the organization of the central apparatus of speech is that of a continuous cortical region occupying the space be-

245

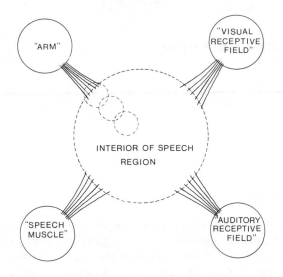

Figure 11.1. A simplification of Freud's (1891) model of aphasia. The four peripheral 'fields' are required for writing, reading, auditory comprehension, and articulation, respectively. Connections to sensory and motor regions in the right hemisphere have been omitted. Crossings of these tracts with those within the left hemisphere were held by Freud to be important, since lesions in such a region are especially prone to be interpreted in terms of 'centres'. The dotted circles represent three lesions of similar size that differ in how central they are within the system.

tween the terminations of the optic and acoustic nerves and of the areas of the cranial and certain peripheral motor nerves in the left hemisphere' (p. 67) (Figure 11.1). He 'refused to localise the psychic elements of the speech process in specified areas within this region' (p. 67) and argued that if

we imagine a moveable lesion of constant size within this association area, its effect will be the greater the more it approaches one of these [other] cortical fields i.e. the more peripherally it is situated within the speech area. If it borders immediately on one of these cortical fields it will cut off the association area from one of its tributaries i.e. the mechanisms of speech will be deprived of the visual, or auditory, or some other element. . . . If the lesion is moved towards the interior of the association area its effect will be more indefinite; in no event will it be able to destroy all possibilities of one particular category of association. (pp. 63–64)

The aim of his argument was to show that rough anatomical concordance between lesions that have fairly similar psychological effects does not entail the existence of specific centres. There are other, and according to Freud, more plausible possibilities.

His psychological arguments were rather vague and couched in terms of a nineteenth-century associationist's approach. It is, though, clear that he was attempting to explain the dissociations that arise in Broca's and Wernicke's aphasia without having recourse to the idea of damage to specific separable processes. Theories like his, which reject the idea of isolable subsystems, have in essence been attempts to explain away the heterogeneity of neuropsychological findings in a fashion that *might* in principle be correct but makes no claim to provide a tight account of individual dissociations. Such explanations therefore tend to be forgotten after a generation – or even less, in Freud's case.[1] They cannot withstand a change in theoretical fashion.

In more recent times, the pendulum has continued to swing between holistic and modular explanations. The incorporation of information-processing ideas into neuropsychology gave a great boost in the modular direction. Indeed, with the ease of explaining a dissociation in terms of isolable subsystems within that conceptual framework, such explanations began to be treated illicitly as almost having the force of a logical inference. This is particularly clear in methodological accounts of the role of double dissociations.

When the importance of double dissociations for avoiding problems of test sensitivity, as discussed in chapter 10, began to be understood in the 1950s and 1960s the principle was couched in terms of concepts like 'tasks' and 'functions'. Thus an early statement of the principle applied to one particular case was given by Teuber (1955) in an influential review article:

To demonstrate specificity of the deficit for visual discrimination we need to do more than show that discrimination in some other modality, e.g., somesthesis, is unimpaired. Such simple dissociation might indicate merely that visual discrimination is more vulnerable to temporal lesions than tactile discrimination. This would be a case of hierarchy of function rather than separate localization. What is needed for conclusive proof is 'double dissociation', i.e., evidence that tactile discrimination can be disturbed by some other lesion without loss on visual tasks and to a degree comparable in severity to the supposedly visual deficit after temporal lesions. (p. 283)

A later more abstract and sophisticated version, again concerned with group studies, was given by Kinsbourne (1971) in a lengthy analysis of neuropsychological methodology:

If a patient group with damage centred at location A is superior to one damaged at B in respect to task P, but inferior in task Q, a double dissociation obtains between these groups. This permits the inference of at least one difference between the two groups specific to location of damage, for P may be a nonspecific task, relating, say, to general intelligence or some other variable in which the groups are imperfectly matched. But then it must be admitted that function Q must have been selectively impaired by a lesion at location A; since the inferiority in performing Q cannot be accounted for by failure of matching on the other task. (p. 295)

These accounts of the principle are indeed concerned primarily with the methodological problems of the relative difficulty of different tasks. In so far as they make any claims about the underlying processes, it is by the use of 'function', a

---

1. Freud's (1891) own position was unsatisfactory. For instance, his theory did not explain conduction aphasia. After cogently criticising Wernicke's (1874) account of the syndrome, he unfortunately concluded that the syndrome did not exist, not having seen such a patient himself.

term little used in information-processing explanations, which have a conceptual framework derived primarily from engineering rather than biology. So cognitive neuropsychologists have tended to rephrase the principle in other terms. Marin, Saffran, and Schwartz (1976) wrote, 'If process X is intact where process Y is severely compromised or absent, and especially if the converse is found in other patients, there is reason to believe that X and Y reflect different underlying mechanisms in the normal state' (p. 869). In this account, the statement is concerned entirely with theoretical constructs. The change from earlier versions is masked by the inclusion of the bland qualifying clause 'there is reason to believe'. Very soon, though, the relation between data and 'mechanisms' or 'systems' was explicitly drawn, and the qualifications were dropped. One author, for instance, was unsubtle enough to write, 'The crucial theoretical point is that the double dissociation does demonstrate that the two tasks make different processing demands on two or more functionally dissociable subsystems' (Shallice, 1979b, p. 191). In such a version, the double dissociation principle becomes a relation between data and isolable mechanisms, given that one assumes that a concept like 'functionally dissociable subsystems' does not tautologically refer to just any part of the overall system that produces a dissociation when damaged. In this example, it was certainly intended to have a more specific sense.[2]

The error in such a formulation can be simply seen if one replaces the phrase 'functionally dissociable subsystem' with a term like *module,* which can be independently defined, as in Fodor's (1983) sense. An argument to justify it could then proceed in the following way: 'If modules exist, then, as has been discussed in chapter 10, double dissociations are a relatively reliable way of uncovering them. Double dissociations do exist. Therefore modules exist.' Presented in this form, the logical fallacy is obvious. To make the inference valid, one would need to add the assumption that dissociations do not arise from damage to non-modular systems.

This additional assumption was never, to my knowledge, explicitly stated, but it was easy to hold implicitly. The only generally discussed alternative to systems with isolable or modular components were 'mass action' ones, which were associated with Lashley's (1950) notion of equipotentiality. A completely equipotential system could not give rise to a double dissociation, since the effects of all lesions on all tasks could be ordered on a single dimension that combined lesion size and task sensitivity. In modern terms, a single performance/resource curve is sufficient to describe all behaviours of the system. Damage to such a system would show 'graceful degradation'; all tasks would become gradually more poorly performed, and equivalently so, as lesion size was increased. More complex alternatives, such as the one suggested by Freud (1891), were not considered.

The inadequacy of these lazy assumptions was exposed by a theoretical analysis made by Wood (1978). He produced an example of a near-equipotential system

2. Other cognitive neuropsychologists explicitly or implicitly took a similar position (e.g. Marshall & Newcombe, 1973; Marin, Saffran, & Schwartz, 1976; Beauvois & Derouesné, 1979). This change in the formulation of the double dissociation principle is a good example of an unconscious conceptual shift in the development of a new scientific paradigm. Until I reread Kinsbourne's (1971) version and mine (1979a), I had assumed that I had merely restated his position.

that, he argued, could give rise to a dissociation if appropriately 'lesioned'. As will be shown later in the chapter, his detailed argument was incorrect. However, his work made it clear that to assume that the set of possible systems divides comfortably into two types – those with isolable components that produce dissociations, and equipotential ones that do not – is potentially dangerous. So the idea that the existence of a double dissociation necessarily implies that the overall system has separable subcomponents can no longer be taken for granted. The transition to the cognitive neuropsychology conceptual framework has clearly brought dangers in its wake.

11.2   Specimen Non-modular Systems

In archaeology, Hodder (1982) had available to him existing societies of an economic level roughly equivalent to that of the ancient ones with which he was concerned. They could be treated as concrete examples for the issue of what physical legacies a society might leave. The neuropsychologist is in a less fortunate position. There are no systems analogous to cognitive ones that have a structure that we already know, except for those that people have constructed. The modularity that such systems exhibit might, as Rosenthal (1984) argued, conceivably reflect the limitations of human thought as much as some absolute superiority of modular systems.

Even if one moves from considering the effects of damage on real systems to how theoretical ones operate, only a few studies have been carried out on how they might be affected by 'lesions' (e.g. Wood, 1978, 1982; Gordon, 1982; Hinton & Sejnowski, 1986). Thus too little information exists for it to be possible to give a general treatment of the range of systems that can give rise to dissociations when 'lesioned'. It is, however, possible to give examples of non-modular systems that can produce dissociations if damaged. Five such systems will be considered (Figure 11.2).

Possibility 1: Continuum of a Processing Space

One type of system that can produce dissociations and even double dissociations when damaged is that based on a continuum of subprocesses. As a concrete example, consider the visual cortex. It is obvious that two patients with scotomas (visual-field deficits) in different parts of the visual field can be conceived of as forming a double dissociation. One might be able to see perfectly at 9° eccentricity but not at 15°, and the other could show the inverse pattern. Yet it does not make much sense to say that the simple cells analysing the input at 9° eccentricity are part of a different isolable subsystem from those analysing it at 15° eccentricity. They do not lie within different discrete functional units. No place between 9° and 15° eccentricity is any more appropriate than any other to select as boundary. Therefore, a double dissociation can arise from damage to two different processes that do not interact but are not themselves units, being merely different sections of a continuum of processes.

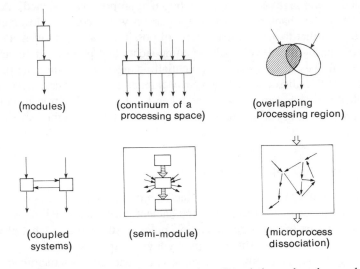

Figure 11.2. Varieties of system that can produce dissociations when damaged.

Put more abstractly, the argument is obvious. The existence of a double disso-ciation gives information about what happens when two regions of the brain are damaged. It can tell us nothing about what happens with damage to regions *physi-cally* between the two or, conceptually, what exists *between* the two processes car-ried out in those regions.

The continuum possibility might seem an obvious and academic one. It does, however, have implications. Consider the abstract–concrete dimension. The double dissociation discussed in chapter 5 could merely reflect damage to different areas of a semantic processing *space,* where the 'space' is not just metaphorical but relates to a multi-dimensional processing space in which the dimensions are physically represented in some way in the brain. The example will be considered in more detail in chapter 12.[3]

Possibility 2: Overlapping Processing Regions

A second possibility is that process A might require regions X and Z of the cortex, and process B might need regions Y and Z, with the cells in the two regions oper-

---

3. Another candidate for an explanation of this type is that of the different levels of unit involved in spelling-to-sound correspondences on the word-form theory, which was discussed in chapter 5. The argument has been put forward that the existence of a form of phonological alexia in which words are read by morphemic spelling-to-sound correspondences would support the position that there are functionally separate lexical and non-lexical phonological reading procedures and be incompatible with the word-form model, in which multiple levels of information are transmitted by one system (see Saffran, 1984). However, if the transmission system were itself viewed as a continuum, one could clearly obtain double dissociations from within the system.

ating in an equipotential way for each process. Then separate lesions to X and Y would give rise to a double dissociation on tasks that stress processes A and B, respectively. Yet, again, X and Y are not parts of two isolable subsystems, since they function as only parts of wholes that overlap. I know of no plausible examples of this type of system. However, it remains a theoretical possibility.

Possibility 3: Coupled Systems

Consider two subsystems, each of which contains a set of units that categorises a different domain of input (see Figure 11.2). Assume that each can categorise its own input effectively. However, also assume that the units that are activated when one of the subsystems categorises an input are strongly connected to complementary units in the other system. If one system were categorising auditory–verbal input at the lexical semantic level and the other, visual input at the semantic level, then this would be a plausible assumption (chapter 12).

An overall system of this type can give rise to a double dissociation in a simple fashion if appropriately damaged. Yet the two parts of the whole system can be highly interactive. If the lag is small between when units in one of the subsystems are activated and when they affect the complementary units in the other subsystem and the interconnections between the two parts are sufficiently strong, then when one part categorises an input effectively, the other can do little more than act as a slave in the process. Each of the two subsystems is not able to categorise simultaneously inputs that do not correspond. They are therefore not computationally autonomous. The two subsystems would not be conceived of as 'modules' in Fodor's (1983) sense.

Whether it is appropriate to consider them as 'isolable' one from the other can be held to depend on one or the other of two conditions. If the function being computed by each of the subsystems can be specified and differs from that being computed by the other, it is appropriate to consider them isolable. The concept of isolability in this sense is a characteristic of a different level of description of the system from that of the detailed mechanism by which subsystems interact and is an all-or-none concept. Alternatively, the concept can be specified in a more molecular and continuous way in terms of the *degree of isolability* of the subsystems; this concept is fairly self-explanatory, but will be defined more formally below. With this approach, which is the one I will adopt, the coupled systems are partially isolable.

Possibility 4: Semi-modules

The relation between a single subsystem or processing region and the rest of the system in which it is embedded can be viewed as on a continuum. One can theoretically consider the mode of operation of its individual elements on a micro-level and ask how much they depend on the output of other elements of the processing region itself and how much on variables that relate to the state of the rest of the system. The greater the disproportion in favour of within-processing region variables, the more isolable it is. The *degree of isolability* of a subsystem will then be the average of the ratio of intra-subsystem variables to extra-subsystem variables necessary for explaining the behaviour of elements of the subsystem on a micro-level. The relevance of this abstract definition is that it makes the idea of a *semi-module* a useful one.[4]

A semi-module would be a processing region with a considerable degree of isolability that receives inputs from many sources but in which a very few types of source – possibly only one – provide qualitatively the most influential input for the subsystem's operation *or* in which the outputs of the region are widespread but primarily affect a small number of other parts of the rest of the system (see Figure 11.2).[5] On the first of these alternatives, a single input from one source would activate the semi-module as much as many inputs from other sources. Damage to the semi-module would tend to affect primarily the efficiency with which the whole system performed one or a small number of types of operation and would therefore give rise to a dissociation. Possible applications of the concept of a semi-module are given in chapter 12.

Possibility 5: Multi-level Systems

A single structure may operate on more than one level, and a dissociation may reflect the existence of damage specific to only one of the levels. Take, for instance, a system that performs a given function in a distributed fashion over a large number of neurons, which has been a common theoretical approach at least since Hebb's (1949) ideas on cell assemblies; this class of models is currently widely used for simulations of cognition (e.g. Hinton & Anderson, 1981; McClelland & Rumelhart, 1985).[6] Assume further, in line with standard ideas on cell assemblies and distributed networks, that the network of neuron-like elements can learn and that the relative flexibility of the system in this respect is describable by a particular parameter.[7] If some form of damage – say, depletion in the amount of some chemical – left this parameter in a non-optimal state, learning would be impaired, and yet the system would be able to perform its steady-state function appropriately. But damage of a different sort – say, a loss of a certain percentage of its elements – might lead to an impairment in the steady-state function of the subsystem, but its learning capacity would be retained. In this case, a double dissociation could be observed between the ability of the system to learn new links between, say, highly frequent inputs and its ability to process rarely occurring inputs. In an abstract sense, two

4. Whether the definition can be formalised more adequately or operationalised is unclear.
5. This definition depends on most of the rest of the system being composed of modules or semi-modules. A possible application of the concept is discussed in chapter 12.
6. Such models are discussed more generally in sections 11.3 and 11.4.
7. In distributed memory models, this parameter determines the rate of alteration of the weights that particular idealised synaptic connections have. As this varies, so does the speed of learning (for an example, see Anderson & Mozer, 1981).

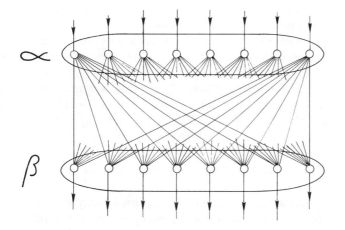

Figure 11.3. The type of distributed-memory system for which the effect of lesions was modelled by Wood (1978). The α units are the input neurons, and the β units, the output.

different processes are being affected by the different types of damage, but the different processes involve the same set of neurons. It would clearly be inappropriate to argue that the two processes are being carried out by 'isolable subsystems'. One could, however, extend the concept of resource introduced in chapter 10 and say that the subsystem had two independent resources.

11.3 Distributed Networks

As the argument in this chapter has developed, the dissociation has become less and less the *necessary* sign of damage to a modular subsystem. All the systems considered have, though, incorporated functional specialisation. Can one continue the argument further and completely dissociate the dissociation from functional specialisation? In recent years, the rising popularity of distributed-network theories of the way in which cognitive processes are implemented has fuelled the argument that one can draw no solid inferences about the functional architecture from dissociations. Thus Allport (1985) argued, with respect to 'the box-and-arrow notation of current cognitive neuropsychology', that 'obviously threatening to this approach, Wood (1978, 1982) has shown how, in a distributed memory system, a clear "double dissociation" between behavioural deficits can be consistent with a complete overlap in the underlying representations' (p. 35).

Wood (1978) considered the effects that lesions would have on a neural net model of the type whose properties had been investigated by Anderson, Silverstein, Ritz, and Jones (1977) (Figure 11.3). The basic psychological element of this model is the association. The aim of the model is to demonstrate that many different associations can be carried in parallel by connections between one set of input and another set of output neurons. Their model is based on two sets of neurons, set α and set β, with each neuron of set α being connected to every one of set β.

Different *patterns* of activation over the input cells stand for the different possible inputs to the systems, and patterns of activation over the output cells correspond to the possible outputs. The system is said to have the capacity to learn a number of associations between different inputs and their corresponding outputs.[8] Wood's analysis was, however, concerned with the operation of the system when learning has been completed. He dealt with a system having eight input and eight output neurons (see Figure 11.3). It stores four different associations in parallel. How well the system can process any individual learned association in this steady-state situation can be calculated. In his simulation, he was interested in the effects of hypothetical lesions.

In the first part of his analysis, he used 100 'randomly selected' sets of 4 input and output associations. He then simulated lesions by eliminating all possible combinations of up to 7 input neurons and up to 7 output neurons. Wood's (1978) conclusion was,

The pattern of results . . . contributes a clear example of mass action. Increasing lesion size produced a systematic decrease in performance of the model for lesions of input and output neurons alone as well as for combined lesions. . . . A lesion of any given input or output neuron produced, on the average, a deficit of similar magnitude to that of any other neuron in the set. (pp. 587–588)

There was no suggestion in this analysis of any type of dissociation occurring as a result of lesions. However, in the second part of his analysis, Wood selected a specific set of associations and a specific lesion intentionally constructed to illustrate an important departure from equipotentiality. In fact, in this example, two of the inputs (III and IV) he selected differ only as far as two of the eight input neurons (1 and 2) are concerned. They are identical as far as the other six input neurons are concerned (Table 11.1). It is therefore hardly surprising that if neuron 1 or neuron 2 is lesioned, the system loses much of its ability to distinguish between the two inputs; it frequently produces the wrong one of the two outputs.

Wood (1978) summarised these contrasting effects in two ways.

When the input vectors are orthogonal or nearly so, lesions of specific neural elements have little or no selective effects on performance. However, when the input vectors are distinguished by the activity of one or few neurons, highly selective lesion effects can be obtained. (p. 589)

This seems a reasonable summary. However, he also says, 'These effects correspond closely to the "double dissociation" result often interpreted as strong evidence for localisation of function' (p. 589), and 'the present results provide . . . evidence of the profound logical difficulties in attempting to infer principles of neural organisation from the results of lesion experiments' (p. 590).

8. For possible procedures see McClelland and Rumelhart (1985).

Table 11.1. *Input and output vectors for Word's (1978) double dissociation example*

	Training inputs					Training outputs			
α Neurons	I	II	III	IV	β Neurons	I	II	III	IV
1	−.196	−.229	.114	.912	1	1.000	−1.000	1.000	−1.000
2	.000	−.459	.912	.114	2	1.000	−1.000	−1.000	−1.000
3	−.196	.459	−.114	−.114	3	1.000	1.000	1.000	1.000
4	.392	.229	.228	.228	4	1.000	1.000	−1.000	1.000
5	.558	−.459	.114	.114	5	−1.000	−1.000	1.000	1.000
6	.558	.000	−.114	−.114	6	−1.000	−1.000	−1.000	1.000
7	−.196	−.229	−.114	−.114	7	−1.000	1.000	1.000	−1.000
8	−.196	.459	.228	.228	8	−1.000	1.000	−1.000	−1.000

Note: The system is held to have learned to produce output I, given input I. The input to or output from a neuron can lie between −1 and +1.

His conclusion about simulating double dissociations seems unwarranted.[9] What is lost in Wood's simulation are individual associations. A dissociation in neuro-psychology is the loss not of an association, but of the ability to perform a certain type of operation. There is an even more serious problem about the claim to have simulated a double dissociation in a distributed-memory system. In whatever way a system operates, if the lesion results in the loss of the input information relevant to a discrimination, then the ability to make the discrimination will inevitably be lost. Yet Wood's special case nearly reduces just to this. The two relevant inputs he chose differ only in how they influence two particular neurons; it is hardly surprising that lesioning one of these neurons has a major effect on the ability of the system to discriminate between the inputs. Thus the 'dissociation' that he obtained can reasonably be viewed as a product of the stimulus set used and the role that *individual* neurons have in the critical dissociation rather than as a consequence of the principle of organisation of the system lesioned.

Distributed-memory systems are of interest because they simulate the possible behaviour of real neural networks. One can presume, however, that any real neural network undertaking some cognitive operation will be composed of millions of neurons. In such a network, no individual neuron is likely to have much importance in determining what output occurs. Thus the implementation chosen by Wood (1978) to assess the effects of lesions, in which he used a network with very few neurons, removes an essential element of real neural networks as far as the implications for understanding double dissociations are concerned.

9. A rather minor criticism is that Wood (1978) has, at best, modelled not a double dissociation, but a single dissociation. Sartori (1988) has given a related example of a 'double dissociation' arising from two lesions in a single network.

A valid demonstration of a double dissociation arising from the effects of two different lesions to a distributed-memory system would need to satisfy two conditions. First, before the lesion is made, the influence of any particular neuron on what output is produced should be small. Second, the neurons affected by the lesion should not be selected by some complex algorithm that is determined by the dissociation to be explained and that is not typical of those that arise naturally. It seems most unlikely that if these conditions are satisfied, a classical or a strong double dissociation could be demonstrated in a properly distributed memory system.[10]

Wood's (1978) second analysis can, however, be put to a more positive use. It is well recognised within the isolable subsystem framework that a possible explanation for a dissociation is that of a disconnection between subsystems. Indeed, the key papers that resurrected the work of the diagram-makers for a modern readership from half a century of neglect were those of Geschwind (1965), in which he emphasised this type of explanation.

Wood's second example illustrates the possibility that within what is basically a distributed network, certain cells may be especially critical for processing particular types of input or for producing certain sorts of output. A network might, for instance, operate on more than one type of input – say, auditory and visual. Even if the cells that provide the entry points for a particular input – say, visual – play a role equivalent to that of any other cell in the network when the *other* type of input – the auditory – is being processed, they will obviously play a disproportionately important role in processing the visual input, for which they provide the entry point. A lesion within this set of cells will differ in principle from a disconnection in having some effect (at least) on the performance of non-visual tasks that use the system, although this may not be detectable. The lesion will, however, have much greater effect on visual tasks. Moreover, the cells onto which the visual input cells synapse directly will also be disproportionately important for tasks involving visual rather than auditory input, unless the network is properly distributed for all cells other than input ones. Any partial 'layering' within the network (see Rumelhart & Zipser, 1985) will lead to the disproportionate effect of a lesion extending farther into the system. Damage within what could be called an 'imperfectly distributed network' will therefore have a tendency to produce dissociations between the processing of different types of input (possibility 6). This type of situation is a possible explanation for certain disorders of semantic memory, to be discussed in chapter 12 as access disorders.[11]

---

10. The reason for the exclusion of trend dissociations is given in footnote 13. A 'properly' distributed memory system would be one in which there is no large variation between different parts of the network in the probability of a randomly selected neuron being important for any given operation. As far as I know, the claim in the text has not been refuted for any existing distributed memory model.

11. For the equivalent disorders arising from lesions towards the output end of a network, a possible name is a 'retrieval' disorder. The relation between 'access' and 'retrieval' disorders *conceived of in this way* and Freud's (1891) arguments, discussed in section 11.1, should be noted.

The primary conclusion of this section is, however, that there is as yet no suggestion that a strong double dissociation can take place from two lesions within a properly distributed network.

11.4 The Degree of Specialisation and the Depth of Dissociations

The architectures discussed in sections 11.2 and 11.3 differ in their degree of specialisation. Modules are highly specialised for particular operations. A region within two overlapping subsystems is somewhat less specialised. Sub-parts of properly distributed neural networks are apparently completely unspecialised. However, as discussed in section 11.3, regions within an imperfectly distributed network can differ in their degree of specialisation, regions 'close' to input neurons being more specialised than those deeper in the system.

Can this concept of degree of specialisation be made more rigorous? In chapter 10, a procedure was developed to compare how well a lesioned system behaved in carrying out different types of task. The variation in observed performance across the tasks is not a suitable measure, since it is confounded by differences in task difficulty. Instead, it was suggested that if performance is measured in terms of the amount of resource required, then the effect of a lesion on the performance of different tasks can be compared more satisfactorily.

Can this framework be used in principle to make inferences about the degree of specialisation of the part of the system affected by a lesion? One possibility is to utilise the variability in the degree of resource loss across a patient's performance of tasks that require the system. The greater the difference in resource losses across the performance of different tasks, the more specialised the region affected by the lesion will tend to be. More formally, the greater is the lower bound for the degree of functional specialisation.[12] The *depth* of an observed dissociation – the difference in resource loss across a critical pair of tasks – becomes a means of estimating the minimum degree of specialisation of that part of the overall system that is damaged.

The answer to the problem of what can be inferred about the normal functional architecture of a system for a dissociation therefore becomes close to a definition. The concept of a *functionally dissociable subsystem* claimed in Shallice (1979b) for what could be inferred has been replaced by the wider concept of the *functional specialisation* of part of a system. Is this concept useful or potentially misleading? With one possible exception and one proviso, the concept fits appropriately all cases considered in this chapter. The possible exception is that of multi-level systems (section 11.2), where it is necessary to think of specialisation as referring to a process rather than a physical part of the whole system. The proviso is that the claim made in section 11.3 is valid – that is, that lesions well within a properly

---

12. This formulation needs to be rather convoluted because it would appear that the complementary relation does not hold. Damage to a highly specialised component might have an equivalent effect on all the tasks that use a system; consider the effect of a fault in the power supply to a computer.

distributed memory system will not give rise to a classical or strong double disso-ciation.[13]

It remains logically possible that specialisation, as defined in this way, could have no functional relevance. In biological systems, this seems implausible. What does remain conceivable is that in particular cases, the pattern of resource specialisa-tion might throw no useful light on what function is responsible for the special-isation. If and when examples of this are found will be the time to begin to consider this possibility. For the present, a reasonable conclusion is that determining the degree of specialisation within a system is a useful guide to system architecture and its functional organisation.

11.5   Specifying the Forms of Functional Specialisation

On the approach presented in section 11.4, the existence of a neuropsychological double dissociation signifies that at least part of an overall system is functionally specialised. Earlier in this chapter, it was pointed out that functional specialisation can take a variety of forms. Fodor's (1983) module is only one end of a range of possibilities. Can neuropsychological evidence help to narrow down the forms that the architecture can take in a given processing domain?

There seem to be a number of possibilities based on the dissociation approach outlined earlier.

A Common Dissociation Site Across Patients

In some functional architectures – the more discrete ones – the possible lines of functional cleavage are limited. In others – in particular, the continuum (possibility 1) – there are an infinite number of possible lines of cleavage. Thus if patients exhibiting related dissociations have the same lines of functional cleavage when many are a priori possible, it is likely that the underlying architecture is organised in a discrete fashion (which includes possibilities 2, 3, and 4). But if patients differ in where in the same domain the functional line of cleavage lies, then this supports the continuum possibility or an imperfectly distributed memory system.[14] An ex-

---

13. The effect of two lesions to a distributed system can easily result in a trend double dissociation. Any given lesion will produce a small resource difference between its effects on two separate tasks, and another lesion could well give a complementary resource difference. If the average resource loss is the same for the two lesions, then the pair of complementary resource differences will man-ifest itself in performance as a *trend* double dissociation. This provides yet another reason why trend dissociations should be rejected as an unsuitable basis for theoretical inferences to normal function on methodological grounds. They do not guarantee a sizeable resource difference.

14. This argument presupposes that one can place the tasks themselves on a continuum. Yet many dissociations concern the performance of qualitatively different operations; consider, for instance, phonological reading contrasted with reading for meaning in the context of the double dissociations between them, discussed in chapter 5. For qualitatively different operations, that dissociations are replicable does not give any particular support to the existence of isolable subsystems. The positive argument for the relevance of replication is restricted to task dimensions that are continua or ordinal ones with a considerable number of steps, such as imageability, duration of memory, and the size of spelling-to-sound translation unit.

ample of this type of argument will be given in chapter 12, when impairments of the semantic system are discussed.

The Pattern of Dissociations Across Patients

This type of argument can be extended to the overall pattern of dissociations across patients. Thus an isolable systems architecture allows for the possibility of a disconnection between subsystems, each of which is functioning normally. This possibility would seem difficult to realise in the overlapping subsystems and imperfectly distributed network architectures and impossible in the multi-level system (possibility 5). Thus the evidence that in deep dyslexia, the input orthographic and output phonological processes are relatively intact, but direct transmission between them is not possible, suggests that these two processes are indeed carried out by separate subsystems.

The Measurement of the Amount of Resource-Loss Difference

For some types of functional architecture, the maximum difference in resource loss that can exist for any two tasks will be limited. This is true, for instance, of overlapping subsystems (possibility 2) and of certain types of imperfectly distributed networks. Thus if any really deep dissociation is observed, such alternatives could in theory be ruled out. For instance consider non-semantic reading patients like WLP or KT, whose orthographic and phonological abilities seem virtually unscathed and for whom semantic processing, even of high-frequency words, is grossly impaired (chapter 5). It would seem very difficult to explain such a deep dissociation on the basis of any theory that held that there was considerable overlap between the structures required for orthographic or phonological analysis and those required for semantic ones. Semantic processes seem likely to be carried out by subsystems separate from those involved in the other two processes.[15]

Correspondences with Other Experimental Paradigms

There are, of course, other procedures available for investigating the functional architecture. If a double dissociation indicates the same lines of functional specialisation as, say, dual-task experiments in normal subjects, the range of alternative interpretations is much reduced. Of the range of functional architectures discussed in this chapter, only the continuum possibility, apart from the modular one, one would predict that two tasks that dissociate in patients should be capable of being

---

15. The argument in the text rules out possibilities 2, 4, and 6. Possibility 3 – coupled systems – seems an implausible candidate for the relation between phonological and semantic processing. The same applies for possibility 5, that one structure operates in two different modes, since the two processes seem likely to be most effective if they operate together in real time.

carried out together in normal subjects.[16] An example of this type of argument was given in chapter 7, where the inference from dissociations that input and output phonological word-form systems are isolable was supported from normal experiments. Two tasks can be performed together, each of which requires one of the two subsystems.

11.6   More Specific Functional Architectures: Cascade and Distributed-Memory Models

The type of approach discussed in section 11.5 is that of using empirical findings to gradually narrow the range of theoretical possibilities; it was advocated by Broadbent (1958), but is rarely adopted. The more frequently adopted alternative is to explore the implications of one theoretical possibility – in this case, for the type of functional architecture – using the empirical findings for theory testing. In the past, neuropsychological investigations usually took as an underlying premise the assumption of isolable subsystems, being concerned with the nature and organisation of these subcomponents of the overall system, as discussed in chapter 10. In fact, there have been few attempts to explore the consequence of findings for other architectures or even for determining the specific type of architecture within the broad class of isolable subsystems. The one example of a specific architecture within the broad class of isolable subsystems that has been used to explain specific findings is the cascade model, in which the output of one of a series of sub-process is held to feed continuously into the next (e.g. McClelland & Rumelhart, 1981).[17] Such a model has been employed to account for observations on anomia, the inability to name from picture or definition or in spontaneous speech (Miller & Ellis, 1987), agrammatism (Stemberger, 1985), agnosia (Humphreys, Riddoch, & Quinlan, 1988), and deep dyslexia (Shallice & McGill, 1978).

Cascade models have two aspects. First, subprocesses at different levels overlap in time. Standard neuropsychological findings that do not involve reaction times do not speak to this aspect of the model. They can, however, speak to the other aspect – that outputs from one subprocess to the next are not all-or-none. Neuropsychological results can definitely be compatible with this assumption. Whether they have yet provided strong support for it is less clear. Consider one example, the attempt

16. This is a considerable simplification. For a discussion of the methodological requirements for inferences from dual-task paradigms to the underlying architecture, see Shallice, McLeod and Lewis (1985). Their most basic assumption is that 'general' interference can be differentiated from 'structural' interference.

17. If a cascade model is 'layered', to use the terminology of Rumelhart and Zipser (1985), it can be viewed as a series of isolable subsystems, each transmitting continuously to the next layer up. The layered cascade model can be compared with what is often thought of as the prototypic type of isolable system – the simple stages model of Sternberg (1969) – in which information is transmitted to later stages only when a stage completes processing. A simple stages model will, in general, be thought of as the more isolable because during the periods when the processing in a stage is being carried out, it is not influenced by the operation of other subsystems. It should be noted that the simple stages model and the layered cascade model are equally specialised.

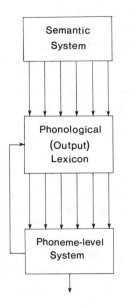

Figure 11.4. Model of the processes involved in word selection and production in speech adopted by Miller and Ellis (1987).

by Miller and Ellis (1987) to explain the paraphasic errors produced in naming, reading aloud, and spontaneous speech by an anomic patient, RD. RD had had a left hemisphere stroke, which had left him with a severe Wernicke's aphasia; his comprehension of spoken speech was very poor and his spontaneous speech was fluent and well articulated, but many paraphasic errors occurred. There were two aspects of RD's anomia with which Miller and Ellis were particularly concerned. The first was the strong effects of word frequency on naming performance (high frequency, 72% correct; low frequency, 24%). The second was the way that the paraphasic errors tended to be phonologically similar to the correct word. This effect was particularly striking when the number of syllables in the actual response and in the correct word were compared. Out of 60 paraphasic errors made to one-, two-, and three-syllable words, for 95% the number of syllables was the same as in the target stimulus.

The findings of Miller and Ellis (1987) on anomia were not in themselves very surprising; frequency effects and literal paraphasias are well-known phenomena in aphasic naming problems. It was the explanation they provided that was both novel and plausible. They argued that these aspects of RD's anomia arise because the flow of activation between the semantic system and the phonological output lexicon is greatly reduced (Figure 11.4). The frequency effect was held to occur because the word-forms in the phonological output lexicon (word-form) system have high resting levels of activation and require only a small input to be produced accurately.

For less frequent words, though, with lower resting levels of activation, the weak input is 'insufficient' to subdue neighboring word-forms, and so only weak activation is passed down to the phoneme level. Phonological approximations to the intended word, containing some correct phonemes and some incorrect ones, therefore occur.

There is, however, a problem with this type of explanation. It is rather unconstrained. The results are targeted against one hypothesis rather than in favour of another. Miller and Ellis (1987) argued that a specific version of the modular position – Morton's (1970) logogen model – could not explain their results. Logogens are held by Morton to have all-or-nothing thresholds, so once the activity level reaches threshold, a full specification of the phonemic structure of the word is available. If the damage preceded the attainment of the phonemic structure, a frequency effect would be expected, but *not* errors that are phonological approximations to the intended word. If the damage was after that point in the flow of information, then phonological confusions should indeed occur, but on high-frequency words as much as on low-frequency ones. However, no argument is presented that some unit functionally equivalent to the phonological output lexicon, using a different algorithm and mechanism from the logogen, could not produce these two types of effect together if it were damaged.[18]

Miller and Ellis argued for a cascade model in which the lesion affects the pathway between the semantic system and the phonological lexicon. Yet might similar effects not be predicted from partial damage to the lexicon itself or the pathway connecting it to the phoneme-level system? Or consider the possibility of a distributed network that received input from the semantic system that was not in cascade form and that produced a specification of word structure as an organised set of distinctive features. What would happen if such a network were damaged? Word frequency would be likely to have an effect, and its output also seems likely to be a phonological approximation to the target. It would obviously depend on how it was damaged, but might it not produce a set of phenomena similar to those observed in RD?

How is the argument provided by Miller and Ellis (1987) to be assessed? Do the findings provide support for one type of architecture, the cascade type, over others? Miller and Ellis did not show that their findings are incompatible with other possible architectures. There is an additional problem about the support their results provide for a cascade model. It is dangerous to rely on post hoc purely verbal deductions about the effects that damage might have in a complex model. There are too many possible interactions that cannot be foreseen. If a simulation of this model were to be carried out and it was shown that damage to a certain component did lead to a particular set of consequences – even if they were only qualitatively specified – the existence of patients with these symptoms would indeed provide positive support

18. In fact, no argument is presented that the results could not be explained on Morton's (1970) model by two lesions: one to the phonological output lexicon, and the other at a later stage. In the argument in the text, I follow Miller and Ellis (1987) in assuming one lesion site, but this is an uncorroborated assumption.

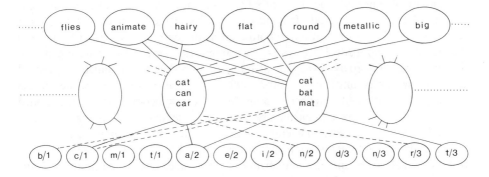

Figure 11.5. Hinton and Sejnowski's (1986) model of reading-to-meaning of individual words. The input units are at the bottom, and the output units, at the top. The semantic feature labels and hidden unit characteristics suggested (e.g. *cat, can, car*) are included for illustrative purposes only. The actual simulation used random 'semantic features'.

for the model. Until that is achieved, the type of analysis given by Miller and Ellis provides only a suggestion that a particular line of research has promise.[19]

A beginning has been made to assess the effects of lesions in another architecture, that in which an individual subsystem is of a distributed-memory type. Hinton and Sejnowski (1986) have simulated reading-to-meaning by a model with three subsystems: an input graphemic one, an output semantic one, and an intermediate one (Figure 11.5). The input subsystem contained a set of 30 graphemic units, each representing a letter in a particular position in words. The output subsystem also contained 30 units, each representing different semantic features. Units in the graphemic subsystem initially activated all 20 intermediate-level units to some extent, and they, in turn, activated all the semantic units. The intermediate level – the 'hidden' units – therefore operated in a distributed-memory fashion. The model was trained with 20 different three-letter word-meaning pairs presented many times in a given order. A learning procedure was used by which the 'weights' of the synaptic connections are altered after any trial in such a way that, on average, a small step is made towards the (unknown) optimal set of weights.[20] After 5,000

19. As an example of the ease with which it is possible to make appropriate verbal predictions about the effects of damage to complex models, consider the account given by Miller and Ellis (1987) of the perseverations that are another aspect of RD's anomia. They argue that 'weak activation reaching the phoneme level will result in a failure to inhibit units for phonemes activated earlier in previous pronunciations of words. Thus phonemes from earlier words and neologisms will tend to intrude into current efforts as perseverations.' This sounds plausible, but without an explanation of how activation is switched off after a word has been produced in the normal state, this explanation is completely ad hoc.

20. The reason for not directly associating input (graphemic) units to output (semantic) units in an analogous fashion to that shown in Figure 11.3 is that it is known that simple two-level distributed networks are incapable of learning certain input–output mappings (see, e.g. Minsky & Papert, 1969; Rumelhart, Hinton, & Williams, 1986). Technically, the system uses the so-called Boltzmann machine learning algorithm (see Ackley, Hinton, & Sejnowski, 1985).

learning trials, a performance level of 99.9% accuracy was achieved by the system!

How the system behaved after individual units at the intermediate level were removed was then tested; in other words, an analogue of a very small lesion was made. The system made 1.4% errors. Two interesting similarities were noted with the behaviour of deep dyslexic patients (chapter 5), although, of course, the overall error rate was very much lower. First, 59% of the errors consisted of the precise meaning of an alternative grapheme string. When it was incorrect, the system tended to produce explicit errors, not merely arbitrary collections of semantic features. Second, these errors were, on average, both semantically more similar and visually more similar to the target word than an average member of the set. The coexistence of both visual errors and semantic errors is, of course, one of the intuitively surprising characteristics of deep dyslexia.

This investigation was not an attempt to simulate deep dyslexia. It indicates, however, that mimicking lesions in systems with complex architectures could be a most interesting theoretical development for cognitive neuropsychology.[21]

11.7 Conclusion

Where has the tortuous path travelled in this and the previous chapter taken us? Chapter 10 concerned the variety of alternative possibilities that need to be considered before deciding that neuropsychological findings should be explained through the *subtraction assumption* – that is, by the operation of the normal system with some components impaired. At each stage in the argument, the elimination of alternative explanations required assumptions that were plausible but not watertight. The bedrock of the approach, it was argued, should be the double dissociation. In this chapter, the security of assuming a modular architecture has been abandoned. It was shown that if the subtraction process is assumed to apply, functional specialisation follows from double dissociations. To determine which form this specialisation takes requires consideration of a range of possibilities. At present, though, the methods for determining which architecture is the most appropriate for a given domain are not that strong.

These arguments have implications both for the concrete inferences drawn from the dissociations discussed in earlier chapters and for the usefulness of the general approach of analysing dissociations. How valid were the concrete inferences made in earlier chapters when viewed from the standpoint of the inferential methodology developed in this part of the book? It would be most laborious to reconsider all the arguments in detail at this stage. The most critical point is that for many of the double dissociations discussed, both the dissociations have been at least strong. Examples are those between span and verbal LTS, between span and speech production, between visual object processing and word reading, between reading-to-

---

21. Another very interesting aspect of the system is its ability to be rapidly retrained if noise has been added to the weights and has much depressed performance. Hinton and Sejnowski (1986) speculate that this effect might relate to 'spontaneous recovery' shown by neurological patients, a process that is not understood.

meaning and reading aloud, between reading non-words and reading irregular words, between non-lexical and lexical (semantic) spelling, and between producing syntax and producing content words in spontaneous speech. In none of these are any of the task-demand, resource, individual-difference, and reorganisation artefacts plausible.[22] It is not easy to assess whether any of the alternative architectures discussed in this chapter would account for any of the double dissociations better than the isolable subsystem position put forward earlier. However, in most of these cases, the overall pattern of complementary dissociations across patients makes the isolable processing system view a plausible one.[23]

Turning to general implications of the discussion in this and the preceding chapter, should one be dispirited by the complexity of the inferences necessary to draw theoretical conclusions from an observed dissociation? This would not be justified. Precise measures that directly reflect significant aspects of the functional organisation of the cognitive system do not exist. Hence any empirical procedure that stands a reasonable chance of helping to uncover the functional charateristics of the system is likely to involve as many assumptions as does the use of neuropsychological findings.

Whether the approach advocated in this book will prove to be theoretically valuable depends on the general nature of the functional architecture of the cognitive system. If it is in some sense modular, the approach is clearly appropriate, although for any particular dissociation, the alternative possibilities discussed here and in chapter 10 need to be considered. The opposite possibility, that there is a general lack of functional specialisation, can be eliminated, given that the argument of this chapter is valid; the variety and prevalence of strong dissociations are sufficient grounds to reject it.

The intermediate possibilities are more difficult to assess. If there is indeed a high degree of functional specialisation but it generally takes a more complex form than a set of isolable subsystems, then neuropsychological evidence should prove fruitful. It was argued in section 11.6 that neuropsychological findings might well prove to be one of a few types of evidence that will allow the nature of the architecture to be much more tightly specified. It is likely that the development of an empirically sound theory of a complex architecture will be a long process. A useful transitional stage would be to obtain the closest theory based on isolable subsystems, since such an approach uses concepts that are relatively easy to articulate and test. Indeed, it is noteworthy that when simulations of distributed-memory models

22. This statement may need to be modified with respect to individual differences. Thus Bryant and Impey (1986) have recently shown that there is a very wide span of individual differences in the ability of normal reading children to read non-words and irregular words. In my view, this is most easily explained in terms of individual differences in the development of different 'routes'. However, without additional evidence, the defence is clearly circular. To what extent the differences are maintained in adult readers is also not known.

23. An exception would be the double dissociation between irregular-word and non-word reading. Here, the continuum view was preferred (chapter 5). Another would be the syntactic and semantic production pair, which was discussed in chapter 7.

– apparently the least modular of models – have been applied to concrete situations, they have generally used sets of units, each of which has a different function. In other words, theorists based the distributed network on a set of isolable subsystems. Any line of evidence that models using isolable subsystems cannot explain should point the way to more complex possibilities. The dissociation would therefore provide the stepping-stone to a satisfactory theory.

This leaves one possibility. Maybe the cognitive system is basically designed on distributed principles, but in the concrete implementation of these principles, regions of measured functional specialisation occur. It could be that the apparent function of these regions of functional specialisation is, in effect, an artefact. To attend to them could lead the investigation away from the basic design principles of the system rather than towards them. Then, but only then, will the analysis of the neuropsychological dissociation prove a snare and a delusion to the theorist. It is a risk worth taking.

From this stage on, these methodological cautions will be abandoned. In general, it will be assumed that a (double) dissociation signifies the existence of an isolable subsystem. Inferential traps and alternative architectures will at times be considered. However, the main aim is to determine whether neuropsychological evidence can throw light on psychological issues deeper and more complex than, say, how the orthographic analysis of words is carried out. Avoiding being deceived by a tempting shadow will be less important than dimly making out the existence of some possible path.

Part IV

Central Processes: Equipotentiality or Modularity?

12   Selective Impairments of Knowledge

12.1   Introduction

One of the major causes of the sea-change in psychology that occurred in the 1960s was that the nature and organisation of knowledge, a topic that had been virtually dormant, began to become a highly active area of research. This increase of interest in the field did not, however, lead to any great degree of agreement. Views became polarised on a range of issues. Are the systems that mediate knowledge in some sense distinct from other cognitive systems, particularly those having the processes that underlie our experience of a memory? Are different types of knowledge the province of distinct semantic systems, or does all knowledge depend on a system that has a common operating principle? Is knowledge mediated by the operation of networks or schemata? Is it based on individual instances, prototypes, or what? Is there a special status for so-called basic level concepts (Rosch, Mervis, Gray, Johnson, & Boyes-Braem, 1976) – the highest level at which all members have many perceptual attributes in common – for example, *dog, knife,* and *apple?*

The wealth of experiments that have been carried out in normal subjects does not exist for neurological patients. Yet the findings that have been obtained are both surprising and highly counterintuitive. In this chapter, I will not attempt a survey. Rather, I will consider whether neuropsychological findings exist that bear on major theoretical issues in the analysis of the cognitive basis of knowledge in normal subjects and, in particular, on its modular structure.[1] I will begin, however, with an even more basic issue – whether there are grounds for assuming that central systems might be organised very differently from peripheral ones.

12.2   Are Central Systems Non-modular? The Case of Acalculia

The position that more central systems may not be modular, even though more peripheral ones are, was elegantly expounded by Fodor (1983), primarily on philo-

---

1. In the earlier part of the book, since the stress was on the possible theoretical relevance of the dissociations, it was natural to introduce each dissociation prior to theoretical discussion. In this section, however, the bearing that neuropsychological evidence has on wider theoretical issues is the theme, and the dissociations discussed are often much more isolated from one another than are those discussed earlier. Theoretical arguments will therefore frequently be used to situate the dissociations.

269

sophical grounds. He argued that only input systems are modular. If one draws the line between input and central systems appropriately, then knowledge would be the product of a diffuse equipotentially organised system. Dissociations within it would not therefore be expected.

Fodor's argument has been very influential. Moreover, the general form of his conclusions is of sufficient importance for my thesis in this and the following chapter that it is relevant to describe it briefly. The core of the argument is a piece of conceptual analysis that is striking but far from clear. He took two highly plausible and seemingly unconnected propositions. The first is that the critical property of modularity is *informational encapsulation*. By this, as was discussed in chapter 2, he meant that a module has access to only certain types of information; much of the information stored in the cognitive system is not available to it. The second is that in science, a theory can in principle be confirmed or refuted by any type of evidence; there are no boundaries on the information that may be relevant.

In a dazzling series of conceptual moves, Fodor linked the two apparently unrelated propositions. Scientific inference is not only in principle conceptually unbounded, but also in practice so whenever an unexpected analogy is used. Thus it cannot be produced by a system composed only of modules, each of which has no knowledge about most of the information stored in the rest of the cognitive system. The next step was to argue that there is nothing special about the thought processes involved in science. Thought in general, right down to the humble level of understanding the meaning of sentences, must not be informationally encapsulated. Finally, and almost implicitly, there is the step, that because qualitatively similar tasks – say, understanding a set of sentences – may be carried out using different procedures on different occasions, there are mechanisms involved in the carrying out of the task on any particular occasion that are not informationally encapsulated. It then follows that the comprehension of sentences depends on a system that is not informationally encapsulated and therefore not modular. The cognitive system is therefore divided into two parts: the input systems, which are modular, and the central systems, which begin at the level of the comprehension of sentences and which are equipotential. Fodor would, no doubt, accept Marshall's (1984a) suggestion that output systems, too, are modular.[2]

---

2. Fodor (1983) attempts to buttress his philosophical argument for the existence of non-modular systems by two semi-empirical arguments. The first is the claim that artificial intelligence has not developed an effective modular theory of thought, an argument that seems historically a little premature. The second is from neuropsychology or, to be more precise, from the table of contents of the September 1979 issue of *Scientific American,* which was concerned with neuropsychology. 'There are, as you might expect, articles that cover the neuropsychology of language and of the perceptual mechanisms. But there is nothing on the neuropsychology of thought – presumably because nothing is known on the neuropsychology of thought. I am suggesting that there is good reason why nothing is known about it – namely that there is nothing to know about it . . . in the case of central processes, you get an approximation to universal connectivity, hence no stable neural architecture to write *Scientific American* articles about' (Fodor, 1983, p. 119)! It has indeed been more difficult to isolate central subsystems than input ones, which might suggest that the former are less modular than the latter. From within the field, it is apparent that even if central systems are modular, they would be

Fodor's philosophical argument is not compelling. However, it certainly shows that it is dangerous to extrapolate unthinkingly from the probable modularity of input systems to the probable modularity of more central ones. It places on the intellectual agenda the possibility that central systems might operate on quite different basic ground rules from input systems. The position that central systems are equipotential, not modular, will therefore be considered not only in this chapter, but also in chapter 14. To assess Fodor's theory empirically, one needs to be able to situate the supposed division between input and central systems, or, as Fodor called it, the observation–inference interface. The main criterion that Fodor used is whether an operation is mandatory, given a particular input. If it is, it is carried out by modular input systems; if it is not, by equipotential central ones. So one cannot *not* see a certain visual display as consisting of objects in three dimensions. One cannot respond in some way to the written word *red* and *not* know, at some level, that it refers to a colour. Using this criterion, processes involved in achieving some, but not all, aspects of the meaning of *individual* words are contained in the modular input systems, as is a syntactic parse of the sentence; but sentence comprehension requires central systems.[3]

Any knowledge process that is dependent on sentence-level comprehension would be central. Is this, in fact, a reasonable boundary for differentiating input and central processes? Is this the upper limit for the functions giving rise to specific dissociations, as Fodor would predict?

Consider doing simple sums as an example of a routine skill that depends on knowledge. For an arithmetic operation to be carried out requires a prior stage of understanding the sum – sentence-level comprehension – which should be central, and the actual computation is not an automatic process. It requires intention, will, and concentration. Even with subtractions as simple as $13 - 5$, Warrington (1982c) found that highly intelligent subjects in their 60s took longer than 3 sec on 10% of trials – clearly longer than an automatic response would take. Also on Fodor's (1983) view, modular subsystems are innate and are not assembled from more basic processes. In fact, developmental research by Young and O'Shea (1981) strongly suggests that a skill like subtraction is acquired in a series of discrete steps and not

much more difficult to investigate, so the argument is not at all compelling. In fact, although the Scientific American failed to consider frontal lobe lesions (chapter 14), for instance, their effects were well known – even in 1979! For criticisms of Fodor's philosophical argument, see Shallice (1984).

3. Fodor (1983) says that recent experiments 'strongly suggest that input processing for language provides no semantic analysis "inside" lexical items . . . the functionally defined level *output of the language processing module* respects such *structurally* defined notions as *items in the morphemic inventory of the language*' (p. 92). However, he also accepts (p. 80) a Collins and Loftus (1975) type of semantic network as being within the language-processing module. Therefore, it would appear that the automatic processes that can be mediated by spreading activation between nodes, each corresponding to an individual morpheme, are not 'semantic analysis' in the sense of the previous quotation. For visual object recognition, he assumes the input system to end at the level of the attainment of the basic category, which he says 'can be made with reasonable reliability, on the basis of the visual properties of objects' (p. 97).

Table 12.1. *WAIS scaled subtest scores for DRC*

Arithmetic	4	Picture Completion	10
Similarities	11	Block Design	12
Digit Span	14	Picture Arrangement	12
Vocabulary	14		

From Warrington (1982c)

by a single maturational process. Therefore, on Fodor's view, there should be no selective deficits of calculation.

The facts of acalculia – disorders of calculation – would appear to be otherwise. Acalculia itself has been treated as a neurological symptom since at least the time of Henschen (1919), who considered it to be functionally largely independent of aphasia, alexia, and agraphia, even though the disorders frequently co-occur (see also Boller & Grafman, 1983). After Henschen, however, acalculia was not a major topic within clinical neuropsychology, being treated chiefly as a subcomponent of the Gerstmann syndrome (see, e.g., Benton, 1977), which was discussed in chapter 2. Number processing has, however, recently begun to attract the attention of cognitive neuropsychologists (see, e.g., McCloskey, Caramazza, & Basili, 1985; Deloche & Seron, in press).

The first detailed analysis of a form of acalculia from a cognitive neuropsychology approach (Warrington, 1982c) concerned the isolation of knowledge of arithmetic facts. The patient, DRC, was a consultant physician, who became severely acalculic following a left parieto-occipital haematoma. A month later, he was scoring at normal level on language, reading, and memory tests. The selective nature of his arithmetic deficit is shown in Table 12.1, which gives the WAIS results. The Arithmetic subtest is at least 2 standard deviations below the other tests, and the set of dissociations is close to being a classical one. It provides strong neuropsychological evidence for an isolable subsystem.[4]

What process would such a subsystem be carrying out? The first sign of DRC's arithmetic difficulty occurred when shortly after his stroke, he was asked to solve $5 + 7$; he replied, '13 roughly'. This type of arithmetic operation was examined quantitatively, and his performance compared with that of five consultant physicians of similar age. The results of a series of tests of very elementary calculations are shown in Table 12.2. These include sums like 4 add 2, 11 add 3, 6 take away 2, 18 take away 5, and 4 multiplied by 3. It is obvious that for DRC, simple arithmetic was no longer the routine matter that he was adamant it had been before his illness.

Within the domain of skills relevant to arithmetic, it was DRC's knowledge of elementary arithmetic facts that was specifically impaired. When tackling the WAIS Arithmetic subtest, DRC had reasoned aloud, and so his ability to perform the

4. The pattern of performance on other demanding subtests rules out a resource artefact.

Table 12.2. *Performance of DRC on simple arithmetic sums*

	Range of number			Errors	Response latency (%)		
Operation	First	Second	Subject	(%)	0–2 sec	3–5 sec	⩾6 sec
Addition	1–9	1–9	DRC	11	74	17	8
Addition	11–19	1–9	DRC	8	55	26	19
			Control	0	97	2	<1
Subtraction	1–9	1–9	DRC	8	72	20	8
Subtraction	11–9	1–9	DRC	18	31	34	35
			Control	0	90	10	<1
Multiplication	2–9	2–9	DRC	9	76	12	12
			Control	0	98	2	<1

Response latency is given in terms of frequency within 3 ranges.
From Warrington (1982c)

appropriate sequence of operations was clear. For instance, given the question that many people fail, 'A man earns £60 a week; if 15% is withheld in taxes, how much does he receive a week?' he said, 'so we do it 10% first, is £6, half of that is £3, equals £9, 60 minus 9 is £51''. This, however, took over 1 min because the individual calculations were very difficult for him. On a variety of other tests that assess number knowledge, he performed normally. For instance, he estimated the number of dots presented in a 2-sec exposure as accurately as controls and was as good in a test that requires estimates of magnitude, such as 'How far is it from London to New York?'

The nature of the dissociation is clearly shown in DRC's performance on Hitch's (1978) test of numerical abilities. This test has three components, each with various subtests:

1. A test of speed and accuracy of elementary arithmetic.
2. A test of manipulation and conversion of decimals, fractions, and percentages in which the numerical element is relatively simple.
3. A test of appreciation of numbers and evaluation of arithmetic expressions.

He was significantly impaired in 4/6 of the subtests of the first type and in none of the others.

The example of DRC's specific acalculia suggests that there are as good neuro-psychological grounds for postulating modularity for certain processes that follow sentence comprehension as for those that lead up to it. It would seem likely that when a particular type of arithmetic knowledge is called on, the processes involved in accessing and retrieving that knowledge are isolable from other thought processes. A similar conclusion seems plausible for other higher processes that are routine. At the very least, this type of finding calls for an alteration to Fodor's (1983) thesis. 'Central' systems need to be subdivided. Part of them at least, seem to be modular (for a related view, see Schwartz & Schwartz, 1984).

12.3 General Impairments of Knowledge

Arithmetic facts are a rather atypical area of knowledge. It is easy to see how they might be retained in some special-purpose subsystem. Should one generalise from this example? Is it plausible that more standard areas of knowledge, such as those concerned with the meanings of words and the functions and properties of objects, are also stored in isolable subsystems?

Individual-case studies of patients whose disorder has been analysed within the context of a modern psychological approach to knowledge – 'semantic memory' – began with a study by Warrington (1975).[5] Each of the main subjects of this study, AB and EM, had a dementing illness that resulted in diffuse brain disease. Warrington argued that their primary functional impairment was one of semantic memory. Related investigations of patients with a qualitatively similar condition arising from a rather similar illness have been undertaken by Schwartz, Marin, and Saffran (1979), on patient WLP, and by Martin and Fedio (1983), in a group study.[6]

The performance of AB and EM on many baseline tests was very well preserved. AB had a verbal IQ of 122, and EM a performance IQ of 117. The primary symptom of the two patients was a blunting of their knowledge of words and of the significance of objects, an impairment that had been observed in a group study of patients with Alzheimer's disease (Irigaray, 1973). In Warrington's investigation, AB's and EM's knowledge of the meanings of words was assessed in a number of ways. One procedure was simply to ask the two patients to define words. As the patients showed no signs of any expressive aphasic difficulty, except for a somewhat limited vocabulary, they were capable of giving succinct and accurate definitions when they knew words. This was particularly striking in AB. Thus he defined *supplication* as 'making a serious request for help'. However, he gave responses such as 'I've forgotten' or 'No idea' to words like *hay, trumpet, needle,* and *cottage.* To *geese,* he said, 'An animal but I've forgotten precisely'. There were strong effects of word frequency on their ability to provide definitions. Thus AB gave adequate definitions for 96% of the A or AA words, but for only 51% of the ones of lower frequency. For EM, the corresponding values were also 96% and 51%.

As both patients could repeat words they could not define, an explanation in terms of auditory perceptual difficulties can be rejected. A production-deficit account can also be rejected because similar difficulties occurred in tasks where definitions did not have to be produced. The patients were asked simple questions about animals or objects, such as for the word *swan:* 'Is it an animal or an object?' 'Is it

---

5. Before the mid-1970s, studies of the semantic difficulties of aphasic patients had taken place (e.g. Weigl & Bierwisch, 1970). Apart from some clinical case studies lacking in quantitative baseline data, they were generally group studies using the fluent/non-fluent division (for a review, see Lesser, 1978) or approached the topic from a specifically linguistic perspective (e.g. Marshall, Newcombe, & Marshall, 1970).

6. The reading of both WLP and EM has been considered in chapter 5. Warrington's (1975) study included a third patient, CR. His impairments were less specific, so I have not considered his data.

Table 12.3. *Percentage errors made by AB and EM at answering two-alternative factual questions (e.g. Is it a bird?) about animals or object names*

	Animal or object?	Animals		Objects	
		Bird?	English?	Indoors?	Metal?
AB	28	25	30	25	45
EM	15	35	40	20	45
Controls	<1	3	6	4	2

Table 12.4. *The visual analogue of the experiment shown in Table 12.3*

	Animal or object?	Animals			Objects		
		Bird?	English?	Two-alternative forced-choice[a]	Indoors?	Metal?	Two-alternative forced-choice[a]
AB	8	35	55	60	20	10	60
EM	3	5	45	35	5	10	40
Controls	1	2	8	7	1	3	0

[a] Two pictures in the same category are presented together, with the question 'Which is the X?'; it therefore requires both specific verbal and visual knowledge.

a bird?' 'Is it found in England?' The results are shown in Table 12.3. As one would expect, the controls found the task very easy, but the two patients had a devastating deficit.

The impairment of the two patients was not limited to auditory–verbal input. They also had a problem with recognising photographs. Thus when photographs of the animals and objects whose names were used in the above test were shown to the two patients and similar questions were asked, both had problems. The results are shown in Table 12.4. AB would appear to be the more affected. Confirmatory evidence was obtained from a task involving the naming or identifying by description of photographs of familiar objects, of which the lowest frequency were items like *scales* or *sledge*. EM made only 8% errors.[7] AB, however, made 53%! This difficulty in identifying objects visually appeared to be at a semantic level. Thus on the Warrington and Taylor (1978) test of matching objects from a conventional and

7. The issue of whether naming can be carried out by a route that by-passes the semantic system is discussed in section 12.7.

an unconventional view, discussed in chapter 8, both AB and EM scored within the normal range (85% and 100%, respectively). Thus there seems good evidence that both patients have a relatively isolated impairment of semantic processing that, however, affects both verbal and visual input.

How selective can such a deficit be? It turns out that the deficit can be very specific indeed. Many other processes can be dissociated from the semantic one.

Consider the ability to reason. In many patients with dementing diseases, problem solving is impaired. Both AB and EM, however, performed extremely well on problem-solving tasks, given that little or no knowledge was required to obtain the appropriate solution. Thus AB scored in the top 5th percentile on Raven's Matrices, and EM scored in the top 10th percentile. Therefore, a striking classical dissociation exists between reasoning ability and knowledge. Semantic systems for word and object knowledge, like those for arithmetic knowledge, are isolable from other higher level cognitive systems.

The contrast between semantic processing and other types of language operations – syntactic, phonological, and orthographic – has been explored in most detail by Schwartz, Marin, and Saffran (1979; see also Schwartz, Saffran, & Marin, 1980a) in the patient WLP, whose reading was discussed in chapter 5. Like AB and EM, WLP suffered from a severe dementing disease. She was left with a gross difficulty in producing content words in spontaneous speech (see quotation in chapter 7). Her difficulty was also present in comprehension. She was given a picture–word matching test using a series of pictures corresponding to 'basic level' terms (Rosch et al., 1976), such as *spoon, apple,* and *cigarette.*[8] For each picture, WLP was shown a set of five written words, which had to be read aloud. She could almost always read the words aloud correctly, and if she made a reading error, the word was repeated to her. She then had to select the picture's name from among the words. She made 36% errors on the picture–name matching task, almost all of which involved the selection of the one semantic distractor in the set of foils. So for the picture of a *fork* she chose *spoon,* for the picture of a *brush* she chose *comb,* and so on. She was able to mime the appropriate use of the objects for which she selected the wrong name, so it would appear that her difficulty lay within the verbal realm.

Despite her severe semantic difficulties, WLP could read words very well, even when they were irregular (chapter 5), and she could apparently repeat them.[9] Her speech was rapid, clear, relatively free of semantic and phonemic distortions, and syntactically fairly intact. Moreover, her comprehension of semantically reversible sentences using various grammatical constructions, when tested by sentence–picture matching, was nearly perfect, and far better than that of agrammatic aphasics (Table 12.5). Therefore, it would appear that within linguistic processing, just as

8. A basic level term is a label for the highest level of the conceptual hierarchy, which is fairly perceptually homogeneous – for example, *spoon.* Thus *kitchen utensil* is a superordinate, not a basic level, term, while *soup spoon* is a subordinate. Basic level terms are much the most frequent spontaneously given responses in picture naming by normal subjects.

9. No details are given of repetition performance. However, as will be shown later, spared repetition has been demonstrated quantitatively for AB and EM.

Table 12.5. *Errors made by WLP and three Broca's aphasics on the comprehension of semantically reversible sentences (a two-alternative forced-choice test)*

	Active voice ($n=24$) (e.g. 'The cow kicks the horse.')	Passive voice ($n=24$) (e.g. 'The car is pulled by the truck.')	Comparative adjective ($n=48$) (e.g. 'The girl is fatter than the boy.')	Spatial preposition ($n=48$) (e.g. 'The square is over the circle.')
WLP[a]	4	4	1	0
Broca's aphasics				
BL	7	17	12	27
VS	2	10	0	26
HT	12	11	19	25

[a] All WLP's errors were on items where she could not correctly select the lexical items when they were tested in isolation.
From Schwartz, Marin, and Saffran (1979)

within thought in general, specific impairments of semantic processing exist. Word-form level processing, both orthographic and phonological, can be spared, and there are strong suggestions that syntactic processing can be relatively intact.

This range of dissociations, within both the problem-solving and the linguistic realms, makes it plausible that knowledge of the meaning of words is effected by a system that is at least partly isolable from other language and thought processes. What form the isolability takes remains unclear. Thus certain of the dissociations, such as the one between semantic and syntactic processing in language, might turn out to be explicable in terms other than the existence of separate 'modules'. For instance, these two subsystems may well be highly interactive, providing a more complex analogue of the coupled systems discussed in chapter 11.[10]

Two other aspects of the semantic memory disorder of these patients are worth noting. First, EM, at least, was highly consistent in her pattern of responding.

10. See, for instance, theoretical discussions related to cohort theory (e.g. Marslen-Wilson & Tyler, 1980). A related dissociation from which a specific theoretical corollary follows is that concerning semantic memory and span performance. Both AB and EM had word spans in the normal range. Moreover, there was no difference in span between words they still knew and words they had forgotten (AB: 4.4 vs. 4.0; EM: 4.6 vs. 4.2)! By contrast, they were significantly worse on nonsense syllables than on unknown words: For AB, the difference was 1.0 item; for EM, 1.8 items. This pair of findings has the theoretical implication that the poor performance of normal subjects on nonsense syllables is not evidence that span has a secondary-memory component, as has been suggested (chapter 3). If this were the case, span for unknown words in AB and EM should also have been impaired. Instead, it would seem that the phonological familiarity of the units involved is the important factor for span.

Coughlan and Warrington (1981) gave EM the same set of 121 words to define on two occasions seven months apart, during which her illness became somewhat more severe. Her responses were classified by independent judges instructed to use a lenient criterion. For example, for *leaflet,* the definition 'a bit of paper' was treated as correct. Despite the variability inherent in the use of a definition rating as a measure, virtually no word that was not known on the first occasion was known on the second. It appeared that if a word became unavailable for her, it remained lost from her vocabulary.[11]

The second aspect concerns what the patients know about individual items. As the disease process advances, knowledge of the superordinate of an item tends to be the type of information last retained (Warrington, 1975). For instance, when EM was presented with 20 words that she had previously identified by definition using a lax criterion, she made only 2% errors on a three-alternative forced-choice decision concerning category membership: Is *cabbage* an animal, a plant, or an inanimate object? But she made 28% errors on attribute decisions: Is *cabbage green, brown,* or *grey?* EM is not alone in showing relative preservation of superordinate information. Martin and Fedio (1983) noted that a frequent type of naming errors in Alzheimer's patients is to give a superordinate. So *asparagus* is named as a *vegetable,* a *raft* as a *boat,* a *pelican* as a *bird,* and so on.

In these patients, once information has become unavailable, it seems to be permanently lost. In addition, information about attributes is more vulnerable than that about the nature of the superordinate. Word frequency has a large effect: On high-frequency items, the patients did well, but on low-frequency ones, they made many errors. Warrington (1975) therefore argued that the information in the store is itself damaged. By analogy with the terminology used in the memory literature (Tulving & Pearlstone, 1966), the information is no longer available, not merely inaccessible.

In earlier chapters, all types of impairment of any particular subsystem were considered functionally equivalent when viewed in contrast to impairments of other subsystems. This position has been captured axiomatically in chapter 10 by the idea of a subsystem having a unidimensional 'resource'. Within semantic memory impairments, however, it has become useful to distinguish a qualitatively different type of disorder from the 'degraded store' ones discussed in this section. The contrast is, in fact, a general one that is potentially applicable to many subsystems. The other type of impairment is to the access process, rather than to the representation in the store itself.[12]

---

11. The contingency coefficient of 0.58 was close to the maximum possible (0.71). Schwartz, Marin, and Saffran (1979) noted a variability in performance in one of the tasks they gave WLP. However, this was a forced-choice task in which the errors involved the selection of a semantically related 'distractor'. The inconsistency can therefore result from guessing between two equally plausible alternatives on the two occasions, and not from a variability in the available knowledge on the two occasions.

12. In the account of the two types of disorder, I will ignore differences in the critical modality of input for the particular patient being considered.

12.4 Access Disorders

On certain computational theories of word comprehension – for instance, that of Rieger (1978) – it is held that accessing the precise meaning of a word is a complex process that requires a number of stages. To give a concrete example of such a process, one might first access broad categorical information – that a *banana* is a food and then that it is a fruit – then major attribute information – that it is roughly crescent-shaped or that it is yellow or that it comes from the tropics – and finally precise attribute information – that its skin can have brown patches or that fritters can be made from it. The more precise the information, the more optional will be access and the more dependent on the sentence context. If the normal comprehension process operates in this way, might it not be possible to contrast disorders of the access process with the 'degraded store' deficits? To use an analogy given by Howard (1985a), the 'degraded store' deficit would correspond to pruning the access tree; the access disorder, to a difficulty in making appropriate choices at each branch point.

Arguments in favour of the existence of access disorders have been based on two methodologies: group studies and individual-case studies. In two group studies of aphasic patients, Milberg and Blumstein (1981) and Blumstein, Milberg, and Shrier (1982) used a single criterion to characterise an access disorder – that material that cannot be directly accessed can be primed. The studies used different modalities of input, but came to similar conclusions.

In their first experiment, Milberg and Blumstein compared a group of Wernicke's aphasics, a combined group of both Broca's and conduction aphasics, and a group of normal controls on a written lexical decision task. The test word was preceded either by a related or by an unrelated word prime or by a non-word prime, to which the subject need make no response. The speed of responding to the test word is shown in Figure 12.1. The error results also show main effects of patient group and priming condition and no interaction between them.

Milberg and Blumstein considered their main finding to be the existence of a semantic priming effect in the Wernicke's aphasic group. This, they claimed, does not support the position advocated by Zurif, Caramazza, Meyerson, and Galvin (1974) and by Goodglass and Baker (1976) that 'Wernicke's aphasics have a deficit in the underlying structure of the lexicon and are operating with restricted semantic fields and/or associative capacities' (Milberg & Blumstein, 1981, p. 381). Instead, they suggested that the failure of the Wernicke's aphasics in a task 'requiring metalinguistic judgments or conscious semantic decisions reflects a deficit in accessing and operating on semantic properties of the lexicon and not an impairment in the underlying organisation of the semantic system' (p. 381). Yet if Wernicke's aphasics generally have access difficulties, might one not expect the effects to be stronger? The Wernicke's group in the Blumstein et al. (1982) study made 33% errors on lexical decision in the related condition, as contrasted with 40% in the unrelated! To interpret the 7% difference as evidence for access problems and to ignore the 33% errors, even in the most favourable condition, seems a one-sided interpretation of the data. These studies do suggest that some Wernicke's aphasics may have

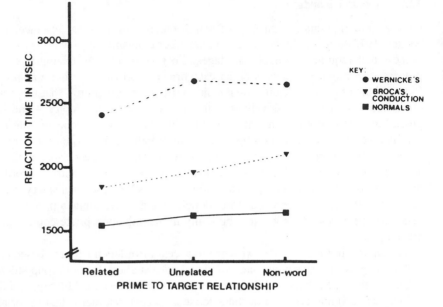

Figure 12.1. Lexical decision latency for words preceded by three sorts of clearly visible primes (related word, unrelated word, non-word) in three groups of subjects: Wernicke's aphasics, Broca's aphasics, and normal controls. From Milberg and Blumstein (1981) by permission of Academic Press.

access difficulties, but hardly that all Wernicke's aphasics do or even that an access problem is the main disorder in those patients who show a priming effect.

The other approach to isolating semantic access disorders is through single-case studies. Again, it is useful to begin with an illustrative example. Semantic access patients, unlike degraded store patients, tend to have a deficit that is specific to one access route. In the case of the first semantic access patient whose disorder was analysed in detail, AR (Warrington & Shallice, 1979), the route to the semantic system that needs to be considered is that by means of reading. AR had had a left parietal abscess drained. He was left with a severe naming difficulty and an acquired dyslexia. Otherwise, his cognitive abilities were unimpaired; his verbal and performance IQs were both in the average range (101 and 107, respectively). However, unlike many acquired dyslexic patients, AR had a grave difficulty in reading individual letters. This made reading, non-lexically, by the phonological route very difficult for him; thus only 27% of three-letter nonsense syllables were read correctly. Thus the set of alternative reading procedures available to him was reduced. AR was rather atypical in another way. His reading of words was relatively little affected by frequency, length, part of speech, or imageability/concreteness. His reading showed at most a trend dissociation over variables that give rise to strong dissociations in many other dyslexic patients.[13]

13. Frequency: frequent (AA) words, 49% correct; 1–50 per million, 37% correct on the Brown and Ure (1969) pool. Length: words read, mean length 5.4 letters; words failed, 5.9 letters. Part of

Table 12.6. *AR's performance (in percentage correct) in two- or five-choice categorisation tasks for words which he could neither read nor indicate their meaning*

	Read or indicated meaning (%)	Other words: categorised correctly (%)
Concrete categories: two-choice	30	78
Concrete categories: five-choice	20	69
Surnames/forenames	15	96
Boys'/girls' names	2	93
Authors/politicians	14	80
Subject/measurement	24	82

If AR's difficulty lay either early or late in the reading process, then one might expect that these variables would have little effect. However, there was no evidence supporting either of these possibilities for the locus of his impairment. For instance, a naming difficulty was not the source of the problem. A number of tests on which he could have performed perfectly if he had been able to understand the written word were poorly carried out (lexical decision, picture–word matching, cross-case matching, and carrying out mimes). On all of them, he scored at the level that would be expected if he had to guess when he could not read the word aloud. For instance, on the first 100 items of the Peabody picture–word matching test, he scored 90/100 when the words were presented auditorily. Given an average reading rate of 42%, one would expect a score of 53/100 with written words as stimuli if he had to guess randomly when he could not read the word aloud. In fact, he obtained 59/100, close to the predicted value. In complementary fashion, there was no evidence directly supporting an early locus for the deficit. Degrading the input by the use of brief tachistoscopic exposures did not lead to any deterioration in performance.

AR seemed to be able to access some aspects of the semantics of a word when attempting to read it. Thus in trying to read *beaver,* he said, 'could be an animal, I have no idea which one', and he commented on his difficulty, 'It seems as if I am almost there, but it seems as if I can't go over the last little bit and finally grasp it.' This phenomenon of partial semantic access came over clearly in a number of tests where he had to select from a limited set the category in which a word fell. He performed very well, even when he could neither read the word aloud nor indicate its meaning by giving a description (Table 12.6).

All these characteristics of AR's reading suggest that his impairment lay within

speech: AA nouns, 54%; AA verbs, 37%; AA pronouns, 68%. Imageability/concreteness: high, 44%; low, 27% – combining various pools – only a trend dissociation.

the semantic domain. However, they do not differentiate his difficulty from a degraded store deficit, except in the important respect that it was limited to one type of input – the written word. If the information in the store is itself damaged, then the effect should manifest itself by whatever route the input arrives at that store.[14] In an analysis of AR's reading impairment, Warrington and Shallice (1979) suggested that four characteristics might be used to differentiate an access disorder from a degraded store disorder.

1. Consistency

In a degraded store deficit, the inability to identify an item should be consistent over testing sessions, as was the case for EM, the patient discussed in section 12.3. However, for an access difficulty, temporary local factors will influence whether an item can be accessed. As had been argued by Weigl (1961), this would lead to a lack of consistency across sessions in which items are identified. AR was relatively inconsistent from one session to another in what words he could read.[15]

2. Depth of Processing

For both types of impairment, it should be easier to obtain the superordinate category than to identify the item. This is based on the assumption that in the understanding of a concept, its superordinate is the first piece of information accessed and the strongest represented. Once the superordinate has been obtained, the types of impairment should differ in the ease with which attribute information can be accessed. This should be very difficult, and, indeed, impossible for many items, for the degraded store type of impairment. So, as discussed in section 12.3, EM made many more errors on decisions about attributes than on superordinates. However, in an access disorder, the accessing of the superordinate should assist in accessing the attribute. Indeed, on the same test as that used with EM, AR performed as well at making a decision about an attribute (75% correct; chance, 33%) of a word he could not identify as he had in the original decision about its superordinate (56% correct).[16]

3. Priming

On the degraded store deficit, if an item cannot be identified, it should not be possible to prime it.[17] On an access deficit, priming would be expected to improve

---

14. This inference presupposes that the information from different access routes arrives at the same store. This issue will be discussed later in the chapter.
15. There was a contingency coefficient of only 0.31.
16. AR, in fact, performed worse on giving the superordinate at this session than on any other occasion during which a categorical judgement was tested.
17. It has not been empirically demonstrated that this property holds in a patient held to be of the degraded store type.

performance, as was discussed with respect to the work of Milberg and Blumstein (1981). Verbal prompts, such as presenting the word *cold* auditorily before the written word *freezer,* improved AR's reading performance in one experiment from 28 to 51%.

4. Frequency

A fourth characteristic suggested as relevant was item frequency. More frequent items presumably have a larger and more redundant underlying representation. So it is natural that item frequency is a major factor in determining which items are lost in degraded store impairments, like those of AB and EM. AR, however, showed relatively little effect of word frequency on reading. It was suggested that for an access difficulty, the variability in performance might be expected to reduce the slope of the frequency function.[18]

5. Rate of Presentation

An additional characteristic was considered an access one by Warrington and McCarthy (1983). Their patient VER, who had another access characteristic (inconsistency) performed at a somewhat better level if there was an interval between her response and the presentation of the next stimulus.

Since the 1970s, an increasing number of patients with impairments within the semantic domain have been investigated in detail. The five characteristics can be used as criteria for provisionally differentiating degraded store and impaired access difficulties for almost all of them for whom enough relevant information is available from single-case studies. Table 12.7 summarises results from patients classified as degraded store – two discussed in section 12.3 and two to be discussed in section 12.8 – and five classified as semantic access. The four patients other than AR classified as semantic access are CAV (Warrington, 1981; see also chapter 5), for written-word inputs; VER (Warrington & McCarthy, 1983)[19] and YOT (Warrington & McCarthy, 1987), for verbal input; and JCU (Howard & Orchard-Lisle, 1984; Howard, 1985a), for visual object access.[20] Across these patients, the five charac-

---

18. It could be argued that AR may have been using a partially damaged phonological route to read words aloud, relying on spelling-to-sound morphemic correspondences. If this were the case, then the support that AR's results give for the use of the four characteristics as operational criteria for a difficulty in accessing the semantic system would become suspect for the consistency and frequency characteristics where semantic processes would not need to be involved. Consistency is, however, the characteristic that, together with priming, has the greatest face validity.

19. VER's aphasia is relevant to the discussion of relateralisation of function (chapter 10). In her case, the study took place 17 months after her stroke. If relateralisation of function were a standard response of the brain to such global aphasic difficulties, it is unclear why such severe aphasias should persist.

20. Two other patients reported – JH (Albert, Yamadori, Gardner, & Howes, 1973), in the written-word domain, and JCB (Deloche, Andreewsky, & Desi, 1981) in the auditory–verbal domain –

Table 12.7. *Performance of patients' categorised as degraded store (above line) and access (below line)*

	Procedure	Consistency (within modality)	Frequency High [A or AA]	Frequency Low [<50]	Priming (P) rate (R) effects	Superordinate–attribute information
AB[a]	Defining	NT	96	51	NT	NT
EM[ab]	Defining	0.58	96	51	NT	Super >> attribute
JBR[c]	Defining	0.61	91	68	NT	Super >> attribute
SBY[c]	Defining	0.4	84	72	NT	Super >> attribute
AR[d]	Reading	0.31	49	37	Strong P	Equal
CAV[e]	Reading	0.23	56	36	Strong P	NT
VER[f]	Word–picture matching	At chance	61	55	Strong R	NT
YO[g]	Word–picture matching	At chance	NT	NT	Strong R	NT
JCU[h]	Picture Naming	NT	58	48	Strong P	NT

Note: The results are based on four procedures: (1) providing a definition for a presented word, (2) reading aloud, (3) word–picture matching using a four- or five-alternative forced-choice procedure, and (4) picture naming. The consistency measures are, in general, contingency coefficients; frequency results are given in terms of percent correct; superordinate/attribute contrast is based on the ability to perform forced-choice tests or the ability to give superordinates for categories where attribute information could not be provided. For more details of measures, see Shallice (1987). NT means 'Not Tested'.

[a] Warrington (1975)
[b] Coughlan and Warrington (1981)
[c] Warrington and Shallice (1984)
[d] Warrington and Shallice (1979)
[e] Warrington (1981)
[f] Warrington and McCarthy (1983)
[g] Warrington and McCarthy (1987)
[h] Howard and Orchard-Lisle (1984)

showed categorical effects somewhat analogous to those discussed for AR, but fewer relevant details are available. In JH's case, it is unclear how critical was his severe naming problem.

The evidence that the impairments of the patients listed in Table 12.7 are of a semantic-access type differs across patients. VER, JCU, and YOT were, for instance, too severely aphasic for direct-naming or reading responses to be used. VER was very severely aphasic for both comprehension and production following a purely left hemisphere lesion. She could not name pictures or read words aloud. However, she could score above chance on picture–word matching tests. On such tests, she showed little effect of item difficulty, except possibly for the most difficult items. She was also very inconsistent in her responses from one testing session to another. A five-alternative forced-choice test was carried out on four occasions. The proportion of items giving each pattern of correct and incorrect responses (e.g. three correct; one incorrect) was very close to that expected by chance if all were equally likely to be accessed. It was not the case that some items were consistently known

teristics that have been claimed to differentiate access and degraded store disorders operate in a relatively consistent way for each patient. Thus the differentiation seems reasonably robust.

12.5 Criticisms of the Impaired Access–Degraded Store Dichotomy

This differentiation between impaired access and degraded store disorders is open to various criticisms. The most direct objection is that patients exist whose impairment is at the semantic level but has characteristics that do not fit either of the two suggested types and cannot be considered to be a mixture of the two. Howard (1985a) has presented one such case: PW, the deep dyslexic patient discussed in chapter 5.

In naming pictures, as in reading words, PW's errors were mainly semantic, as in a picture of a tiger being named as 'lion'. Also, when his error responses were presented again auditorily, together with the picture, and he was given the instruction 'Is this the best name for the picture?' he frequently said, 'Yes'. Thus his difficulty would appear not to be just an output one. He was highly consistent, but he showed no effect of word frequency; the correlation was a mere 0.01. Thus one characteristic is of the access type; the other, a degradation one.

One possible way of resolving this paradox can be obtained from PW's being relatively unimpaired when compared with the patients discussed earlier; his naming of pictures was 77% correct. A small degree of degradation might be expected to lead to loss of only limited attribute information, even for low-frequency items. Whether this would be sufficient to produce a semantic error would depend on the existence of a closely similar distractor, which might be unrelated to frequency, particularly for concrete items. More extensive degradation would, however, lead to a general pruning of the attribute tree for lower frequency items and the retention of little more than superordinate information for them. Thus the word frequency criterion could be viewed as relevant for only sizeable degrees of degradation of the store. This means of resolving the paradox is not particularly convincing. Howard (1985a) himself, though, provides no alternative explanation of PW's pattern of performance. Whether item frequency is a satisfactory criterion for differentiating the two types of impairment remains an unresolved issue.

The opposite type of criticism of the degraded store–impaired access dichotomy can also be made, that it is too crude. Theoretically, access disorders might arise because of a quantitative or qualitative reduction in the input received by the store, through a malfunctioning of the process of compiling the precise representation or

---

and the rest were guessed fairly randomly from trial to trial. These effects were also observed in YOT.

For JCU, as for VER, non-verbal tests of her visual identification ability suggested that it was not responsible for the difficulty in relating visual and verbal material. In her case, it was discovered that naming could be facilitated by the provision of a first-letter cue. As with VER, the pattern of performance across items was very inconsistent; no core group of known items appeared to exist.

even through a lack of stability in the system. Should all these be conflated? Also, some of the differentiating characteristics, such as rate and priming, would give a similar pattern for disorders that combined both access and storage aspects as for purely access disorders. Indeed, VER, JCU, and YOT were global aphasics who almost never produced the correct response without the use of a forced-choice or cueing procedure. Is it appropriate to treat them as qualitatively equivalent to AR and CAV, who could identify a reasonable proportion of items without aid?[21]

No conclusive answers can be given to these questions at present. To attempt to make a finer differentiation within access disorders on theoretical grounds alone would be premature, in the absence of a well-established model of the semantic access process. Moreover, with the single exception so far of PW, applying the different criteria gives compatible answers. The dichotomy therefore remains a useful way of ordering the highly complex set of semantic memory impairments.

12.6   The Structure of Semantic Memory I: The Elements

Can neuropsychological evidence guide us on how semantic memory is locally structured? Many types of theory now exist: network theories (e.g. Collins & Quillian, 1969; Norman & Rumelhart, 1975; Anderson, 1976, 1983); feature theories, both hierarchical (e.g. Katz & Fodor, 1963) and parallel (e.g. Smith, Shoben, & Rips, 1974); theories derived from computational semantics (e.g. Miller & Johnson-Laird, 1976; Rieger, 1978); and complex hybrids, such as the parallel distributed processing position of McClelland and Rumelhart (1985). On Marr's (1982) metatheoretical framework, which was discussed in chapter 2, they are all theories on the algorithm or mechanism level. Therefore, from the arguments developed in that chapter, making a selection among them is not the type of issue for which neuropsychological evidence is best suited. However, it might provide suggestions.

The most relevant result from the study of degraded store deficits appears to be the saliency of superordinate information. For instance, both AB and EM were much better at saying whether a word was an animal name or an object name than in deciding which of two names matched a photograph of the item. If anything is retained about a word or an object it is not the supposed kernel of the 'basic level' concept of Rosch et al. (1976), but its superordinate. This finding suggests that the basic level is less important than previously thought. It does not refute any class of model, but it is much less simply compatible with some than with others. As far as earlier network theories are concerned, the finding is not a particularly natural one. A more principled explanation can be derived from the more advanced network theory of Collins and Loftus (1975). They argued that when an exemplar of a cate-

---

21. Another difference between AR and CAV, on the one hand, and VER, JCU, and YOT, on the other, is that the latter trio had no intact access routes to their verbal system. Intuitively, the deficits of the second set of patients may be more simply explicable in terms of generally unstable central representations or mixed access/degradation difficulties rather than as a combination of access difficulties.

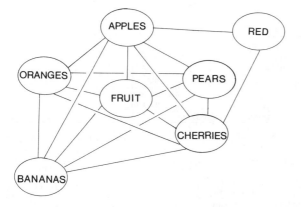

Figure 12.2. Differing relation of a superordinate (fruit) and an attribute (red) to a category member (apples) on Collins and Loftus's (1975) theory. The strength of activation passing down a link is inversely related to the distance between the two nodes in the diagram.

gory is activated, activation will spread to other items of the same category and from each of them, in turn, to the superordinate. The superordinate therefore receives indirect activation in a number of ways in addition to the direct activation through the so-called Isa link (Figure 12.2).

There are, by contrast, theories that explain findings of this sort more directly. One such is Rieger's (1978) computational model (see also Rieger & Small, 1979). Rieger argued that the network approach is not capable of capturing the specific context-dependent subtleties of a word's meaning. He gives as an example the word *take*. It can mean 'starting out to select an object or move it with one' (*John took the book*), 'to get an idea or acquire information' (*John took the advice*), 'to swallow a medicine' (*John took the pill*), 'to vent an emotion' (*John took out his anger*), 'to escort' (*John took out Mary*), 'to start a process' (*John took out an advertisement*), 'to begin a habitual activity' (*John took to alcohol*), 'to begin liking something' (*John took to the puppy*), and so on. Rieger argued that the meaning of a word like *take* is represented by an 'expert' program that selects among the alternative senses depending on syntactic information and semantic information from the subject and object of the verb; it is represented by a hierarchical sense net (Figure 12.3).

In Rieger's model, the expert programs for all the words in, say, a clause 'run' together, exchanging information. The type of information that the *take* expert requires from its neighbours to distinguish different senses at the choice points in the sense net is categorical information.[22] Therefore, even for concrete nouns with a very limited set of meanings, such as *spider,* it would be useful if the first type of

22. This process is related to the procedure developed in linguistic theory by Katz and Fodor (1963) using the concept selection restriction.

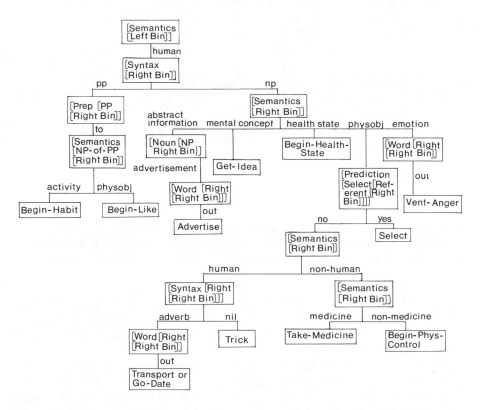

Figure 12.3. Rieger's (1978) model of the sense net of the verb *take,* which his system accesses in a top-down fashion. The Right Bin refers to the next unit to the right in the clause and the Right Right Bin, to the following one; *pp* stands for prepositional phrase and *np,* for noun phrase. Reprinted from Rieger (1978); *Discourse Processes 1:*267, by permission of Ablex.

information accessed is its categorical status.[23] Such an approach would fit with superordinates being first accessed and also last degraded.

The final set of theories are those in which meaning is represented by an unstructured set of propositions or features. For such theories, the preservation of superordinates seems anomalous.[24] It can, however, be assumed that a superordinate is

23. A supporting argument can be obtained from acquisition. Keil (1981) has suggested that a critical aspect of a child's learning of new terms is giving them a position on the *predictability tree* – essentially, the hierarchy of superordinates of nouns. Position on the tree determines what type of adjectives or verbs go meaningfully with the nouns.

24. Howard (1985a) has, however, presented an ingenious argument on this point: 'Having partial (and subordinate) semantic information and a reasoning system will often permit the deduction/induction of superordinate information but rarely give subordinate information. . . . The ability to make category judgments therefore reflects the hierarchical nature of entailment relations, rather than hierarchically-organised semantic representations' (p. 408). This explains the performance of de-

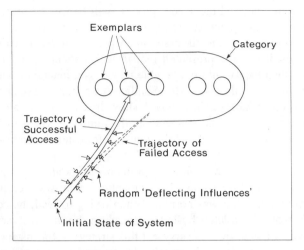

Figure 12.4. The trajectory of a successful and a failed access in the semantic space of a distributed network. The failed access, however, still arrives within the region for the correct category.

learned through the conflation of the common elements of the exemplars. The exemplar may well have a representation that has more elements in the same state as its superordinate than the number in which it differs from a co-ordinate (for examples, see McClelland & Rumelhart, 1985). In this case, random damage to elements will impair the co-ordinate decision prior to the superordinate one.

According to this distributed model, elements need not be explicitly accessible units of knowledge. Indeed, it is becoming standard to conceive of them as quasi-neurons that are in an on or off state and that receive inputs both from the input signal and from their fellow elements, the latter being initially random (Hinton & Anderson, 1981). Those stable states of the system towards which the pattern of activity of the elements tends to move, given appropriate inputs, correspond to the concepts that the system can identify. Within this framework, access can be conceived of as the attainment of a series of increasingly close approximations to the 'correct' state of the elements as the effect of the input signal gradually wins out over the random influences (Figure 12.4).[25] Thus as required by Rieger's (1978) theoretical arguments, effective knowledge about a superordinate is obtained prior to effective specific information about the concept; the superordinate corresponds to a region of the space within which the individual exemplars lie.

The distributed-model approach has one further advantage. If the input signal to the network is weak, then the effect of the random influences on each element will

graded store patients in category judgement tasks. However, it does not fit well with their actual behaviour. Why do they not say that a *goose* is something that *walks* and is *white*, if that is what they know about it? Why, instead, do they infer that it is a living thing?

25. For an example of a simulation of such a process, see Hinton and Sejnowski (1986).

be more difficult to overcome, and the access process will be slowed or may even be aborted.[26] In certain access patients, the input to the semantic system is weak. The evidence comes from a syndrome discussed in chapter 4 – letter-by-letter reading. In that chapter, evidence was presented that if such patients could not read words letter-by-letter, then they would not be able to access semantic or phonological information. Two recent studies – of ML (Shallice & Saffran, 1986) and of JG, TL, JC, and AF (Coslett & Saffran, in press) – show that this is not always the case. The way these five patients read was essentially similar. I will therefore describe the performance of one, ML, who, following a left posterior cerebral artery stroke, had a measured verbal IQ of 130!

ML was not aphasic, having no word-finding problems in spontaneous speech or in response to auditorily posed questions. The semantic system was certainly not degraded; auditory comprehension was normal. When trying to read, he could almost always identify words by a letter-by-letter procedure, but he was very slow. When he did not have sufficient time to carry out this strategy – for instance, with the 2-sec exposures used in testing – he nearly always denied knowing what the word was and could only very rarely guess it. He was given a set of categorical decisions about words, being instructed to say if he knew what the word was; as with AR, if he could name or identify the word, it was eliminated. Yet unlike the letter-by-letter patients discussed in chapter 4, at this exposure duration, he was able to make correct categorical decisions on 90% of trials in discriminating whether cities or countries were in Europe or the rest of the world, on 85% for discriminating living things from objects, and on 83% for differentiating pleasant and unpleasant words. ML's overall pattern of performance with 2-sec exposures resembled that of an access disorder.

When performing lexical decision judgements with restricted exposure durations, ML again performed well above chance, even though again he could identify virtually none of the words. However, he had much more difficulty rejecting orthographically regular distractors that differed from a word by one letter (e.g. *cancas*) than rejecting otherwise matched non-words that differed by two letters (e.g. *hoitor*) (47% vs. 13% false positives). The more similar the non-words were to specific words, the more difficulty he had with them. It appears that the output of the visual word-form system is less well differentiated than for normal subjects and hence suggests that the semantic system receives a quantitatively reduced input. Thus in ML's case, an explanation of an access disorder as arising from the semantic system receiving a reduced input as illustrated in Figure 12.4 is plausible.[27]

26. If the state of the system comes close to any of its stable states, it will tend to move towards this stable state because a stable state acts as an 'attractor' or 'energy minimum' of the system. Thus an incorrect state can be accessed, and this will correspond to a semantic error. In this respect, the distributed model approach is preferable to the hierarchical one, which has been criticised because it seems to predict that an access failure should lead to the production of a superordinate and not to other forms of semantic error (see Coltheart, 1980c; Howard, 1985a).

27. Warrington and Shallice (1979) rejected an explanation of AR's semantic access disorder as arising from reduced output from the visual word-form system. Our argument was that the effects found in

The phenomena found with semantic memory disorders, surprising though they are, are therefore explicable by more than one theory. They fit well with the distributed memory models discussed in chapter 11.

12.7 The Structure of Semantic Memory II: Modality Specificity

When you recognise that a quill pen has roughly the same function as a biro, when you use an object of either sort to write, when you know that it is lighter than a hammer, or when you hear or use the word *pen* in speech, to what extent do they all rely on a single central representation of meaning? Since 1970, there has been an extensive debate within cognitive psychology on this issue. Some argue that items are represented at the 'semantic' level in a single amodal system (Chase & Clark, 1972; Seymour, 1973; Potter, 1979). To others, separate systems for verbal, visual, and maybe other modalities are involved (e.g. Paivio, 1971) or even these and an abstract one, too (Anderson, 1980). At present, the evidence from studies of normal subjects is far from clear-cut (see Te Linde, 1982; Snodgrass, 1984; Glucksberg, 1984).

A number of lines of nueropsychological evidence are relevant. Warrington (1975) pointed out that semantic memory patients can be more severely impaired for visual input than for verbal, and vice versa. Thus WLP could use objects correctly when she could no longer identify words (Schwartz, Saffran, & Marin, 1979). If the patients' deficits are *entirely* of the degraded store type, then this would point to the existence of separate storage systems. The most solid quantitative evidence on this point comes from Warrington's patient EM. As discussed in section 12.3, she was extremely consistent, had much greater difficulty with attribute information than with superordinates, and showed strong frequency effects; she represents as pure a degraded store deficit as has been described. She, however, was much more impaired for decisions based on verbal input, for which her consistency had been measured, than for ones based on visual input (Table 12.8). Moreover, her overall performance was, if anything, worse than that of AB, given verbal input; with visual input, it was far better. Warrington explained this contrast in terms of the two patients' having different degrees of damage to two semantic systems – visual and verbal.

Interpretation of such effects depends critically on the validity of the inference that the impairment is a pure degradation one. Potentially stronger evidence for separate systems comes from another type of syndrome, the modality-specific aphasias.

AR were much larger than the 'tacit' semantic phenomena found in normal subjects under, say, visual masking conditions (e.g. Marcel, 1983a), which can also be explained in terms of reduced input received by the semantic system (see Shallice & McGill, 1978). However, given the arguments earlier in this section that semantic access effects lie on a continuum, it seems entirely possible that quantitative differences in the input signal (to the semantic system) are responsible for the greater magnitude of these effects in patients than in reduced viewing conditions in normal subjects. It should be noted that Coslett and Saffran (in press) prefer an explanation of the syndrome in terms of right hemisphere processing.

Table 12.8. *Percentage correct performance of two semantic memory patients in identifying by description (or for a picture by naming) from 40 concrete words and their corresponding clear line drawings*

	AB	EM
Picture	48	93
Word	68	65

From Warrington (1975)

The modality-specific aphasias are among the most obscure, complex, little investigated, and yet controversial syndromes in neuropsychology. Their essential characteristics are that naming from one modality alone is impaired, but there appears to be no agnosic difficulty in that modality. Thus in optic aphasia, first described by Freund (1889), the naming of visually presented objects is impaired, but objects can be named from touch; the syndrome cannot be a loss of the names of the objects. Yet the patient can identify objects presented visually, if identification is assessed by, say, demonstrating use. The syndrome can therefore be defined in terms of two dissociations: a dissociation between impaired naming for one modality of input and intact naming for other input modalities, and a dissociation within the impaired modality between naming performance and some non-verbal means of demonstrating the intact identification of the stimulus (at the semantic level).

In view of the counterintuitive nature of the syndromes, it is hardly surprising that scepticism was the normal response in the days when syndromes were investigated in a purely clinical way. The standard argument was that the patient in fact had an agnosic or more general aphasic difficulty (see, e.g., Kleist, 1916). Recently, however, there have been a number of studies of a small number of individual patients that have been of a much higher quality than the earlier investigations – studies of optic aphasia (Spreen, Benton, & Van Allen, 1966; Lhermitte & Beauvois, 1973; Assal & Regli, 1980; Beauvois, 1982; Poeck, 1984; Gil et al., 1985; Coslett & Saffran, personal communication), of auditory aphasia (Denes & Semenza, 1975), and of bilateral tactile aphasia (Beauvois, Saillant, Meninger, & Lhermitte, 1978).

To illustrate the general characteristics of this type of disorder, consider the last of these, bilateral tactile aphasia, which was described in the remarkable patient RG, who was also the first recorded case of both phonological alexia and lexical agraphia (chapters 5 and 6). Apart from these specific problems, the patient had no aphasic difficulties. In visual-naming tasks that included naming 50 pictures of objects that were difficult to recognise, the patient made only 3% errors, all of which were immediately corrected. In naming familiar sounds (e.g. telephones ringing, cats miaowing), the patient made 1% errors. However, when he was blindfolded, RG made 33% errors in naming from touch objects that are very familiar (e.g. cup, pair of scissors) and was very slow. Errors tended to be semantic (e.g. a box of matches→some cigarettes, a glove→slippers). Yet if the subject was asked to demonstrate the use of the object, he made only 1% errors, and did this very much more quickly than producing the name.[28]

Optic aphasia for objects shows a related pattern of findings, the three most critical studies being those of JF (Lhermitte & Beauvois, 1973), GJ (Gil et al., 1985), and CB (Coslett & Saffran, personal communication).[29] In these patients, a pattern of findings complementary to that found in RG with touch was obtained. Thus in naming objects or pictures from vision, GJ made more than 35% errors in three different series. Yet when 21 objects were presented for naming from vision, and from touch, and for indicating use, a selective deficit in visual naming is clear. She again made 38% in naming from visual presentation, but no errors at all in the other two conditions. As with the study of bilateral tactile aphasia, classical dissociations have been obtained. The pattern of errors produced by both JF and GJ was a mixture of semantic and perseverative errors and occasional visual ones, with semantic ones predominating.

The modality-specific aphasias have also been explained in terms of the semantic system having a more complex architecture than that possessed by a single homogeneous system. Separable verbal, visual non-verbal, tactile non-verbal, and auditory non-verbal systems have been held to exist, with communication between the verbal semantic system and a modality-specific part of the system being impaired (Beauvois, 1982) (Figure 12.5). Thus in optic aphasia, the deficit was held to lie in the transmission of information from the visual semantic system to the verbal semantic one. However, a number of objections to this account have been raised.

The first is that one of the dissociations claimed for the syndromes – that of miming versus naming – arises from a resource artefact (chapter 10); in particular, it has been argued that the miming task used to establish that a modality-specific semantic system works satisfactorily is a less demanding test of semantics than is naming (e.g. Howard, 1985b; Riddoch, Humphreys, Coltheart, & Funnell, 1988). It is argued that mimes are ambiguous to interpret; for instance, a semantic error of *shoe* for *boot* would be much more difficult to detect as an error in miming than in naming. This account, though, is insufficient to explain the large difference between miming and naming performance in, say, bilateral tactile aphasia. Only 1% of the mimes were in error. The semantic errors that occurred in naming would often give rise to clearly different mimes. Take, say, *cap*→*jockey* or *glove*→*slippers*. In addition, 30% of the naming errors were perseverative. It is difficult to understand why perseverations did not occur with the mimes if mimes merely provide a less sensitive measure of the same underlying process.

28. Good performance on demonstrating the object's use occurred only when a strategy of avoiding verbalisation was strongly suggested to the patient. His mouth was taped as an *aide-mémoire*.
29. An exhaustive study of optic aphasia for colours exists (Beauvois & Saillant, 1985). However, its relevance to the issue of the possible multiplicity of semantic systems is unclear.

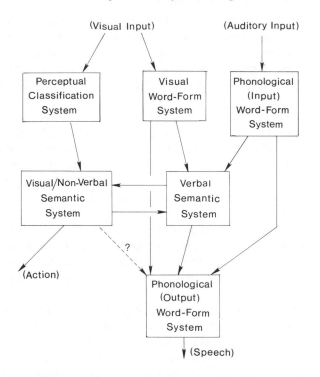

(Visual Input)   (Auditory Input)

| Perceptual Classification System | Visual Word-Form System | Phonological (Input) Word-Form System |

| Visual/Non-Verbal Semantic System | Verbal Semantic System |

?

(Action)

Phonological (Output) Word-Form System

(Speech)

Figure 12.5. The multiple semantic systems model. It is normally assumed that the route marked by ? does not exist. Auditory and tactile non-verbal systems are not shown.

Two alternative explanations that accept the syndrome as a valid entity have been put forward by Ratcliff and Newcombe (1982)[30] and by Riddoch et al. (1988). Both sets of authors hold that there is only a single semantic system, but they add a different transmission route. Ratcliff and Newcombe suggest that transmission routes exist from perceptual classification systems directly to naming systems, by-passing the semantic system. They also propose that in naming, the mapping from the semantic system onto the phonological output word-form system is 'fuzzy'. So on their theory of optic aphasia, a lesion to the non-semantic naming route will produce semantic errors in naming, but leave non-verbal identification performance intact.

The claim that there are naming routes that by-pass the semantic systems is not supported by strong evidence.[31] It is not clear why they should exist. How often, for instance, does one name objects from touch? Normally, they are identified and

30. Ratcliff and Newcombe's (1982) explanation was applied specifically to optic aphasia. If the theory does not also explain the other modality-specific aphasias, its plausibility is clearly lessened. I have therefore treated it as a way of explaining all the modality-specific aphasias.
31. It has been argued by Heilman, Tucker, and Valenstein (1976) and by Kremin (1984) that some patients can name objects but do not know what they are. For criticisms of these claims, see Howard (1985a) and Shallice (1987).

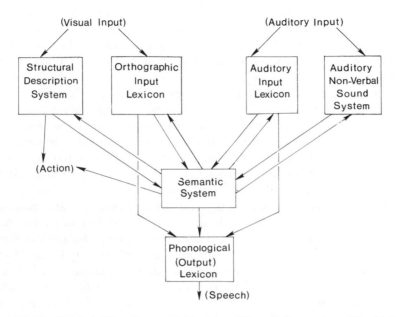

Figure 12.6. The Riddoch, Humphreys, Coltheart, and Funnell (in press) model, which contains only one semantic system.

then used non-verbally. Also, it needs to be assumed that in the absence of the non-semantic route satisfactory naming cannot be achieved. Ratcliff and Newcombe's position on this was derived from the theory of deep dyslexia put forward by Newcombe and Marshall (1980a), according to which semantic representations map onto output phonological word-form systems in a 'fuzzy' fashion. Various criticisms of this idea have already been discussed in chapter 5. Therefore, overall, the Ratcliff and Newcombe theory does not seem particularly plausible.

The additional route proposed by Riddoch et al. (1988) is one between a perceptual classification system, which they refer to as a structural description system, and a system that controls action (Figure 12.6). In a test of indicating use, they argue, this route is all that is needed; one does need to be able to *identify* the object at a truly semantic level. In fact, *identification* can be shown by other non-verbal means. Thus Coslett and Saffran (personal communication) used a test similar to Warrington and Taylor's (1978) function-matching test, discussed in chapter 8. They asked an optic aphasic patient, CB, to indicate which of three items (e.g. *pencil, sheet of paper, knife*) presented were functionally related. CB scored at 81% on this test, which Coslett and Saffran consider to be normal for a person of his age (67). Use of, say, a *zip* and a *button,* two of the items that were functionally related, involve quite different actions, so the preserved performance of CB on this test cannot be explained in terms of the route postulated by Riddoch et al.

It may be that Coslett and Saffran's test does not demand complete visual identification, so that a semantic access type explanation of CB's naming problem might be a possibility. However, for a number of neuropsychological phenomena, the Riddoch et al. explanation needs to make additional assumptions that would be most difficult to test.[32] While it has not been refuted, it does not seem that plausible a possibility.

Let us assume that these explanations of the modality-specific aphasias in terms either of impairment to a hypothetical non-semantic naming route or of reliance on direct connections between structural descriptions and action can be rejected. Then the group of findings suggest that different modality-specific semantic processes are dissociable. What, in turn, does this entail? Our visual semantic representations are far more complex than just the representations of isolated objects or actions; consider how one interprets a silent film. On the verbal side, as argued in section 12.6, the unpacking of sentence meaning into features or propositions and, particularly, the determining of word sense are processes that are probably very different from the visual ones, at least for a first pass at comprehension. The way that semantic elements are integrated into understanding is quite different in the two domains. Consider how the scene represented by the sentence *Tom arrived to take Mary out for the evening* would be represented on film. The elements that need disambiguating would be entirely different in the two cases – between the different senses of *take out*, say, in the verbal case, and the different reasons why a teenager might stand diffidently on the doorstep in the visual one.

Consider the problem in another way. What sort of processes have been assumed to lie within the semantic domain? They form a very wide set. For a visually presented object, they include the sensory qualities not directly observable, the other objects that might be expected in its vicinity, the appropriate ways of using it, its function, the behaviours it is likely to have, one's emotional attitude to it, as well as a host of more abstract possibilities.

Some of these 'sub-semantic' processes, such as the objects likely to be found in its vicinity and appropriate ways of using it, seem unlikely to be frequently accessed from verbal input. Some of the semantic aspects of objects, though, may be as frequency accessed from verbal input as from non-verbal – their function, for instance – and when one moves to abstract properties, a distinction between verbal and non-verbal semantic domains becomes much more difficult to sustain. Indeed, if one considers a purely verbal semantic system, it has been strongly argued that it provides an insufficient basis for adequate comprehension operating alone; it acts as an input to other semantic systems (Johnson-Laird, 1983). Overall, it seems fairly implausible that verbal semantic processes and these visual ones are totally autonomous from each other, that they form tight Fodorian modules. They seem to

---

32. Riddoch, Humphreys, Coltheart, and Funnell (1988) also argue that a patient of theirs who showed the optic aphasia pattern of performance did not have intact semantic access from vision. However, their patient was far less good at indicating use (25% errors) than GJ. Moreover, their tests of semantic access involved language and so would be contaminated by the optic aphasia. If their patient represents intact 'miming without meaning' then GJ must be employing other means to achieve perfect miming performance.

be more plausibly viewed as coupled subsystems.[33] The issue is, though, best deferred until after the discussion of category specificity.

12.8 The Structure of Semantic Memory III: Category Specificity

There is a separate type of evidence for computational sub-domains within the semantic system that is even more counterintuitive: the existence of impairment specific to particular semantic categories or different types of semantic operation. There have long been suggestions within the clinical literature that even more specific dissociations exist within the semantic realm. Nielsen (1946), for instance, described a patient who had considerably more difficulty identifying inanimate objects by sight or touch and foods except by taste than identifying living things, and a second patient who showed the reverse dissociations. A similar observation was made by Hécaen and Ajuriaguerra (1956). They described a patient who found animals easier to identify than objects. An even more surprising claim was made by Yamadori and Albert (1973). Their patient was said to have had a specific difficulty in understanding the meaning of the names of common objects found in a room. When asked to point to a wall, he said, 'W-A-L-L, wall, W-A-L-L, wall. . . . I have to double check later', and similar difficulties were obtained for *chair, bed, light, door,* and *floor.* But he was said to have had no difficulty understanding the meaning of names of tools, utensils, or clothing, although he did have one with parts of the body.

All these observations took the form of the clinical judgement of the investigators, together with a number of examples of the claimed phenomenon. No quantitative support for the dissociations was produced. Given how counterintuitive the claims were, it is only too easy to be sceptical. To judge from the way they dropped from the consciousness of those working in the field, scepticism was the standard response.

The first quantitative attempt to investigate this type of category specificity was made by Goodglass, Klein, Carey, and James (1966). They tested 135 aphasic patients for their ability to comprehend six types of word: body parts, objects, actions, colours, letters, and numbers. They found that a surprisingly high number of patients showed some dissociation in their ability to comprehend particular semantic categories. However, the small number of items tested in each category (six) make the results rather difficult to assess.

A later group study by Wilkins and Moscovitch (1978), while not on category specificity per se, provided support for the idea that patients might differ on which semantic operations they found most difficult. They showed that patients with left temporal lesions had significantly more difficulty than patients with right temporal ones in making a series of rapid decisions about whether stimuli were living or manmade, but there was no such difference for judgements of size. Moreover, the effect

---

33. This leaves unresolved the issue of the characteristic error pattern that occurs in the modality-specific aphasias. I will return to this in chapter 13.

Table 12.9. *Performance of four semantic memory patients on identifying by verbal description the meanings of concrete and abstract words of frequency less than 50 per million*

	Concrete	Abstract
AB[a]	24	85
SBY[b]	50	94
EM[a]	56	45
JBR[b]	65	71

Note: Two show an abstract word superiority; the other two do not.
[a] Warrington (1975)
[b] Warrington and Shallice (1984)

occurred in the same fashion whether the stimuli used were words or drawings. It appeared that the left temporal group had a semantic-processing deficit on the more abstract of the two decisions. However, since the stimuli were presented at the fierce pace of 1 per 750 msec, it remains possible that the difficulty lay in producing the words *living* and *man-made* rather than in making the semantic decision itself.

In the mid-1970s, quantitative investigations had also begun to be made of category specific deficits in individual patients. AB was one of Warrington's (1975) original 'semantic memory' patients (see section 12.3). He performed far better when asked to define abstract words than concrete ones (Table 12.9). Thus he defined *vocation* as 'what one's job is'; *pact,* as 'friendly agreement'; and *arbiter,* as 'He is a man who tries to arbitrate. Produce a peaceful solution.' Yet to *hay,* he said, 'I've forgotten'; to *poster,* 'no idea'; and to *needle,* 'forgotten'. A similar effect was obtained in a patient, SBY, reported by Warrington and Shallice (1984), and an analogous dissociation in word reading was described in chapter 5 for patient CAV (Warrington, 1981). Thus we have the striking finding of a superiority in processing abstract words compared with correct ones, which in the case of AB and SBY appears to arise at the level of the semantic representations themselves.

Quantitative accounts of even more specific dissociations were soon to be reported. Dennis (1976) studied an epileptic girl who had had a left temporal lobectomy to remove the epileptic focus. Clinically, it was noted that she had problems naming body parts, frequently producing a circumlocution such as saying for a *left wrist* stimulus, 'the left arm on your fingers beside'. On formal testing, she named only 12/20 (60%) of pictures of body parts, by contrast with 35/40 (88%) of pictures of other nouns of comparable frequency, thus showing a just significant difference between body parts and other stimuli. More pronounced difficulties with body-part

Table 12.10. *Percentage performance of FC on three different tests of availability of five categories*

	Colour	Object	Country	Body part	Animal
Naming (visual)	0	10	65	50	5
Naming (from description)	0	10	75	0	5
Auditory–visual matching[a]	85	95	100	35	85

[a] 10 alternative within category forced-choice
From McKenna and Warrington (1978)

comprehension have been obtained by Ogden (1986) and Semenza (personal communication).

Another striking category specific effect was obtained by McKenna and Warrington (1978). Their patient, FC, who had a left temporal lobe tumour, performed extremely poorly on three different standardised naming tests, obtaining only one correct on each of the tests. It was noted that he tended to give the names of countries in his response. So to a photograph of Mahatma Gandhi, he said 'India'. A comparison was therefore made between his ability to process five different categories of high frequency (AA) words. Picture–word matching, naming from visual presentation, and naming from description were used. The results are shown in Table 12.10. An isolated preservation of country naming was observed.[34]

Presented with strange dissociations of these sorts, it is natural to try to explain them as artefacts. Thus Brown (1981) argued that this last effect arose because FC was a sales manager and therefore was especially familiar with the category country! Actually, it does not seem at all plausible that the shape of India on a map should be more familiar then, say, the colour red, even to a sales manager! The possibility that category specific effects arise through some artefact is, however, more easily addressed in the most detailed investigations that have been carried out of two contrasting semantic domains: the identification of living things and foods, on the one hand, and that of man-made artefacts, on the other (Warrington & McCarthy, 1983, 1987; Warrington & Shallice, 1984; Hart, Berndt, & Caramazza, 1985; Sartori & Job, 1988; Silveri & Gainotti, personal communication).

The most extensive of these investigations (Warrington & Shallice, 1984) concerned four patients, all of whom had lesions arising from herpes simplex encephalitis, a disease that tends to lead to maximal damage in the medial temporal lobes (Illis & Gostling, 1972). Patients with similar impairments have been studied by Sartori and Job and by Silveri and Gainotti. Two of the originally studied patients had severe expressive dysphasias and were more generally impaired than the other

34. Semenza and Zettin (in press) has recently observed an even more dramatic proper-name dissociation. The patient was virtually normal at naming objects, colours, etc., but could produce hardly any proper names in naming situations.

Table 12.11. *Identifying and naming by JBR and SBY of three categories of stimuli with two modes of presentation (results combined over three experiments) (in percentages)*

| | a: Visual | | | | | | b: Auditory | | |
| | Living things | | Foods | | Objects | | Living things | Foods | Objects |
	Identify	Name	Identify	Name	Identify	Name		Identify	
JBR	6	6	20	20	80	54	8	30	78
SBY	7	—	25	—	68	—	5	25	59

From Warrington and Shallice (1984)

two. The two patients with the less general impairment had verbal and performance IQs that indicated considerable sparing of intellectual abilities (JBR: 101, 103; SBY: 95, 93). The most striking aspect of the behaviour of these two patients was their vastly better ability to identify by description – and, in one case, to name – pictures of inanimate objects than ones of living things or foods, when they were matched for frequency (Table 12.11). Identification was measured by whether judges considered that the description given by the patient had 'grasped the core concept' of any given word. A similar pattern of results was found when the patients were asked to describe the meaning of object-name, food name, and living-thing words (Table 12.11). The results are also the same when familiarity, too, is controlled.

The results cannot plausibly be attributed to any greater difficulty in describing food and living-thing words because a similar pattern of results occurs with other testing procedures. For JBR, actions appropriate to objects were compared with ones appropriate to foods (such as *spaghetti* and *banana*); performance on the objects was much superior (65% vs. 20% correct). Also in a five-choice picture–word matching test, the three patients tested were significantly superior in matching objects than either foods or living things.

Could it be that objects are in some sense generally easier to process for the semantic system or some other relevant system; this might be a structural description system, as suggested by Riddoch et al. (1988), which would have to be accessible in top-down fashion from the semantic one (to account for the word results) (see Figure 12.6). In fact JBR and SBY were normal on the unconventional views test, held to stress this system (chapter 8). A resource-artefact argument of this sort is most convincingly ruled out by the existence of a double dissociation. The patient VER (Warrington & McCarthy, 1983), the global aphasic whose semantic access characteristics were described in section 12.6, in fact showed the complementary pattern of difficulty across categories. She was significantly worse at performing five-choice picture–word matches for objects (58%) than for foods (88%), and at two-choice for objects (63%) than for animals (86%) and flowers (96%). YOT

(Warrington & McCarthy, 1987), who had an access difficulty similar to that of VER, also performed similarly. With five-choice picture–word matching, she performed significantly worse with objects (65%) than with animals (86%), flowers (86%), and foods (93%).

This contrasting pattern of dissociations was explained when initially obtained in terms of a different semantic process being required for analysing the function that a thing has than for the sensory features it possesses. To distinguish two objects – say, a jug from a vase – what is critical is whether they serve the appropriate function; the actual sensory features may vary considerably. However, to distinguish, say, a strawberry from a raspberry, the sensory features are the critical characteristics because there is virtually no functional difference. So it was argued that the herpes patients had retained the functional-specification semantic system but had lost knowledge of sensory features; indeed, they described objects in terms of their function. By contrast, Warrington and McCarthy (1983) argued that VER had retained some access to sensory features, but not to function.

Interesting support for the idea that the herpes encephalitis patients had a specific difficulty with sensory-quality information, even for auditory–verbal input, was provided by Silveri and Gainotti. Their herpes patient, LA, showed characteristics similar to those studied by Warrington and Shallice (1984). In addition, they gave the patient a verbal test with animal names in which they were defined using perceptual attributes – 'A black and white striped wild horse'→ *zebra* – or by a metaphorical expression or function – 'Man's best friend'→ *dog,* or 'The farm animal which bleats and supplies us with wool'→ *sheep.* LA was only 9% correct with perceptual types of question, but 58% correct with metaphorical or functional. Moreover, when presented with objects to define, LA very frequently (66% of occasions) described their function.

That the differentiation between a functional specification subsystem and a sensory-quality one may not be the complete answer was suggested by a study of Hart et al. (1985). They analysed a patient, MD, who had had a left hemisphere stroke. When tested, he was no longer aphasic, as assessed on the Boston Aphasia Battery (Goodglass & Kaplan, 1972). However, he had a highly selective naming difficulty. Using colour photographs, he made 39% errors naming different fruits and 33% errors on vegetables, but with all other items presented – a total of 229 – he made only 3% errors. Thus he failed to name *peach* and *orange,* but was correct on *abacus* and *sphynx.* Moreover this 'other' group included 13 food products other than fruit and vegetable. MD's naming difficulty also extended to naming from auditory definitions and tactile input. Thus only 2/10 fruit and vegetable items were named from definition, by comparison with all of 10 other items.

There is a second problem for the explanation in terms of a distinction between separable subsystems for functional specification, on the one hand, and sensory qualities, on the other. It comes from an additional observation made by Warrington and McCarthy (1987) on YOT. When YOT was given large man-made objects (e.g. *tank*) in a five-alternative forced-choice procedure, he was correct on 78% of trials, roughly the same as for foods (83%) and significantly higher than for indoor objects (e.g. *brush*) (58%). This is the same dissociation as that observed clinically by Yamadori and Albert (1973). Large man-made objects, though, have functions, and Warrington and McCarthy argued that they are as varied in their sensory qualities as are indoor objects, although no quantitative evidence was presented on this point. Thus the preceding dictotomy does not explain the selective preservation of this category. Warrington and McCarthy suggested that performance differences might exist between large man-made objects and indoor objects because the outdoor objects are not manipulable.

How is one to understand all these category specific effects? They can occur as semantic access deficits (e.g. VER), as degraded store deficits (e.g. JBR),[35] or as naming deficits (e.g. MD). They can also occur for a bewildering variety of categories. There seem to be patterns in which categories go together in being either selectively impaired or preserved. Yet the combinations are far from simple. Moreover, there are strong suggestions, although it is yet to be conclusively proved, that some types of impairment appear in both a 'wider' or a 'narrower' form.[36]

Instead of conceiving of the semantic system as a set of discrete subsystems (functions, sensory properties, and so on), therefore, it may be more useful to think of it as a giant distributed net in which regions tend to be more specialised for different types of process. For an object, these might include the representations of non-visible sensory features; knowledge related to relevant actions; knowledge related to what would be found near it; somewhat more abstract aspects, such as knowledge related to an object's function; more spatial ones, such as its geographical location; and even more abstract operations, such as how it was manufactured and its chemical constituents. The specialisation could arise because of the different pattern of connections – outside the semantic system itself – used by each particular process. Warrington and Shallice (1984) suggested that the coding of functional specificity may take place in a partially separable part of the semantic system because of the pattern of connections made with other subsystems, particularly those subserving action and intention. This idea that the pattern of dissociations within semantic categories might reflect the connections made with systems outside the semantic system has also been advocated by Allport (1985) (Figure 12.7) and, in much more detail, by Warrington and McCarthy (1987).

Warrington and McCarthy point out that the idea is compatible with Lissauer's (1890) original conception of associative agnosia! They argue that different processing channels may have a different 'weighting' in the identification process, even within, say, visual perceptual input. On a distributed network approach, such a developmental process can be viewed as one in which individual units (neurons) within the network come to be most influenced by input from particular input chan-

---

35. JBR had a contingency coefficient of 0.61 for the similarity of his performance in two picture-defining tasks, close to the maximum possible (0.71).

36. No detailed investigation of names of fruits and vegetables in comparison with names of other food items has been carried out with the herpes patients, and Hart, Berndt, and Caramazza (1985) did not examine MD's performance with living things. Thus it cannot be conclusively stated that MD's impairment is the narrower.

non- linguistic   attribute- domains

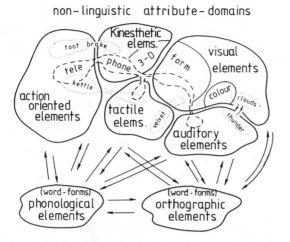

Figure 12.7. Allport's (1985) model of the accessing of semantic representations in word comprehension. Reprinted from Allport (1985) by permission of Churchill Livingstone.

nels and, in turn, come to have most effect on particular output channels. Complementarily, an individual concept will come to be most strongly represented in the activity of those units that correspond to the pattern of input–output pathways most required in the concept's identification and use. The sets of units that are most critical for a related group of categories would then come to form semi-modules, to use the conceptual framework of chapter 11.[37] The capacity to distinguish between members of a particular category would depend on whether there are sufficient neurons preserved in the relevant partially specialised region to allow the network to respond clearly differentially to the different items in the category.

The basis on which differentiation among processing regions within the semantic system would develop would include the most favoured modality of input for the process. Modality-specific pre-semantic classification systems would, thus, come to be more closely linked to some of the processing regions within the overall semantic system. So 'visual semantic' and 'verbal semantic' could be thought of as partially specialised subregions, and the modality-specific effects discussed in sec-

---

37. This would entail that damage to a partially specialised region should not produce classical dissociations because all processes using the system would use all its parts *to some extent*. Classical dissociations have yet to be observed for impairments within the semantic system. To account for the pattern of dissociations observed, it is probably necessary to assume that if a concept's representation in one partially specialised region increases, its representation in others will tend to decrease. This would certainly be computationally efficient overall. Without this assumption, it is difficult to see why adding a characteristic (manipulability) should decrease how well it can be identified, as has been claimed to be the case in YOT. A second complex problem that remains unexplained is that the major double dissociation observed sensory quality versus functional specificity has involved qualitatively different types of disorder (e.g. access vs. degradation).

tion 12.7 could be subsumed within the general framework.[38] Category specific naming difficulties might be explicable in terms of damage to sub-zones of particular specialised regions lying more towards the output part of the system. However, for explanations of this sort to be more than a speculation, a simulation of the hypothetical semantic system would be required.

12.9   An Application of Category Specificity: Agrammatism?

As its name implies agrammatism is normally viewed as a disorder of syntactic operations. It is commonly characterised as an inability to use inflections and function words appropriately, and a reduction in both the length of utterances and the range of syntactic constructions used. In chapter 7, it was shown how it is implausible to view all disorders of this type as arising from a deficity to a subsystem common to both comprehension and production.

Many agrammatics tend to omit main verbs. Can this problem be viewed as a syntactic disorder? Two recent studies suggest that in at least some 'agrammatic' patients, the deficit is best viewed within the lexical semantic sphere, possibly as another category specific semantic disorder. In the first of these studies, Miceli, Silveri, Villa, and Caramazza (1984) compared how well three groups of subjects – 5 agrammatic aphasics, 5 anomic patients, and 10 normal controls – performed on two naming tests. To be included as an agrammatic aphasic, a patient had to misuse or omit inflections and function words and to have a reduced length of utterance. The anomic aphasics had to make naming errors or circumlocutions, avoiding the use of a word by the use of a more laborious expression, and to make no agrammatic errors. The patients were compared on a test of naming pictures of objects and one of naming pictures of actions. The patients had to respond with the single word (noun or verb) most appropriate to the picture. The scores of three of the patients are shown in Table 12.12. Four of the five agrammatic patients were worse on action naming than on object naming, and the relative superiority of object naming was greater than for any of the controls. By contrast, four of the five anomic patients were better on action naming than on object naming, again with the relative superiority being greater than for any control subject.[39]

It might be possible to interpret the greater difficulty the agrammatic patients had in naming actions as a syntactic difficulty, even when only single verb labels are used. It could be argued that to name an action requires a number of stages. A proposition (the depicted action) must be constructed, with its corresponding arguments (the person or object involved); from this, a sentence frame must be generated, and then the predicate and arguments given lexical form. So a syntactic problem might be the root cause.

Such an explanation is not plausible for the agrammatic difficulties of ROX, a

---

38. Coupled subsystems, the characterisation used in section 12.7, is one form of partially specialised subregion.

39. It can be seen that CDA and ML$_2$ form a cross-over double dissociation.

Table 12.12. *The performance (% correct) of one agrammatic aphasic (CDA) and two anomic aphasics (AA and ML₂) on different naming tests (in percentages)*

	Object naming	Action naming
CDA	71.4	50
AA	10.7	59.1
ML$_2$	37.8	75
Controls	91.5	95.8

From Miceli, Silveri, Villa, and Caramazza (1984)

patient suffering from cortical atrophy who was studied by McCarthy and Warrington (1985). His spontaneous speech was dysfluent and characterised by a marked reduction in the use of substantive verbs. It was also noted that like the patients reported by Miceli et al., ROX was very poor at naming common mimable verbs (e.g. *kick*) (30 to 57% on different tests). By comparison, he scored at the average or superior level on graded-difficulty naming tests, which required his being able to produce correctly nouns such as *shuttlecock, pagoda,* and *mitre.* With the verbs, ROX tended to make semantic errors; for instance, he said 'pulling' for a picture of *pushing,* and 'caught' for one of *throwing.* Such semantic errors are not obviously explicable on the syntactic account of the verb difficulty in agrammatism. More critically, a similar phenomenon occurs in comprehension. Picture–word matching tests using common but semantically related verbs (e.g. *eat* and *drink*) were performed significantly worse than tests with semantically related nouns (e.g. *seal* and *walrus*) (74 vs. 99% correct).

ROX's difficulty was not just limited to verbs. He had difficulty comprehending prepositions. In addition, he performed poorly on four-choice abstract-word–picture matching tests (57% correct). It therefore seems plausible to view his difficulty in verb comprehension and production as the consequence of damage to a region of the semantic system possibly neighbouring those involved in comprehension of function and other yet more abstract relations. The view of McCarthy and Warrington (1985) was that his *syntactic* difficulties in spontaneous speech were the outcome of his using a strategy that attempts to compensate for his semantic impairment. The superordinates *being, having,* and *making* were the only verbs that remained *semantically* available to him.

12.10 Conclusion

The chapter began by considering Fodor's (1983) position on the split between input and central systems and his assumption of a total change in mode of operation as one moves from one domain to the other. Processes that use the semantic system would seem to be near the borderline that Fodor considers to exist between input and central domains. It is clear from the discovery of so many dissociations that the semantic systems are far from being functionally homogeneous. It would, though, probably be inappropriate to describe them as internally modular. They may well differ from 'input' systems in the sharpness of their internal functional specialisation. Instead, the functional specialisation within the semantic systems may technically be only partial, even though it is much stronger than was previously thought. This would be the case if semantic operations were the province of a large distributed network that was far from being an equipotential system. A consequence would be that the binary contrast that Fodor drew between types of cognitive systems – the modular and the equipotential – would be too limited to account for the types of cognitive systems that exist. His conceptual arguments for the equipotentiality of the 'central' systems could also fall. A partially specialised distributed network would not be informationally encapsulated and so could be a possible foundation for creative thought operations.

13 The Allocation and Direction of Processing Resources: Visual Attention

13.1 The Problems of Parallel Processing

The modular model of the mind that is suggested by cognitive neuropsychology research contains a conceptual lacuna. The existence of many special-purpose processing systems, each of which can operate autonomously, would not seem sufficient to produce coherent and effective operation for the whole system. Does this function itself require special-purpose units?

Another aspect of the functional architecture, in addition to modularity, needs to be considered in responding to this question. It has been widely assumed in theorising on cognitive processes that all the routine cognitive and motor skills that we have are controlled by more or less program-like entities, such as 'productions' (e.g. Newell & Simon, 1972) or action or thought 'schemata' (Schmidt, 1975; Rumelhart & Ortony, 1977). It is presumed that just as the mind contains representations of a finite but large and extensible set of words, so it contains a large but finite set of action or thought schemata. What would any individual thought or action schema control? There would be an enormous variety of operations. Take, for instance, how to use a table knife for cutting, for pushing, or for spreading food; how to subtract one number from another; how to rotate an object mentally; and so on. Moreover, schema control would be on multiple levels; so the schema for making a sandwich could call those for cutting bread and for spreading butter.

The hierarchy of schemata can be divided into two broad levels. The higher level corresponds to what Schank and Abelson (1977) called 'scripts' and Schank (1982), 'memory organisation packets' (MOPs); the standard example is the overall organisation of an activity that goes through several stages, such as having a meal in a restaurant. A characteristic of such a higher level script, or MOP, is that selection of such a unit does not commit any particular processing subsystem to operate at any specific time. An activity like paying the bill may be realised in a variety of ways; one may count out coins, write a cheque, sign a credit-card form, or select a voucher, and these do not require the identical set of processing systems.

This chapter will, however, be concerned not with this level of units but with lower level schemata to which I will restrict the term *schema*. It will be distinguished from a script or MOP in that operation of a *schema* in this sense places a particular pattern of demands on the mosaic of functionally specific subsystems that

307

can, for the present purposes, be assumed to operate as Fodorian modules. Thus the schema controlling the writing of a word to dictation requires specific subsystems to be operative – at the very least, the use of the phonological word-form system and a variety of graphemic output systems. The schemata concerned with steering can require visuo-spatial and manual control systems as well as object-recognition systems used for identifying the road's edge, holes, and solid obstacles.[1]

From the dual-task experiments discussed in chapter 7, it is clear that more than one independent schema is capable of controlling the processing systems it requires at the same time. Yet in computer technology, the operation of multiple systems in parallel is known to have potential dangers.[2] For instance, a subsystem can take as an input a state of affairs that another is at that time changing, or two subsystems can produce incompatible outputs so that each blocks the operation of the other; they can also select different aspects of a complex state of affairs as relevant, so that their outputs are not properly comparable.

An analogue of this state of affairs can be observed in patients with lesions of the corpus callosum, which connects the two hemispheres. In these patients, conflicting movements can at times be observed. Thus Smith and Akelaitis (1942) reported a patient who 'performed curious antagonistic reactions, such as attempting to put on an article of clothing with the right hand and pulling it off with the left' (p. 529). Another 'displayed persistent movement antagonisms for a short period after the operation, such as picking up a deck of cards, putting it down and picking it up' (p. 529). Similar observations have been made by Gazzaniga, Bogen, and Sperry (1962), by Logue, Durward, Pratt, Piercy, and Nixon (1968), by Bogen (1985), and, in 'split brain' animals, by Trevarthen (1965). It would appear that coherence of behaviour is not totally preserved by lower level mechanisms.

How, then, can effective coherent thought and action be maintained? In normal

---

1. The concept of schema has been much used in psychology (e.g. Bartlett, 1932; Rumelhart & Ortony, 1977; for a connectionist account, see Rumelhart, Smolensky, McClelland, & Hinton, 1986). In artificial intelligence, *schema* is now used as a general term for a specific collection of a large set of facts, together with specifiable variables (see Charniak & McDermott, 1985). My usage is somewhat more directed in that this 'collection' not only has the function of being an efficient description of a state of affairs – as in, say, Bartlett's usage – but also is held to produce an output that provides the immediate control of the mechanisms required in one cognitive or action operation. The usage is therefore more analogous to Piaget's (1936) view than to Bartlett's original concept.

   The distinction between processing systems (or modules) and schemata is that the former are held to correspond to dedicated hardware, while the lowest level of the latter are thought of as the first level of control process operating on the hardware. From the discussion in chapter 12, it would follow that processes that interact in any unusual combination with other subsystems and are very well practised – reading is an example – develop into separable subsystems. Reading, however, also involves a variety of schemata; consider the differences among reading aloud, 'skimming' a text, proof-reading, and so on, which presumably involve overlapping sets of processing systems. It is unclear to what extent the processes underlying an activity like steering a car, which involves visuo-spatial → motor control, are isolable from other activities requiring visuo-spatial motor control, such as occur in playing many games. I have assumed that they are not. If they were, then the final example would need to be rendered at a more abstract level.

2. See Johnson-Laird (1983) for a straightforward introduction.

psychology, the revival of attention as an active field of research was bound up with the problem of how effective use is made of limited processing capacities. This would seem to make theories of normal attention an appropriate starting place. There is, however, a major complication. The view of the cognitive system first espoused in information-processing psychology had as a principal component the general-purpose limited-capacity single channel (Broadbent, 1958). This is conceptually far removed from the mosaic of special-purpose subsystems postulated in cognitive neuropsychology. Many modern attentional theories still incorporate a general-purpose limited-capacity system with various refinements. Take Shiffrin and Schneider's (1977) influential theory, which is couched in terms of associative networks, a conceptual approach also difficult to map onto the modular one. It has an analogue to single-channel operation – controlled processing. One possibility for coherent schema operation in the spirit of limited-capacity theory or Shiffrin and Schneidere's model would be a single control system that keeps track of all the subsystems required by each schema being effected.

Centralised control of the operation of complex information systems does, however, produce severe computational problems. An example can be found in the automated control of large industrial operations, such as the manufacture of steel, a process that, like the cognitive system, contains many highly specialised processes. Thus Kahne, Lefkowitz, and Rose (1979), in a review of the use of centralised control programs in such operations, pointed out, 'In order to manage the resources of the control computer and to allocate them among the competing control tasks in real time, elaborate executive programs had to be developed' (p. 62). At the time they wrote, such executive programs tended to account for 30 to 40% of all the computer instructions executed, nearly as many as for all the specialised processes. This large 'overhead' dramatically affected the performance of the entire system. The time from the sensing of an external stimulus to the time the control program is able to respond is between 20 and 80 times longer than the basic response time of the computer. Centralised control is thus very expensive in processing capacities and, more critically, greatly slows the speed at which the system can respond. The trend in industrial operations has been towards decentralised control of complex systems.

Decentralised control obviously necessitates some means of measuring the priority that a possible operation should have, so that it can be compared with the priority of operations that might compete with it. The use of local priority measures alone, however, does not cope with the range of more global problems that affect parallel computing systems. In considering these, two states of affairs need to be separated. First, there are groups of subsystems that operate in a fairly tightly interconnected and fixed fashion, but in which control problems can arise because individual subsystems have more inputs than they can process at a time or because different subsystems operate at different speeds. Examples are the subsystems for visual perception that are involved in the transition from the level of the 2½D sketch to that of perceptual classification and identification, and the interaction among phonological, syntactic, and semantic processing systems in language. In both these cases, the subsystems operate frequently in the same combination. The most obvious way of dealing with any control problems involved would be to have a specialised control unit for each combination.

The second type of situation is the demand made on subsystems when more than one type of cognitive and motor skill is triggered. In this case, the combination of subsystems that might be called on to operate together at any particular time would be very large. The problems that might arise due to the interference in attempting to satisfy multiple task demands could vary greatly. A different type of control system would seem to be required. This second type of situation and second type of control system are discussed in chapter 14. In this chapter, I will examine whether there is any neuropsychological evidence for the existence of the first type of attentional control unit in one particular case – visual perception.

13.2   A Special-Purpose Attentional Control Subsystem: Vision

In our visual world, we are surrounded by a plethora of objects, virtually all of which could, under some particular circumstance, be relevant for a possible action. In cognitive psychology, there has been much discussion over the past 30 years of how many of these objects can be effectively processed by the higher levels of the visual perceptual system at any one time (e.g. Broadbent, 1958; Treisman, 1960; Deutsch & Deutsch, 1963; Allport, 1977; Duncan, 1980; Treisman & Gelade, 1980). It is, however, difficult to understand why a facility for multiple-input identification should develop at higher levels of the perceptual system when the lower levels seem to be designed to process only single inputs in detail; acuity falls off very sharply from the fovea. It therefore seems more likely that only a very limited number of objects – maybe only one – can be analysed at higher levels at a time.

From the results of experiments on normal subjects, theorists have speculated that earlier levels of the visual systems might operate in parallel across simultaneously presented stimuli, but later processes might operate more sequentially with the transition from one stage to the other, requiring one or both of active selection or emphasis of some stimuli or exclusion of others (e.g. Posner, 1980; Treisman & Gelade, 1980). A system that can process only a very limited number of objects to a level sufficient for identification would require a rapid system for allocating that capacity in order to analyse effectively those objects within sight that are potentially the most relevant.[3]

3. A more complex computational argument for an attentional control system in vision has been presented by Watt (1987). Following Wilson and Bergen (1979), he argues that a number of spatial filters of different size are used in the visual analysis of a scene. A variety of dimensions, in addition to size, need to be determined using the filters; they include orientation, curvature, and blur. As many visual illusions show, the processing of *particular* dimensions can adapt to particular circumstances. So conflicts among the different types of representation will occur and need to be resolved; Gregory and Heard (1981) called this the process of border-locking. The computational complexity of this process increases rapidly with the number of elements being analysed. Watt therefore proposes that the computational difficulty is best dealt with by beginning with the grossest spatial analysis of the relevant part of the scene and increasing the resolution of the spatial analysis over time until a figure is identified. The control of this process would be a function of visual attention. It would be much more difficult to apply it to two objects simultaneously.

That such a system exists is obvious from one of its more peripheral manifestations – eye movements. Physiological work on this so-called second visual system strongly suggests that there are specialised systems to control the use of peripheral processing capacity. For instance, Wurtz, Goldberg, and Robinson (1982) have discovered that cells in the superior colliculus show an enhanced response 50 msec after a spot comes on the screen if it is to be the target of an eye movement.

That a visual attention system might do more than simply control the position of receptors is suggested by the way that in particular cortical areas, single-cell recordings of the effects of visual stimuli have been shown to be influenced by the attention of the organism, independently of eye movements. Two such areas are posterior parietal cortex (Brodmann's area 7) (Wurtz et al., 1982) and part of extra-striate cortex (V4) and infero-temporal cortex (Moran & Desimone, 1985). A visual attention system might then plausibly be thought of as having a second type of function, concerned with the selection from the information that is processed spatially in parallel of that which is to be processed relatively sequentially at a higher level. At least two different neuropsychological syndromes relate to this aspect of visual attention. The most widely studied of these syndromes – those concerned with so-called visual neglect – are a complex and probably heterogeneous group. I will therefore begin with a simpler disorder, which is functionally more homogeneous and which has properties that map well with those of normal experiments – attentional dyslexia.

13.3 Attentional Dyslexia

Attentional dyslexia appears to be a disorder of the control system concerned in the parallel-to-sequential translation process. It has so far been described in only two patients: FM and PT (Shallice & Warrington, 1977b). Both patients had tumours deep in the left parietal lobe, but their expressive speech functions were intact. Neither patient was demented, both scoring at average level or above on the Digit Span and Similarities subtests of the WAIS as well as the Vocabulary subtest.

The two patients were initially investigated because of similar clinical observations. After reading a single word correctly, each was unable to name its constituent letters perfectly even with the word still present; apparently bizarre errors were often made in this seemingly simple task. The effect was not due to a problem in reading individual letters in isolation; indeed, it was not even specific to letters, but was due to a difficulty in identifying more than one item in a visual category. Thus for letters, words, and familiar shapes, if a single item had to be identified, the error rate was very low; but if a number of items were presented on the page and had to be identified one after the other, the error rate mounted considerably (Table 13.1). It might be asked why the patients, who had already read a word, did not use their knowledge of its spelling to produce the letters. In fact, FM actually claimed that he *saw* the letters incorrectly, and so when asked what the letters were, he naturally said what he saw.

A difficulty of this sort could conceivably be arising at quite a number of levels. At what level is the impairment? First, we are not dealing here with a form of the

Table 13.1. *Percentage errors made by two attentional dyslexic patients in naming visual stimuli in different size arrays*

		\multicolumn{3}{c}{Array size}		
		1	3, 4, or 5	25
Letters	FM	8	22	44
	PT	0	29	52
Words	FM	8	18	—
	PT	0	18	—
Line drawings	FM	0	16	—
	PT	0	22	—

visual disorientation syndrome discussed in chapter 8. The patients could always point correctly to the letter they were attempting to identify. In addition, both could scan rapidly for a fixed target letter in a vertical column of letters.

There were two findings that suggested a more specific perceptual location for the deficit. One procedure used was to flank a target symbol by four other symbols of the same category that were of a different colour and did not have to be reported – for example, HJ*Y*CR. Even though only one response had to be produced, interference was considerable (Table 13.2). If, however, flanking was by a member of a different visual category, then the interference effect dropped almost to nothing. When flanking was by digits, FM made significantly more errors (15%) if the target was itself a digit than if it was a set of dots that had to be counted (4%). If the interference was occurring in the response production process, as much interference would be expected in the latter situation because the same response has to be produced.

A further interesting finding occurred when multiple words were presented. The most typical error was for a letter from the same position in a neighbouring word to 'migrate' into the target word. For instance, *win fed* was read as *fin fed*. For FM, when a letter from another word in the visual field was inserted into a target word, it was from the same position in the other word on 13 of the 14 occasions, significantly higher than chance (estimated at 51%). Errors of this type where the phonological correspondence of the letter changed were frequent; this makes it unlikely to be occurring in the speech production system as a form of Spoonerism. A visual-processing origin is more plausible.

A closely similar phenomenon is now known to occur in normal subjects when they are attempting to report one of a set of words that are briefly presented (e.g. for 200 msec) and followed immediately by a 'pattern mask', made up of strokes that are parts of letters (Allport, 1977; Shallice & McGill, 1978; Mozer, 1983). Letters in the *same position* in another word tend to be perceived in the target word. Thus if *ward hark* were presented, *hard* would be liable to be perceived, but not

Table 13.2. *Percentage errors made by two attentional dyslexic patients in naming one centrally placed letter on a card (the "flanking" experiment)*

	Single	Flanked by numbers	Flanked by differently coloured letters
FM	8	12	27
PT	0	2	27

dark. Thus Mozer, who used elegant controls for guessing, found that 25% of all errors were 'true migration' errors. Moreover, the word-reading errors in attentional dyslexia and the migration errors that occur in brief masked exposure of multiple words with normal subjects have other properties in common.[4]

A number of different ways of explaining the migration errors found in normal subjects have been proposed (see Shallice & McGill, 1978; Mozer, 1983; McClelland, 1985; Treisman & Souther, 1985). Although the explanations differ, there is a strong family resemblance among them. Thus all except for that of Treisman and Souther adopt a cascade type of model of the word-reading process (chapter 11). All except for that of McClelland see migration errors as arising at the parallel-to-sequential focusing of the flow of information through the visual perceptual system.[5] Attentional dyslexia would appear to be explicable in terms of damage to the mechanism that controls this focusing.

On our approach, an attenuating filter analogous to the one proposed by Treisman (1960) and for which there is some neurophysiological support (Moran & Desimone, 1985) reduces the output of letter-level analyses outside the appropriate 'window' in the visual field (Figure 13.1). An impairment of the filter control mechanism would allow output from the 'parallel' levels of analysis of stimuli in parts of the visual field other than the target word to also activate units at the word-form level. Moreover, in its normal operation, the setting of the filter to the appropriate size of window must occur in real time and presumably depends on the prior activation of figure–ground units in the visual system. Thus when subjects are required

4. The visual similarity between the initiating and the recipient words is also known to be important; however, this has been shown for the letters that are the neighbours of the migrating one in normal subjects and for the target and migrating letters in the patients (see Shallice & McGill, 1978). A further similarity is that in both cases, the illusion is the production of what Mozer (1983) terms 'copies'. If two stimuli are to be identified, there is not a switch of components between them, but one component occurs in both responses. The subject presented with *live lone* will be more likely to see *love lone* than *love line*.
5. McClelland's (1985) model is conceptually considerably more complex than the other three. In his model, more than one input may be processed at the lexical level at a time. However, it will remain an open theoretical question whether impairment to this system could account for the properties of attentional dyslexia until the syndrome has been simulated on his model in the same way as have the migration errors found in normal subjects.

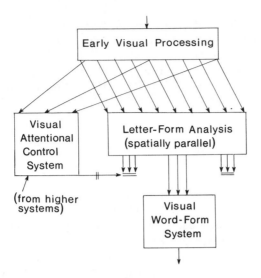

Figure 13.1. A simple model of attentional control of visual perception. The situation represented is during the analysis of the centre one of three three-letter words.

to report one of two briefly exposed stimuli, the filter may typically initially be set to include both words. In this case, too, letters outside the target region would also activate word-form units.[6]

The idea that a visual attention control subsystem exists that determines the size and locus of the 'window' over which the output of parallel lower level analyses is not attenuated is far from being the only possible candidate for explanation. It does, though, help to explain why attentional dyslexic patients have difficulty whatever the type of visual input, given that multiple exemplars are present in the visual display, and why similar phenomena occur in normal subjects with visual masking.[7]

13.4   Neglect as a Pathology of Attention

Of the disorders that arise from neurological disease that relate to attention, much the best known is unilateral neglect. It can take many forms, but some of its manifestations are among the most dramatic of all neurological disorders. The patient

6. The idea that the window decreases to the appropriate size after the initial presentation of multiple stimuli fits with the suggestion of Watt (1987) (see footnote 3). The effect of similarity of context (see footnote 4) arises because the lexical unit corresponding to the similar context error receives activation from both the target and the visually similar distractor. Thus when *hark* and *ward* are presented, *hard* receives relatively more activation than it does when *hark* and *weed* are presented, and so is more likely to be inappropriately detected. Damage to the attenuating filter control mechanism would, of course, increase the probability of such errors.
7. It also fits with the results on 'illusory conjunctions' in normal subjects (Treisman & Gelade, 1980). An interesting alternative is Crick's (1984) proposal that activation of a thalamic centre has the effect of linking the neurons on different processing levels, which are simultaneously active, into a tempo-

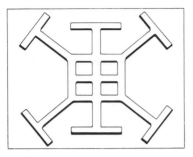

Figure 13.2. One of the two tactile mazes used in the tactile searching test. The subject's forefinger was initially placed in the centre of the maze; the target marble was at the end of one of the four lateral arms. Reprinted from De Renzi, Faglioni, and Scotti (1970) by permission of Masson Italia.

may, for instance, detect a target number on one side of a small array of numbers as rapidly as a normal subject, but fail completely for a minute or more if it is moved only a few inches to the neglected side – typically the left. When drawing, he or she may draw only the right side of objects. When reading, he or she may ignore or misread the beginnings of words. Such patients can even deny that a left limb – say, a paralysed arm – is theirs.[8]

Is neglect to be explained in terms of a disorder of attention control, and, if so, at what level? A wide range of theories of neglect have been proposed. One position that was often held was that its cause was a primary sensory disorder – a result of the loss of information from, say, the left visual field – in the setting of a dementing illness (see, e.g., Bender & Teuber, 1947; Battersby, Bender, Pollack, & Kahn, 1956).

This explanation is now generally considered insufficient. For instance, De Renzi, Faglioni, and Scotti (1970) used a tactile maze in which a marble was placed in one of four positions, the subject having eight trials in all (Figure 13.2). The maze being used on that trial was placed behind a curtain, and the subject had to search for the marble by moving a forefinger along the alleys of the maze. Normal subjects were divided into two groups, each of which used one hand or the other consistently. There was a tendency for normal subjects to search from left to right (Table 13.3).

Four groups of patients were tested, having left posterior, left anterior, right posterior, and right anterior lesions, respectively.[9] The patients always searched

rarily active cell assembly. Crick's idea has the advantage that it might help to explain the perseverative errors that occur in the modality-specific aphasias (chapter 12). The anatomy of attentional dyslexia fits with the locus of the visual attentional control centre being thalamic.

8. Many reviews of the literature on neglect exist. Probably the most comprehensive are those of De Renzi (1982) and Heilman, Watson, and Valenstein (1985).

9. The two left hemisphere groups were divided according to whether or not they had a visual-field defect, and the two right hemisphere groups, similarly. A visual-field defect is typically found with a lesion to the posterior parts of the hemisphere.

Table 13.3. *Mean search time (in seconds) in the tactile maze task of De Renzi, Faglioni, and Scotti (1970)*

| | | Side of marble | |
	Hand used	Ipsilateral	Contralateral
Normal subjects	L	30	32
Left-posterior group	L	28	36
Normal subjects	R	30	22
Right-posterior group	R	27	38

with the hand on the same side as their lesion, which would not be affected by any sensory or motor loss. If the marble was on this side of the maze, they found it as rapidly as control subjects who used that hand. However, if it was on the opposite side, both left and right hemisphere patients were significantly slower. The results of the more severely affected posterior groups are shown in Table 13.3. Errors showed a similar effect. The deficit on the contralateral side cannot be explained by sensory loss because the patients used their unimpaired arm throughout.

Patients with neglect frequently have a so-called spatial agnosia – a difficulty in appreciating the spatial relations between points, lines, and objects – because both disorders tend to be found after right posterior lesions. This has led unilateral neglect to be considered a consequence of a more general visuo-spatial processing difficulty (e.g. Brain, 1941; see also Gainotti, Messerli, & Tissot, 1972). However, patients with severe spatial agnosia but no neglect have been reported (McFie, Piercy, & Zangwill, 1950). In addition, it is not clear why a general visuo-spatial processing difficulty should affect only one side of space.

Two types of theory of the origin of neglect are fairly widely held at present. The first group of theories considers it to result from some impairment of attentional systems (e.g. Heilman & Watson, 1977; Mesulam, 1981; Posner, Walker, Friedrich, & Rafal, 1984). The second assumes that neglect is a cognitive deficit involving a mutilated representation of space (e.g. De Renzi et al., 1970; Bisiach, Luzzatti, & Perani, 1979). Thus De Renzi et al. argued that in their tactile-maze task, the subject must rely on his or her recollection of the outline of the maze and of the already explored areas in order to achieve a good searching strategy, which is to say that the spatial ability called for by the tactile task is a representation and not a perception of space. The relative empirical status of the two theories, the conceptual relation between them, and even whether they are attempting to explain impairments in the same group of patients were unclear until recently. The theories will be discussed separately because their relevance for understanding normal function differs considerably.

The simpler of the two types of explanation is the attention one. The idea that neglect might stem from a disorder of attention is quite old (e.g. Poppelreuter, 1923). The first study to link neglect empirically with the modern cognitive psy-

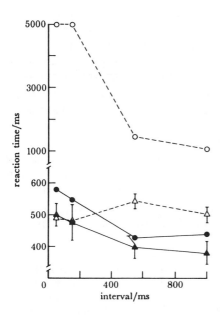

Figure 13.3. Median reaction times of a right parietal patient on targets presented to the left and right visual field in 'valid' and 'invalid' conditions. Circles represent left targets; triangles, right ones. The filled shapes are data from the valid condition; the open ones are data from the invalid condition. A median RT of 5 secs indicates that most targets were missed. Reprinted from Posner, Cohen, and Rafal (1982) by permission of the Royal Society.

chology of attention was that of Posner, Cohen, and Rafal (1982). They utilized a paradigm developed by Posner and his colleagues (see Posner, 1980) to study the spatial orienting of attention. In this paradigm, a cue, a 1° hexagon, is exposed for 300 msec 10° to the left or right of fixation; it is followed by a target either on the same side of the fixation point or on the opposite side. The subject's task is simply to respond to the target as quickly as possible. The subtlety in the design concerns the relationship between the cue and the target. The target occurs on the same side as the cue on 80% of trials, and on the other side on 20% of trials. The RTs in the invalid cue condition are slower. This is presumed to arise from the time taken for attention to be directed to the other side of the visual field.

Posner et al. (1982) used this procedure with five patients who had right parietal lesions, each having been diagnosed clinically as having extinction and visual neglect without hemianopia.[10] The results obtained for one of the five patients, RS, are shown in Figure 13.3. The most striking results occurred when the target was presented to the left visual field – the 'neglected' side. In the invalid (20%) cue condition, when attention was already directed towards the right, the target was

10. Extinction is a clinical phenomenon closely related to neglect in which a stimulus in the abnormal visual field can be perceived in isolation, but becomes imperceptible if presented in combination with a stimulus on the normal side. Unfortunately, neuropsychological details on the patients were not provided.

missed completely on most trials when it was presented close to the cue in time. By contrast, when the cue-onset to target interval was only 50 msec, the response to the 'left' target in the valid (80%) cue condition was only a little slower than if the cue and target were presented to the 'good' right visual field. As this interval is too short to allow any eye movements, the sensory input for a stimulus presented to the left visual field must provide enough information on which to base a response; the results in the invalid cue condition cannot be explained in terms of sensory loss alone.

The explanation given by Posner et al. for the overall pattern of results is that the slowing that occurred in the normal subject in the invalid cue condition due to attention having been directed to the other side was greatly exaggerated for RS if the cue instructed him to attend to the right. The plausibility of this attentional explanation is reinforced by the finding that the pattern of results is unaffected if the peripheral attention-catching cue is replaced by a central arrow pointing to left or right. Posner et al. (1982) continued that

the delay in processing an event on the uncued side is due to a slowing in the time for the event to enter a general attentional system responsible for detecting the event. The fact that under conditions where the uncued event is slowest one can find a complete inability to be aware of the event in some parietal patients provides support for the idea that such latency shifts are a sign of systems responsible for awareness in normal persons. (p. 196)

In this explanation, Posner and his colleagues drew on the position put forward by Posner and Klein (1973) that a general limited-capacity system is responsible for awareness. That this is too simple a conceptual framework from which to explain neglect is shown by a later study by Posner, Inhof, Friedrich, and Cohen (1987). The logic of this investigation was that if a general-purpose limited-capacity system responsible for awareness is what is impaired in neglect, then its capacity should be depleted yet further if the visual-orienting task has to be performed together with a second task utilising entirely different processing systems. In this situation, the invalid-cueing decrement should become considerably greater. The secondary task used was phoneme monitoring – listening to a list of words and detecting every occurrence of a particular phoneme. For cue–stimulus intervals of longer than 100 msec, parietal patients did show a much larger effect than normal subjects of having to carry out two tasks at the same time (Figure 13.4). Yet the speed-up in reaction time provided by a valid over an invalid cue is no different in the single-task and dual-task conditions.

To explain this pattern of results, Posner and his colleagues (1987) put forward a position similar to the one taken in section 13.1. The enlarged effect of the validity of the cue they found in parietal patients was explained as a consequence of damage to a visuo-spatial attention system. They held that when another task must be carried out at the same time, the cue is processed more slowly by a higher general-purpose attention system, used both to 'command' spatial orienting and to monitor. It therefore takes longer for the cue to be utilised by the visuo-spatial attention system (Figure 13.5). But once the information about the cue has arrived in that control

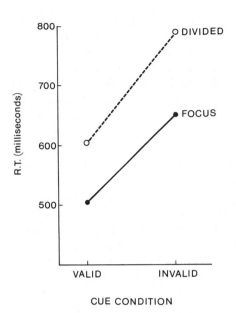

Figure 13.4. Performance of right parietal patients in single (focus) and dual (divided) task situations. From Posner, Inhof, Friedrich, and Cohen (1987); *Psychobiology 15:*112; reprinted by permission of Psychonomic Society, Inc.

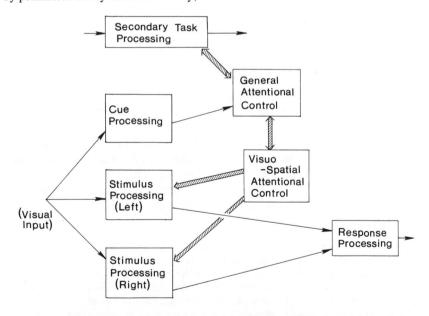

Figure 13.5. The model of Posner, Inhof, Friedrich, and Cohen (1987) for the interrelation of two levels of attentional control in their task. The hatched arrows relate to attentional control processes; solid arrows, to information-flow between processing systems.

system, it produces the same effect as though there were no secondary task. The difference in RT between valid and invalid cueing therefore remains unaffected by the secondary task. Additional support for this explanation can be obtained from the results when the cue–stimulus interval is very short (100 msec). At this speed, normal subjects show the normal cue-validity effect, but parietal patients do not. Posner and his colleagues argued that the cue has not been processed by the general-purpose attention system sufficiently rapidly to influence the distribution of processing by the visuo-spatial attention system before the target stimulus has been detected.

In neglect, then, as in attentional dyslexia, there seems to be an impairment to an attention system specific to visuo-spatial processing. Consider the vivid metaphor of the attentional focus in vision being like a zoom lens (Egeth, 1977).[11] The visuo-spatial attention system would be the control system for the lens. The two syndromes considered fit neatly with this position. Neglect, or at least those of its aspects so far considered, can be regarded as a defect in the activating process necessary to pull the attentional focus away from a previously set region of space. For attentional dyslexia, the deficit is in the ability to restrict the attentional focus to a particular region of space. In both cases, though, one seems to be dealing with a deficit not to any general-purpose limited-capacity attention system but to a special-purpose attentional system which the former system – if it exists – partly controls.[12]

13.5   Neglect Dyslexia

To read text, it is necessary that the attentional focus be limited to each word in turn. Otherwise, reading would be continually derailed by the occurrence of migration errors – the type of error that occurs in attentional dyslexia. Presumably, the visuo-spatial attentional control system utilises the primitive pattern of words and spaces on a page to determine the positioning and focusing of its 'zoom lens' for each word.

What would happen if the focus, as determined by the visuo-spatial control system, and the area of visual space from which information is present do not match? Attentional dyslexia has been given as one example of such a mismatch. Another dyslexic syndrome may be explicable in a related fashion. This is neglect dyslexia, in which the patient makes visual errors that consistently affect only one end of a

---

11. It would have to be a very special sort of lens because the attentional focus appears to be an object and not a region of space (Duncan, 1984). If two objects occupy a similar part of space, in that one overlies part of the other, it is an object to which attention is focused, not the region of space. This shows that the control system must receive at least some of its input from the figure–ground level of processing or above. This complication will be ignored in this chapter.

12. Posner and his colleagues have also been concerned about the processes underlying the deliberate movement of the attentional focus as well as those concerned with initiating such a movement. They argue that deliberate attentional movements are slowed, just as eye movements are, in patients with progressive supranuclear palsy, which produces degeneration of the superior colliculus and surrounding structures (see Posner, Cohen & Rafal, 1982).

word. In the more common form, the errors affect only the beginnings of words. Two papers, however, describe patients who made errors at the ends of words (Warrington & Zangwill, 1957; Friedrich, Walker, & Posner, 1985).

Three studies have been published in which a detailed analysis of neglect dyslexia was made. Kinsbourne and Warrington (1962a) described patients with lesions that included the right hemisphere. All made errors in which the initial letters of words were deleted (e.g. *ran→an*) or, more typically, were replaced by other letters (e.g. *wine→mine, enigma→ stigma*). Three of the patients had a hemianopia. However, Kinsbourne and Warrington argued that was unlikely to be a critical factor because errors continued to occur when information was presented tachistoscopically to the intact half-fields. The authors also noted a tendency for the errors to be of the same length as the words they replaced, suggesting that at least some analysis of the neglected letters was occurring.

These effects have been investigated in more detail by Ellis, Flude, and Young (1987) in patient VB, and by Costello and Warrington (1987) in patient JOH. As a result of a series of right hemisphere strokes, VB's Performance IQ was depressed to 84, but her Verbal IQ remained at 120. VB had a left homonymous hemianopia and showed neglect on a number of tasks, such as deleting crosses from an array and counting lines of dots. The latter deficit occurred not only in vision, but also when the input modality was touch; in this case, the stimuli were raised metal discs.

VB's neglect dyslexia showed itself clearly when she read single words exposed for 2 sec. In this situation she made about 15% errors. The probability of an error occurring was not affected by variables relevant to the central dyslexias – the frequency, length, imageability, syntactic class, or regularity of the words. Moreover, when she made an error she understood the target as the word said in error. All these effects point to the impairment being at an early stage of the reading process. Neglect dyslexia, therefore, falls under the class of dyslexic disorders referred to as the peripheral dyslexias (chapter 4).

Ellis et al. defined a neglect point for an error if it was identical to the target to the right of that point but diverged *completely* to the left of it. Thus in the error *yellow → pillow,* the neglect point lies between the *i* and the *l.* In a large corpus of errors made by VB in reading individual words, 66% had neglect points of this type, 26% of the errors were other real-word errors (e.g. *whom → thumb, abhor → labour*), and 8% of the errors were non-words.[13] Table 13.4 shows the relation between the length of the target words and that of the errors. There are frequently as many letters to the left of the neglect point in the error as there are in the target. Even when a word was misrecognised, information about the appropriate number of letters to the left of the neglect point appears to have been available.[14]

---

13. Occasionally, VB was given non-words to read, so the existence of non-word errors is not noteworthy.

14. This effect is not an artefact of word construction, with the patient guessing when the non-neglected set of letters does not form a word. A list of words was devised with the property that the first letter could be both deleted and replaced so as to produce another word (e.g. *soiling → oiling* or *boiling*). Of the 41 neglect errors that occurred using these stimuli, only 27% were the deletion errors that would be predicted by this explanation; 73% were substitutions.

Table 13.4. *The relation between length of target and length of error in VB measured from the 'neglect point'*

		Numbers of letters to left of neglect point in target				
		0	1	2	3	4+
Number of	0	—	15	3	0	0
letters to left	1	16	79	16	1	0
of neglect point	2	2	10	7	3	0
in error	3	3	1	3	2	0
	4+	0	0	0	0	0

From Ellis, Flude, and Young (1987)

Ellis et al. also established that the neglect effect is not a direct consequence of the hemianopia by presenting VB with cards on which a word composed of 1-cm-high capital letters was positioned 1 cm to the right of a red digit. VB's task was to read the digit and then the word. For the digit to be read correctly, which it was, the word must be in VB's intact visual field. Yet even with unlimited exposure durations, she made 12% errors, 90% of which were of the neglect type.

In the discussion of attentional dyslexia, it was suggested that the letter-form level of the processing of words encodes the relative positions of letters within a word (see Figure 13.1). Ellis et al. argued that in neglect dyslexia, information about letter position is preserved, but information about letter identity is lost. Thus when *train* is read as *slain,* letter-form analysis provides the output $-(1)$, $-(2)$, $a(3)$, $i(4)$, $n(5)$, and the attentional focus admits both types of information from all five positions. A subtly different possibility is that the letter-form system provides the output $t(1)$, $r(2)$, $a(3)$, $i(4)$, $n(5)$, but a reduced attentional focus restricts the input to the visual word-form system to the last three letters. On the first explanation, control of the attentional focus has not adapted to the loss of identity information; on the second, it is itself directly impaired. In either case, the attentional focus is inappropriately controlled.

The existence of errors slightly different in length from the target – for example, *barrel* → *quarrel* – does, however, require one to assume that the position of a letter in a word is not coded simply as its ordinal position in a left-to-right scan. A third possibility, which is more complex but perhaps somewhat more plausible, is that the ordinal position of each letter in the string is doubly coded, both in terms of its distance from the beginning of the word and in terms of its distance from the end. In both cases, the weight that the letter provides for the identification process would decrease as its distance from the relevant end of the word increases. Then it could be argued that in neglect dyslexia, one or other of these codings is lost. For neglect of the left, this would be the first set of codings.

JOH (Costello & Warrington, 1987) is a considerably more complicated patient. He had a left parietal tumour, which had spread across the corpus callosum to affect the right hemisphere as well. This had left him with impaired WAIS IQ performance (verbal, 87; performance; 73) and various manifestations of neglect. He had a right hemianopia but a neglect of the left end of words! Thus as far as his neglect dyslexia was concerned, any problem due to his hemianopia could be discounted. In other respects, his dyslexia had certain similarities to that of VB. Sixty-three per cent of his reading errors had neglect points of the same type as those shown by VB, and length of target was correlated with length of response. However, his reading showed the surprising characteristic that the longer the word, the more likely he was to read it correctly. Thus 86% of six- or seven-letter words were read correctly in comparison with only 66% of two- or three-letter ones, and additions were six times as common as deletions. One might conceivably argue on the basis of the third possible account advanced earlier that the information available coded from the end backwards is greater for long words than for short; so it is more resistant to being obscured if there is additional noise in the system.[15] However, neglect dyslexia has not been sufficiently explored for any explanation to be at present more than a speculative possibility.

13.6 Neglect as a Disorder of Spatial Representation

The other major strand in modern work on neglect is the idea that it consists of a disorder in the representation of things on one side of space. As early as 1913, Zingerle argued that in severe neglect, the patient's representation of the body is apparently confined to the right half only. The idea that a possible way to account for neglect is as a disorder in the representation for what lies in the left part of space was resurrected by the study of De Renzi et al. (1970). It became popular with the dramatic studies of Bisiach and his colleagues in Milan in the late 1970s (Bisiach & Luzzatti, 1978; Bisiach et al., 1979).

One of these studies, that of Bisiach et al. (1979), was a group study of 19 patients with right hemisphere lesions, all of whom showed clinical neglect in that they omitted to cross out one or more 1-cm circles in a 23 × 18 cm display. In the experiment, the patients had to view two cloud-like shapes that passed rapidly behind a narrow slit and decide whether they were the same or different. One-third of the pairs were the same; one-third differed on the left, and one-third on the right. The shapes took 2 sec to pass behind the slit, and there was a 1-sec interval between them. Detection rates were not very high, even for the control subjects (Table 13.5). However, the interaction between subject group and side of difference was significant.[16] As the stimuli passed continuously behind a vertical slit, an explanation in terms of an attentional disorder affecting stimulus *registration* of different parts of the field can be ruled out. Bisiach et al. argued that to perceive a moving cloud under these circumstances, a translation has to be made from a temporal dimension into a representational spatial one. They suggested that the left side of this representation may to some degree fade in unilateral neglect.

15. The number of competitors is also smaller for long words than for short ones.
16. This result has been replicated by Ogden (1985b).

Table 13.5. *Percentage of differences detected in the different conditions of the experiment of Bisiach, Luzzatti, and Perani (1979)*

	Side of difference	
	Left	Right
Control	48	47
Brain-damaged	34	44

In this experiment, the neglect phenomenon investigated was in the visual domain. Neglect is not, however, limited to perceptual representations. In a brief note, Bisiach and Luzzatti (1978) reported asking two patients with neglect of the left to describe from memory the square in front of Milan cathedral. The square has a roughly equal number of landmarks on two opposite sides. When asked to report how it would appear when viewed from the end opposite to the cathedral, the first patient reported five buildings and streets on the right and none of those on the left. When, however, asked to report the view from the other direction, as though she had her back to the cathedral door, she reported seven buildings and streets, again all on what would be her right. There was, of course, no overlap between the set of landmarks reported on the two occasions. A second patient produced the same phenomenon to a reduced degree and also showed it when describing his own study.

The same procedure was used by Bisiach, Capitani, Luzzatti, and Perani (1981) in a group study. The results produced strong confirmation of the clinical investigation (Table 13.6). The patients with neglect reported far fewer of the landmarks that would have been on their left in the imagined scenes, and this was the case for both perspectives. Sunderland (1984) obtained a similar finding, although the degree of neglect of the left shown by the right hemisphere lesion patients in his study was not correlated with visual neglect in other tasks. In addition, he pointed out a problem for certain interpretations of the view that neglect arises from an impaired representation of left sided features in the patient's image of the scene. In a second condition, Bisiach et al. specifically asked their subjects to describe the left side of the square when viewed from the particular perspective and then to describe the right side. In this cued recall condition, neglect did not occur. Sunderland argued that this finding supports a hypothesis put forward by Baddeley and Lieberman (1980) to explain neglect – that it arises from a defect in the mechanism that scans the left part of the inner screen to retrieve information and not from damage to the representation itself.

There is, however, another syndrome for which the possibility of neglect operating on an image seems even clearer. This is neglect dysgraphia, a disorder described in a phonological agraphic patient, ORF, by Baxter and Warrington (1983). As discussed in chapter 6, a patient with phonological agraphia can write or spell

Table 13.6. *Group study of Bisiach et al. (1981) on the Cathedral Square of Milan*

| | | Free condition | | | |
| | | First view | | Second view | |
Subjects	Number	L^a	R^b	L	R
Control	41	4.0	3.8	4.8	5.1
No neglect	22	4.2	3.4	3.0	3.3
Neglect	15	1.1	4.6	1.2	3.1

[a] The number of landmarks reported on the left
[b] The number of landmarks reported on the right

only by use of orthographic knowledge of words. The phonological agraphia of ORF arose from a right hemisphere stroke, the patient's speech being lateralised to the right.[17] ORF could no longer write, but he could spell aloud. As he was totally unable to spell two- or three-letter nonsense syllables, the non-lexical spelling procedure appeared to be inoperative. ORF's word spelling was far inferior to that of PR, the phonological agraphic patient described in chapter 6, but he, too, described his attempts to spell as like reading off an image. In addition, though, ORF said that the letters on the right side were more clear than those on the left. This is reminiscent of the fading of left-side representations suggested by Bisiach et al. (1981) as occurring in neglect.

Quantitative investigation of his spelling ability showed an effect of word length but not of either word frequency or word regularity, the latter finding giving further support to the idea that the phonological spelling route was not being used. There was, however, a strong effect of the position of the letter within the word. Surprisingly, it was the beginning of the word that gave most difficulty to ORF (Figure 13.6). This is quite the opposite pattern to that found, for instance, in children. ORF performed in an almost identical fashion when spelling backwards, giving the last letter first, as when spelling in the standard forward fashion. This gives striking confirmation of his introspection that he was spelling off a visual image, as people who lack such imagery ability find it far easier to spell forwards than backwards.

It appeared that the patient's disorder arose from a combination of three different features. ORF had his language functions, including certain aspects of his writing skills, in the right hemisphere and also had strong imagery. Finally, he suffered from neglect when attempting to use imagery to circumvent certain of his writing difficulties. This combination of characteristics will undoubtedly prove to be a very infrequent combination, so that neglect dysgraphia will almost certainly prove a

17. The repetition performance of ORF was discussed in chapter 7, where baseline details are provided (see Table 7.4).

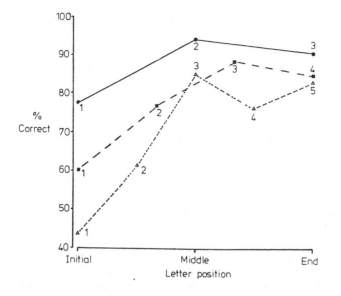

Figure 13.6. Performance of ORF on spelling aloud three-letter (circles), four-letter (squares), and five-letter (triangles) word stimuli. Reprinted from Baxter and Warrington (1983) by permission of the *Journal of Neurology, Neurosurgery and Psychiatry*.

very rare syndrome. ORF may remain unique. However, his syndrome strongly supports the idea that internal representations as well as perceptual input can be affected by neglect.

13.7   Impairments of Attention and Representation: Are They in Conflict?

In sections 13.5 and 13.6, two different accounts of neglect were given. At first glance, it would seem that neither theory can explain the phenomena that support the other. It is also far from clear that the phenomena described exist in the same set of patients. A patient with severe neglect, like those with whom Bisiach and his colleagues work, would not be likely to carry out Posner's cue-validity task properly, even in the valid cue condition; the cue would be neglected when it was on the left.

In fact, the two explanations given do not necessarily conflict. In the account of visual imagery given by Hinton (1979), the information in the visual image is represented computationally at the level of the 2½D sketch – to use Marr's (1982) terminology. This is a level of visual processing in which information is still represented spatially in parallel. The theory of visual imagery developed by Kosslyn (1980) has a component with similar characteristics – his 'surface matrix'. Moreover, on Kosslyn's theory computations that operate on images depend on an operator FIND, which is used to inspect the image and its relevant parts. If the level of representation involved in an image is that suggested by Hinton, then it would be natural for the FIND operation to use the visuo-spatial attentional control system discussed in earlier sections of this chapter. If this control system were faulty, this could have an effect when imagery was being used as well as in direct perception. This would be equivalent to the explanation of the initial Square of Milan findings that was suggested by Baddeley and Lieberman (1980).

It is increasingly clear that if one treats perception and imagery as processes best described by a complex flow diagram, there may well be a number of different types of impairment, each of which could manifest itself as neglect. It is noteworthy that ORF, the neglect dysgraphic patient, showed no clinical sign of neglect. The possibility therefore exists that neglect could fractionate in the same way that clinical syndromes like aphasia and dyslexia have already done.

The neglect dyslexic patient JOH (section 13.5) provides dramatic evidence that this is the case. It will be remembered that although he had a hemianopia that affected the right visual field, he neglected the left ends of words in reading. However, in visuo-spatial tasks, such as copying figures and bisecting lines, he neglected the right. Thus in 17/18 lines bisected, he placed the mid-point to the left of the actual centre of the lines, implying that the right end was being neglected. Any account of neglect that assumes that a single attentional focus cannot be moved adequately to one particular side appears doomed as a general theory!

The study of neglect is at present in a fascinating phase. The existence of a visuo-spatial attentional control system is the aspect of attention that has been most fruitfully explored in studies of the normal subject (e.g. Posner, 1980; Treisman, 1986). Much of the neuropsychological evidence, like that obtained from normal subjects, supports the existence of such an attentional control system specialised for the control of information flow between perceptual subsystems and distinct from a general cognitive resource-allocation system. However, as the study of JOH demonstrates, the phenomena of neglect are not all simply explained on the basis of such an approach. We will see in chapter 16 that there are complex issues of how certain neglect patients conceive of events that occur on their left. Whether they will prove minor anomalies for the attentional control system view or will enforce a paradigm shift remains to be seen. At present, though, the overall view of attention presented at the beginning of this chapter receives some, if limited, support from the neuropsychological evidence on visual attention control.

14   The Allocation of Processing Resources: Higher-Level Control

14.1   Classical Views on Frontal Lobe Function

Initiation of an action sequence can occur in an unintended fashion. This is well shown by the existence of certain types of action lapses called 'capture errors' (Reason, 1979; Norman, 1981), as, for instance, William James's (1890) famous example of going upstairs to change and discovering himself in bed. Such errors tend to occur when one is preoccupied with some other line of thought, as Reason (1984) has shown. Action initiation is occurring in parallel with some other activity. Unintended actions do not, though, occur only when they are inappropriate. They can be both appropriate and unmonitored.[1] This fits with the suggestion made early in chapter 13 that the control of which subsystems will be devoted to what task is often carried out in a decentralised fashion.

Actions such as these can be contrasted with ones that are preceded by 'an additional conscious element in the shape of a fiat, mandate or expressed consent', to quote William James (1890). When we decide or choose or intend or concentrate or prepare, decentralised control of the operation of particular subsystems does not appear to be the sole principle operating. How does the control of either of these types of action relate to the discussions on congitive control at the beginning of chapter 13? Such phenomenological contrasts by themselves provide only a very shaky basis for theorising. Can neuropsychology offer any additional guidance?

One set of neuropsychological syndromes, those associated with frontal lobe lesions, seem relevant. Problems of decision, intention, concentration, and so on have often been considered to arise from lesions to frontal lobe systems. From the nineteenth century on, there has been a school of thought that the frontal lobes are the seat of the most critical higher level control operations and that a lesion to these structures gives rise to a disorder of these functions. Typical of this type of inter-

---

1. In Shallice (1982), the example was given of my walking into a room I knew well and suddenly noticing that I was making a pulling movement with my arm, which I did not understand. I eventually realised what was obviously at some level 'known' – that the light switch in that room was controlled by a cord, which had got hooked up in a cupboard door. As the action was so mystifying at the time, it indicates that initiation and execution of this action was not normally controlled by a conscious intention to execute it.

328

pretation is the way that Bianchi (1922) illustrated the effect of large frontal lesions in the monkey:

The monkey which used to jump on to the window ledge, to call out to his companions, after the operation jumps on to the ledge again, but does not call out. The sight of the window determines the reflex of the jump, but the purpose is now lacking, for it is no longer represented in the focal point of consciousness. . . . Another monkey sees the handle of the door and grasps it, but the mental process stops at the sight of the bright colour of the handle; the animal does not attempt to turn it so as to open the door, but sits on it. Evidently there are lacking all those other images that are necessary for the determination of a series of movements coordinated towards one end. (pp. 184–185)

Bianchi (1922) characterised his monkeys as having lost the ability to coordinate the different elements of a complex activity. Investigations of human frontal lobe disorders have produced related accounts. Thus Burdach, as early as 1819, called the frontal lobes 'the special workshop of the thinking process' (quoted in Rylander, 1939, p. 14). Harlow (1868) argued that lesions there resulted in loss of planning skill. Goldstein, after working with soldiers who had received injuries to the frontal lobe in the First World War, argued that such patients had 'disturbed attention, increased distractibility, a difficulty in grasping the whole of a complicated state of affairs . . . well able to work along old routine lines. But they cannot learn to master new types of task; in new situations . . . at a loss' (quoted in Rylander, 1939 p. 20).

Throughout this century, related positions have coexisted with a contrasting view that the frontal lobes have few, if any, intellectual functions, or at least no special role in the adult (e.g. Pfeifer, 1910; Feuchtwanger, 1923). This dismissive view of the intellectual functions of the frontal lobes was reinforced when the initial investigations using IQ test measures showed that patients with frontal lesions performed at a level in no way inferior to patients with posterior lesions (Hebb, 1945). Later research has borne out Hebb's observations that frontal lesions do not have a disproportionate effect on IQ test performance. This was most dramatically demonstrated in the late 1940s in psychometric studies of psychiatric patients on whom a drastic prefrontal leucotomy had been performed; they did not show much deficit on IQ measures (see Mettler, 1949).[2] Indeed, a relatively frequent result for tasks of the WAIS IQ test type is to find a relative preservation of performance for frontal lobe groups by comparison with patients having more posterior lesions. This has been obtained for tumour patients (e.g. Smith, 1966) and for epileptic neurosurgery patients (Milner, 1975). It should be noted, however, that the results do not indicate that frontal lobe lesions have no effect on WAIS scores. Milner's patients showed an average loss of 7.2 IQ points after frontal lobe surgery. In a very large consecutive series of mixed aetiology, Warrington, James, and Maciejewski (1986) found

---

2. In fact, most of the tests used, even in the more detailed studies carried out at that time, were of fairly routine cognitive skills, such as those assessed in WAIS subtests. With the advantage of hindsight, the minimal effect of leucotomy on the tests used is not that surprising. For an informative history of the use of frontal leucotomy as a psychosurgical technique, see Valenstein (1973).

that patients with left frontal lesions scored insignificantly worse than those with left temporal or left parietal lesions on both Verbal and Performance IQ. For right hemisphere lesions, the complementary pattern was observed.

At the time that Hebb made his observations, Goldstein's (1944) counterclaim that standard IQ tests do not allow higher level deficits to manifest themselves was considered special pleading. Since then, though, the pendulum of neuropsychological opinion has swung Goldstein's way. Thus in more recent reviews, Jouandet and Gazzaniga (1979) characterized the frontal lobes as a system that sequences or guides behaviour toward the attainment of some immediate or distant goal, Fuster (1980) argued that their 'superordinate function' is 'the formation of temporal structures of behaviour with a unifying purpose or goal' (p. 126). Damasio (1985) considered the dorsolateral sector of the frontal lobes crucial for 'the coherent organisation of mental contents on which creative thinking and language depend, and that permit, in general, artistic activities and the planning of future actions' (p. 369).

As Duncan (1986) pointed out in a recent review, such ideas do not constitute a theory in the sense of the models discussed earlier in the book. The ideas on which they are based are everyday-language ones; no link is made with information-processing concepts. Moreover, there is a fairly large gap between these ideas and the empirical studies that have been carried out on patients with frontal lobe lesions. Hebb's (1945) empirical point remains valid; many patients with frontal lobe lesions do not manifest the dramatic deficits that one would expect, given the global characterisation of the function of the underlying system.

Why, then, should there have been a decline in popularity of Hebb's rather negative position on frontal lobe function? One of the key factors was the publication of Luria's work on frontal lobe disorders (see, e.g., Luria & Tsvetkova, 1964; Luria, 1966). Luria's position that the frontal lobes contain a system for the programming, regulation, and verification of activity is much more in keeping with ideas in cognitive science than are most of the other accounts. Moreover, his analysis was supported by descriptions of the behaviour of frontal patients on many interesting tests. For instance, such a patient may be presented with a problem such as 'There were 18 books on two shelves and there were twice as many on one than on the other. How many books were there on each shelf?' A frontal patient of Luria's, having repeated the question correctly, carried out the operation $18 \div 2 = 9$ (corresponding to the first clause) and then followed it by $18 \times 2 = 36$ (corresponding to the second clause), being quite satisfied with the result.

Luria's work, original and insightful as it was, can be criticised on a number of grounds. The patients on which his theories were tested often had lesions extending outside the frontal lobes (see Hécaen & Albert, 1978; Canavan, Janota, & Schurr, 1985), and patients with lesions involving frontal structures often have little or no difficulty with his tests. This is not a critical fault for a purely processing account of the disorders studied (chapter 9), provided that the deficits of individual patients are described in a quantitative fashion and their performance is compared with that of control patients. This was, however, frequently not the case in Luria's reports.

Case studies of frontal lobe disorders within Luria's theoretical framework are

Table 14.1. *The baseline characteristics of three of the patients studied by Lhermitte et al. (1972)*

	L$_2$	G	S
Lesion	Left frontal haematoma	Left anterior cerebral occlusion	Left frontal trauma
WAIS IQ	77	83	88
Progressive matrices percentile[a]	<25%	<25%	<25%
Binois-Pichot[b]	113	98	102
Wechsler Memory	83	87	89
Language	Much reduced	"Abundant enough"	Normal

[a] A non-verbal test of 'general intelligence'.
[b] A vocabulary test.

not limited to his own studies. Some studies are methodologically more satisfactory than his. Thus Lhermitte, Derouesné, and Signoret (1972) studied four patients, for three of whom the baseline characteristics are shown in Table 14.1. From the table, it is clear that all had relatively severe intellectual deficits. They are not therefore a typical cross-section of patients with lesions to the frontal lobes.

If one looks in detail at the performance of the patients, there are a number of clear signs that their deficit is at the programming level. For instance, they were asked to copy the Figure of Rey, a complex design used to test constructional skills and memory. When L$_2$ was presented with the design broken down into six separate stages with only a small section of the total figure to be added at each stage, the figure was fairly satisfactorily reproduced – nearly all the features were correctly inserted. When, however, he was presented with the figure to copy without any additional structuring, his performance was defective; very few features were re-cognisable and even these were misplaced. The effect of providing a program for the initial copying was also seen in his reproduction of the design from memory. When it had been provided, he scored at the 60th percentile; without it, the copy had no single detail correct. Behaviour of a qualitatively similar but less severe type was produced by patients G and S, both being in the lowest 10th percentile on retention if no structuring was provided.

It could be argued that the deficit on this task might be a subtle agnosic one in the perception of complex figures. However, a similar difficulty occurred with the Block Design subtest of the WAIS and is similarly aided by the provision of a program (see also Derouesné, Seron, & Lhermitte, 1975). More critically, a related pattern recurs in a totally different type of task – the solution of written arithmetic problems. For instance, with 'The son is 15 years old; his father is 25 years older; his mother is 5 years younger than the father. What is their combined ages?' Patient

G first added 15, 20 – a transcription error – and 5, and then announced that 40 was the 'total age of the father, the son and the Holy Ghost', thinking that he had solved the problem and producing the sort of irrelevant verbal association that can occur in a frontal patient. By contrast, tasks that require little programming could be satisfactorily carried out by all three patients. For instance, L_2 scored at the average level on the Digit Span, Picture Completion, and Similarities subtests of the WAIS (Derouesné, personal communication).

The behaviour described in these patients fits qualitatively with a disorder in the programming, regulation, and verification of activity. It gives the impression of routine programs being run off without adequate selection, monitoring, and control. However, a concept like 'programming' can be applied to describe different levels of the control of action and thought. When, for instance, one carries out an action like lighting a cigarette or cutting a slice of bread, one can be said to program the outflow to the effector systems. Indeed, theorists of motor control have used related ideas to describe the functions of the basal ganglia (see Marsden, 1982; Paillard, 1982). Intuitively, it would seem that this is not the level of programming that is impaired in the patients described by Lhermitte et al. (1972). However, for the concept of a system for the programming, regulation, and verification of activity to be useful, clear qualitative distinctions between different referents for programming need to be drawn. In particular, one needs to consider what is implied in assuming the existence of a single such system that can operate in all thought and action domains.

14.2   The Supervisory Attentional System and Contention Scheduling

The initial consideration of frontal lobe disorders has moved rather far from the discussion of different modes of attentional control in section 14.1. The two issues, however, relate to different aspects of a model developed by Norman and me (1980, 1986), which can be viewed as an attempt to anchor the overall theory that Luria applied to 'frontal functions' within a cognitive science conceptual framework. Our model was based on two main premises. The first, introduced at the beginning of the chapter, is that the routine selection of routine operations is decentralised. The second is that non-routine selection is qualitatively different and involves a general-purpose Supervisory System, which modulates rather than dictates the operation of the rest of the system.

In chapter 13, it was suggested that the basic units underlying action or thought are a very large but finite set of discrete programs and that this hierarchy can be divided into two broad levels. The higher level programs would correspond to what Schank and Abelson (1977) called 'scripts' and Schank (1982), 'memory organisation packets' (MOPs). No particular processing module is committed at specific times because a MOP is operative. The lower level programs – thought or action schemata – are, however, ones which either directly place a particular pattern of demands on the mosaic of functionally specific subsystems or do so when certain specific circumstances arise. Thus schemata that control steering a car require visuo-spatial and manual processing systems and appropriate recognition systems. The *source* schema for driving will call particular *component* schemata in well-defined circumstances. If a traffic light turns red when you are at a certain distance from it and travelling at a certain speed, you start braking. The activation of the braking component schema can be overridden, but the routine action, 'the default option', is to brake. Similarly, the default option when in the middle of subtracting one large number from another is to subtract the appropriate digit on one line from the one above, or under well-specified conditions to make a carrying manipulation.[3]

We follow much psychological theorising in assuming that each schema has a level of activation dependent on the triggering inputs it receives. Selection of a schema occurs if its level of activation exceeds a given threshold; once selected, it remains active even if its level of activation falls, unless it attains its goal or is actively inhibited by a competitor or by any higher level controlling schema. Schemata are independently activated by triggers and are in mutually inhibitory competition for selection, but which of their fellows they inhibit and by how much depends on the particular processing systems they require (Figure 14.1).[4] Selection of a schema has a variety of consequences:

1. The sub-routines of the program – or, in the present terminology, the component schemata of the source schema – are activated so that they, too, can be selected if the appropriate trigger conditions arise. When the driving schema is selected, the component schemata for braking, signalling, and switching on windscreen wipers are activated, so they can be selected if necessary.
2. For lower level schemata, selection leads to a particular arrangement of transmission routes between processing subsystems being switched in. So the two schemata 'repeat an utterance' and 'write from dictation' require the use of different outputs of the auditory input word-form system.
3. The selection of a schema frequently requires that variables connected with the goal of the schema be set. Catching a ball requires the catching action to be elicited for the expected position of the ball, and not for that of a passing butterfly.[5]

---

3. The version of Norman and Shallice's theory presented here is a modification of that originally described. In particular, the distinction between MOPs and schemata is not present in the original version (1980). The distinction between source schemata and MOPs concerns how rigidly they control the activation of lower level systems. The driving source schema and the paying-the-bill MOP differ in this respect. However, I do not intend to draw a rigid division between MOPs and source schemata. Activity at one level will always be controlled by some source schema. Above that, there may be a hierarchy of systems that are increasingly flexible in the controls they effect over lower level systems. Where one draws the boundary is to some extent arbitrary.
4. This type of selection procedure can be treated as a physiologically plausible analogue of the artificial-intelligence simulations of cognition based on decentralised selection of thought operations – in particular, so-called production systems (Newell & Simon, 1972). The mutually inhibitory competition becomes an analogue of the conflict-resolution procedures used in such simulations (see Mc-Dermott & Forgy, 1978). Triggering of schemata is frequently mediated by language in humans; this corresponds to language operating as a 'second signal system' (see Luria, 1973).
5. Schemata may, in addition, need to modulate the operations of processing subsystems that they utilise. Thus the same specific spatial processing subsystem may well be required both for judging the orientation of a line and for performing a Shepard and Metzler (1971) type task of the mental rotation of a figure. The different schemata would, however, use the processor in different ways. A consequence is that many schemata will themselves control the lower level attentional control systems discussed in chapter 13.

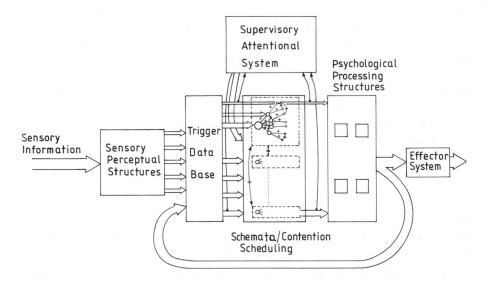

Figure 14.1. Norman and Shallice's model (1980, 1986). The figure illustrates the control processes operating on the isolable subsystems and processing regions, rather than their on-line operation. The *psychological processing structures* unit represents the bulk of the on-line operation of such systems. Their outputs are indicated. They receive control input (shown) as well as processing input from sensory/perceptual structures (not shown). The *trigger database* represents those outputs of the isolable subsystems that have a control function. In the unit labelled *schemata/contention scheduling,* source schemata are represented by the apex node of each tree structure, and component schemata, by lower nodes. Excitatory links are labelled by a + and inhibitory ones, by two parallel lines.

This process of routine selection between routine actions or thought operations is termed 'contention scheduling'.[6] There are, however, a number of grounds why it is not likely to provide a sufficient basis for explaining all levels of the selection of thought and action operations. In artificial intelligence work on problem solving, it has been found necessary to add to a system that routinely executes whatever solution plan is in operation, a planning component that operates in a different fashion and learns from its mistakes (e.g. Fahlman, 1974; Sussman, 1975; for reviews, see Boden, 1977; Charniak & McDermott, 1985). Moreover higher level control programs, such as MOPs, do not operate over a time span of seconds, nor do they have the same modular processing entailments as schemata. The way in which they are selected seems likely to be the province of a different mechanism,

6. It would seem natural for this chapter to include a discussion of possible disorders of contention scheduling. It is not, though, clear if in a modular system operating generally under decentralised control, a process like contention scheduling needs to be the province of a single isolated subsystem. However, in Norman and Shallice (1980, 1986), it was suggested that contention-scheduling functions might be carried out by the basal ganglia, at least for selection of action (see also Robbins & Sahakian, 1983).

which does not sacrifice flexibility for speed of operation. Moreover, a one-level account of action selection, based on contention scheduling alone, gives no explanation of the phenomenological distinction between 'willed' and 'non-willed' actions, with which this chapter was introduced.

We therefore argued that there is an additional system – the Supervisory System – which has access to a representation of the environment and of the organism's intentions and cognitive capacities. It is held to operate not by directly controlling behaviour, but by modulating the lower level contention-scheduling system by activating or inhibiting particular schemata. It would be involved in the genesis of willed actions and required in situations where the routine selection of actions was unsatisfactory – for instance, in coping with novelty, in decision making, in overcoming temptation, or in dealing with danger.[7] Damage to this system, which results in reliance on contention scheduling alone, was held to give rise to the symptoms classically associated with frontal lobe disorders. Grafman (1985) has recently suggested that frontal lobe systems perform cognitive operations at a level equivalent to that of 'scripts', or MOPs. This would dovetail well with this view. The Supervisory System would be the domain in which operations involving MOPs occur.

14.3 The Supervisory System Approach: Individual-Case Studies

The idea of a Supervisory System modulating a lower level system that directly controls action and thought operations is far from novel. A related concept was, for instance, suggested by MacKay (1966a). Most relevant for the present applications, Norman and Shallice's (1980, 1986) model can be seen as an information-processing realisation of Luria's theory, with the Supervisory System corresponding to his system for the programming, regulation, and verification of activity.

A gross impairment to such a system would provide a plausible account of the disorders observed in the patients of Lhermitte et al. (1972), discussed in section 14.1. An impairment of the Supervisory System would also account for the problem of a patient reported by Eslinger and Damasio (1985) who had a milder disorder but one that was still incapacitating in practical terms. EVR, an accountant, had a large orbito-frontal meningioma removed. When tested more than six years after the operation, his IQ was over 130, and he performed well on a very wide variety of tests,

---

7. Our model was developed to explain phenomena in the field of attention, both experimental and phenomenological. This chapter will be concerned with only the neurological implications of attention. The idea of a general-purpose supervisory unit has obviously some similarities to the limited-capacity single-channel notions (e.g. Broadbent, 1958; Duncan, 1980) and, more particularly, to the controller of Shiffrin and Schneider's (1977) 'controlled processing'. The Supervisory System, however, differs from these other two conceptions in one major respect. On their respective theories, most cognitive tasks require the use of the single limited-capacity channel or controlled processing. The Supervisory System is required for only the less routine tasks. The properties of the action lapses, such as 'capture errors', discussed earlier in the chapter, can be explained more easily on the present model. They are held to occur when the Supervisory System is concerned with cognitive operations distinct from both the captured and the capturing actions.

including some – to be discussed later – that are sensitive to frontal lobe damage. On all the tasks that he attempted, his performance was satisfactory.[8]

Despite this excellent performance on a range of quantitative tasks, his ability to organise his life was disastrously impaired. He left an accounting position to go into partnership with someone who had been fired from the firm he previously worked for. He went bankrupt and then drifted through several jobs, being fired from each. Employers complained about disorganisation and lack of punctuality, but his basic skills, manner, and temper were appropriate. His wife sued for divorce. He remarried against the advice of relatives, and this marriage ended in divorce two years later. Deciding to go out to dinner would take hours, as he discussed each restaurant, seating plan, menu, atmosphere, and management; he would even drive to see how busy the restaurants were, but even then could not decide. Thus even though short quantitative tests could be performed satisfactorily, the supervisory organisation of his activities appeared to be very impaired.

At the other extreme are the states of akinesia, a failure to initiate action. Damasio and Van Hoesen (1983) reported a patient, J, who had a stroke that affected the medial parts of the left frontal lobe. The patient lay quietly, following the doctors with her eyes, but said nothing and asked no questions. The patient could repeat sentences and carry out commands; for instance, the Token Test was performed normally. After three weeks, spontaneous syntactically correct utterances had returned, but J could not use speech in the service of an intention. For instance, she could not provide an account of her illness or family life, and when looking at pictures, she could not describe what she saw, although questioning indicated that she recognised what was in them. Voluntary action, too, seemed impaired. She later described herself as having had nothing to say, that she had no will to reply to questions. This is just what would be expected if the Supervisory System had been disconnected from the contention-scheduling system.

14.4 Frontal Lobe Group Studies

Unfortunately, few quantitative single-case studies of frontal lobe syndromes exist. From the perspective of the theory being discussed, this is perhaps not too surprising. To describe a disorder reliably and quantitatively by psychological procedures, repeated testing is required. One counts or averages performance over a series of situations. This has the implication that if a deficit were to manifest itself only in novel situations, then it would be correspondingly difficult to measure in a single subject. Counting presupposes equivalence at some level of abstraction across situations, the opposite of what is required by novelty. Thus the measurement of the ability to cope with novelty is subject to an analogue of the uncertainty principle of quantum mechanics. The more accurately a subject's response to a type of situation can be measured, the less what is measured is an ability to cope with novelty.

---

8. The one exception was on the Wisconsin Card-Sorting Test, to be discussed in section 14.5, on which he obtained the maximum number of categories. However, his 10 errors included 6 perseverative ones, and this is a 'frontal' sign.

This argument does not entail that if the general-purpose Supervisory System theory of frontal lobe function were correct, then single-case studies of frontal lobe disorders would not be possible. Absolutely novel situations are not the only ones in which such patients should have difficulties. The argument does suggest, however, that frontal lobe functions may be one area where group studies in which group membership is determined by lesion location are especially useful, since in a group study, only a small number of measurements need to be made of the performance of each patient.

Effective group studies are, however, subject to severe practical difficulties, as was discussed in chapter 9. There are additional problems for testing the Supervisory System model by means of studies that contrast frontal lobe groups with other groups. The frontal lobes are large structures and have functions other than supervisory control. For instance, the motor strip, frontal eye fields, and more anterior parts of the language areas are part of the frontal lobes, as anatomically defined. More critically, any task that requires the Supervisory System will also involve other processing components that would be more posteriorly located. To obtain a greater impairment from a frontal group than a posterior group would therefore entail that the resources required by the supervisory aspects of the task outweigh those required in on-line processing.[9]

Group studies of frontal lobe function are not very frequently carried out. There is an order of magnitude fewer of them than, say, group studies of aphasic patients. Yet despite the methodological problems, it has become clear over the past 20 years that the frontal lobes are not as silent as was thought in, say, the 1950s. Specific frontal lobe impairments have been described in a steady trickle of studies.[10]

It is possible to give a plausible account of the cognitive deficits observed in these studies in terms of an impairment of the Supervisory System, but other explanations are far from being excluded. As an example, consider the task used by Petrides and Milner (1982) with young epileptic patients who had undergone surgery limited to one lobe. The subjects received a series of cards, on each of which was the same set of six stimuli, but with the position of the stimuli varying randomly from card to card. The subject had to go through the pack of cards, turning cards over one at a time and pointing to one stimulus on each card, but could not point to any particular item more than once. The experiment continued with three new sets of cards, having 8, then 10, and finally 12 stimuli on each, with the same general rule applying. The combined results when the stimuli were representational

---

9. One type of aetiology that is, by contrast, most appropriate for studying frontal functions, as Milner and her colleagues have demonstrated, is lobectomy to remove an epileptic focus. The problem that all tasks are loaded on on-line processing requirements as well as supervisory ones is not so severe a problem for Milner's methodology, since she typically contrasts frontal lobe lesions with lesions in the temporal lobe, which spare the language area. The deficits of this group are primarily on memory tasks.

10. In this chapter, an exhaustive review of these studies will not be attempted. They are comprehensively covered in Stuss and Benson (1984, 1986). Another excellent review, although principally of the animal literature discussed later in the chapter, is Fuster (1980).

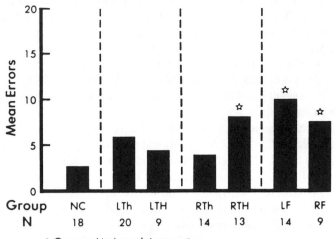

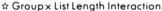

☆ Group × List Length Interaction

Figure 14.2. Mean total errors for all list lengths on the subject-ordering task using representational drawings (LF: left frontal; RF: right frontal; LTh: left temporal lobe with small hippocampal involvement; LTH: left temporal lobe with extensive hippocampal involvement; RTh and RTH: the right hemisphere equivalents of the previous two groups; NC: normal controls). The Group × List Length interaction is for each patient group compared with controls. Reprinted from Petrides and Milner (1982); *Neuropsychologia 20:*258; by permission of Pergamon.

drawings of common objects are shown in Figure 14.2. Both left frontal and the right frontal groups were impaired, by comparison with the controls. The right temporal group, with extensive hippocampal involvement, was impaired too; this is not surprising, given that such patients generally have difficulty with non-verbal memory tasks. The result clearly indicates that the frontal lobes are far from being 'silent' in a group study, if the right type of task is chosen.[11]

Intuitively, it seems that the task involves a planning or programming component, as Milner, Petrides, and Smith (1985) pointed out. Moreover, it is compatible with such an explanation that after a left frontal lesion, a deficit should arise, what-

11. It can be argued that a more appropriate statistical comparison would be that among patient groups rather than that between each patient group and the controls. Patients may show a deficit on a task for reasons unrelated to their specific lesion – for example, due to their drug regimes. Unfortunately, although this procedure is technically correct, it is especially conservative for frontal lobe lesions. As pointed out earlier, a task sensitive to frontal lobe lesions is likely to have functional components that have a more posterior localisation. To obtain a frontal lobe deficit with this methodology, the 'frontal' functional components not only must exist, but also must be greater in their resource demands than the 'posterior' functional components. On the theory being discussed here, the situation is not equivalent for posterior lesions; the 'frontal' functional components of 'routine' tasks are generally minimal. As deficits are not obtained with frontal lobe groups of this type on many other tasks (see Milner, 1975), the frontal lobe deficits on this task and the relative preservation shown by the left temporal groups makes the results sufficiently impressive for them to be used for theoretical inferences.

ever the nature of the material – concrete words, abstract words, drawings, or abstract designs.[12] As with almost all other complex tasks developed in neuropsychology, however, a detailed analysis of the processes required by the task is lacking. To provide solid evidence that the task has a major programming component is very difficult. One possible procedure would be to use the methods of Newell and Simon (1972) – to produce detailed simulations of models of task performance and to compare them with protocols of normal subjects; this, though, would obviously require an extensive research program. Can one, instead, obtain more direct predictions from the model about the types of task where difficulties would be predicted to arise following frontal-lobe lesions?

14.5 The Supervisory System and Frontal Syndromes

There are a number ways in which one can produce predictions about tasks that would be expected to show a frontal lobe deficit on the basis of the model. First, one can consider the way in which contention scheduling is held to operate and hence infer the type of tasks that would be difficult for such a system to carry out unaided by the Supervisory System. Second, one can take tasks selected on a priori grounds because they would appear to make strong demands on a Supervisory System that performs the types of function assigned to it, such as reacting to novelty.[13]

Of the properties of contention scheduling, two seem particularly relevant. First, because it is a process that carries out only 'routine' operations, its triggering parameters will depend on the reinforcement history of the organism and so will change only slowly. If on one trial, a particular schema is strongly activated by triggers, it will continue to be relatively strongly activated on the following trial, given that the same triggering stimuli occur, regardless of what has resulted from the selection of the schema. The system controlled by contention scheduling alone should behave in a rigid fashion. Second, when the stimulus situation does not produce strong trigger-schema activation, then in the absence of the Supervisory System, contention scheduling will tend to be easily and briefly captured by irrelevant aspects of the environment. One should see an analogue of the action lapses of the capture-error type found when normal subjects are distracted. Thus depending on the pattern of trigger-schema relations, a system of contention scheduling without supervisory control may show one of two apparently contradictory types of behaviour. Behavioural rigidity (a tendency to perserverate) should occur in some situations; in others, a distractibility and a tendency to be side-tracked by irrelevant associations.

---

12. By contrast, the right frontal lesion group showed only a mild impairment on the two non-verbal versions of the task. The left hemisphere has long been known to have the dominant role in the control of voluntary actions; it is left hemisphere lesions that give rise to apraxia (Liepmann, 1900; Kimura & Archibald, 1974).

13. A third possibility, suggested by Baddeley (1986), is an empirical one. Any task that is especially difficult to perform in combination with tasks with which it has no structural overlap presumably requires the Supervisory System, and so would be expected to give rise to a frontal deficit.

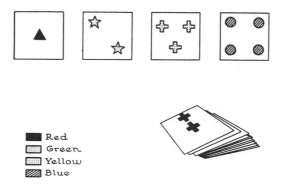

Figure 14.3. The stimuli used in the Wisconsin Card-Sorting Test. Reprinted from Milner (1963); Archives of Neurology 9:91; © 1963, American Medical Association.

Behavioural rigidity is, indeed, one of the best established characteristics of frontal lobe patients (for reviews, see Walsh, 1978; Stuss & Benson, 1986). It is well seen in performance on the Wisconsin Card-Sorting Test of Grant and Berg (1948). This is the test for which the existence of a frontal deficit has been most solidly established empirically with patients having a variety of aetiologies: lobectomy for epileptic foci (Milner, 1963), consecutive series of patients with unilateral lesions (mainly tumour patients) (Drewe, 1974; Nelson, 1976), and prefrontal leucotomy patients (Stuss et al., 1983).[14] Four 'key' cards are placed in front of the subject (Figure 14.3). A pack of 'response' cards is then presented to the patient, one card at a time, and each card must be placed with one of the four key cards. Subjects are told that the key card with which any response card should be sorted is determined by a rule that the experimenter has in mind. After each response card has been sorted, the subject is told whether or not the correct key card has been chosen. The task of the subject is to determine the rule for sorting. For any given response card, one of the key cards will agree with it on the dimension of colour, another on the dimension of shape, and a third on the dimension of number.[15] Whatever rule fits the patient's first response is initially considered correct. After the patient has followed this rule correctly for a certain number of trials, 10 and 6 in different versions, the rule is changed, and responding in accordance with the previously correct rule is treated as an incorrect perseverative response. The rule changes through a maximum of two cycles of the three alternatives or until the pack is used up.[16]

14. With missile-wound patients, however, Teuber, Battersby, and Bender (1951) found that patients with frontal lesions were less impaired than those with posterior ones. However, they used a procedure in which rule changes occurred at intervals, whether or not a rule had been consistently correctly obeyed.
15. This is strictly true only of the version developed by Nelson (1976).
16. In earlier versions, the patient is not informed that a change of rule has taken place. In Nelson's (1976) version, the information is given in order to reduce the stress for the patient. The results of the two procedures are similar.

Table 14.2. *A comparison of the results on Wisconsin Card-Sorting in Milner's (1963) study of the patients with dorsolateral frontal lesions and a control group having unilateral lesions somewhere in the other three lobes*

| | | IQ | | Wisconsin | |
	Number	Pre-	Post-	Categories obtained	Perseverative errors (%)
Dorsolateral frontal	(18)	103	95	1.4	52
Controls	(35)	107	98	4.7	13

The results of Milner's (1963) original study were dramatic. Physiological psychologists have argued for functional differences between the dorsolateral and the orbital parts of the frontal lobes (for a review, see Fuster, 1980). Milner therefore subdivided her frontal lobe patients into two sub-groups according to the site of their lesions within the frontal lobes. All her patients had had neurosurgery as a treatment for intractable epilepsy stemming from a localised epileptic focus. The subgroup with dorsolateral frontal lesions had great difficulty in switching to a second category, and a very high proportion of their errors were perseverations of the previously correct rule (Table 14.2).

The studies of Drewe (1974) and Nelson (1976) contrasted patients having lesions that were apparently confined to the frontal lobe with patients having posterior lesions. They obtained a frontal deficit qualitatively similar to that obtained by Milner.[17] Stuss et al. (1983) studied patients with orbitofrontal lesions – a group in which Milner had found little deficit – and did find an impairment, but only on the second set of 64 cards out of a total of 128 used.

To what is the impairment on Wisconsin Card-Sorting in patients with frontal lesions to be attributed? Motivational factors, such as lack of involvement in the test, seem an implausible answer. Frontal patients frequently work slowly through the test and can become distressed by their inability to perform it. Although, as far as I know, no formal test has been made of the possibility, it is clinically evident that frontal lobe patients who have difficulty with the Wisconsin could follow any of the three rules used – matching by colour, by shape, or by number – if so instructed when they first see the test. They can, after all, carry out much more complex tasks than that as shown by the near-average score obtained on WAIS IQ in Milner's study.

It is sometimes argued that to draw any theoretical conclusions from the persev-

17. In Nelson's (1976) study, the difference in total categories achieved between frontal and non-frontal patients was not significant. A significant difference in the percentage of perseverative errors was, however, obtained. Cicerone, Lazar, and Shapiro (1983) have obtained a significant frontal deficit using a closely related hypothesis-testing task.

erative behaviour of frontal lobe patients on a task like Wisconsin Card-Sorting is inappropriate (see, e.g., Hécaen & Albert, 1978). Many types of patient, it is argued, perseverate; for instance, aphasics do, and so can patients with agnosic difficulties. However, this argument ignores the level at which perseveration takes place. As Sandson and Albert (1984) have pointed out, perseveration is a loose description of behaviour and can qualitatively be of different types. Perseveration in, say, paraphasic errors can be attributed to the malfunction of some particular special-purpose module used by schemata. It can be seen as an extreme form of priming of the module. This is not the case for frontal patients on a task like the Wisconsin, who show what Sandson and Albert call stuck-in-set perseveration. In this variety, it is the schema controlling internal programming that remains fixed; there is no malfunction of the mechanisms being used to carry out the schema. Moreover, it is this type of perseveration – that of the schema controlling internal programming – that one would expect if a Supervisory System is damaged.

The explanation that Milner preferred in her 1963 paper was one based on theories developed by physiological psychologists to explain somewhat analogous behaviour found in monkeys with dorsolateral frontal lesions. Animals with dorsolateral frontal lesions have difficulty learning a reversal in the correct and incorrect stimuli in a discrimination learning task, and 'the older the habit, the more familiar the discriminanda, the greater the difficulty that the frontal animal ordinarily shows in reversals' (Fuster, 1980, p. 44). This was explained by the loss of the ability to inhibit 'central sets' (e.g. Rosvold & Mishkin, 1961; Mishkin, 1964). In fact, a 'central set' corresponds to behaviour controlled by a single schema. Thus Milner's account and the Supervisory System one have considerable similarity. Yet the concept of a deficit in inhibiting central sets is certainly the simpler, and it accounts just as well for the behavioural-rigidity findings.

The complement of the perseveration at the schema level found in some frontal patients is a tendency for schemata to be triggered inappropriately by stimuli. In its more extreme form, this corresponds to a condition described clinically by Lhermitte (1983) as 'utilisation behaviour'. In Lhermitte's procedure, an object such as a glass is brought within reach of the patient. The patient grasps it. A bottle of water is then placed on the desk. The patient grasps this object, too, and then pours water from the bottle into the glass and drinks it. Analogous behaviour is found with other objects. Lhermitte (1983) describes five patients, all with localised lesions involving the frontal lobes, who exhibit utilisation behaviour. Lhermitte has never observed the behaviour in normal subjects or patients with posterior lesions.

A simple explanation of the disorder would be that the patient misinterprets the doctor's intentions. Indeed, Lhermitte's patients often later explained their behaviour by saying that they thought they had to use the objects. Lhermitte rejects this explanation by pointing out that the patient can be told not to grasp or use the objects, and yet the behaviour remains unchanged if the patient's attention is diverted for about 30 sec.[18]

18. Unfortunately, no details are given of the patients in whom the recurrence of the behaviour was observed. The simple misinterpretation explanation cannot therefore be conclusively ruled out.

Utilisation behaviour fits well with how contention scheduling should operate when it is not subject to Supervisory System control and when no other strong triggers are available. A less extreme type of behaviour that also fits is distractibility. In the animal literature, there is now considerable evidence that frontal animals are distractible and that they are hyperactive in a novel situation (see Fuster, 1980). For instance, it has long been known that frontally lesioned animals have a deficit on the delayed-response group of tasks, in which the animal must retain a goal position or information on the correct stimulus over a delay period of 30 sec or so. This impairment now seems likely to be an attentional disorder. Minimising distractions reduces the disability (e.g. Malmo, 1942; Konorski & Lawicka, 1964; Bauer & Fuster, 1978). Moreover, the general level of activity of the frontal animal shoots up after 10 sec, after which performance tends to decline rapidly (Bauer & Fuster, 1976).[19]

In clinical accounts of frontal lobe patients, mention is frequently made of distractibility (e.g. Rylander, 1939). There are, however, few relevant experimental studies. Knight, Hillyard, Woods, and Neville (1981) studied the performance on a selective-attention task of 13 patients with lesions of varying aetiology, all of which were confined to the frontal lobe. The patients had to discriminate in the auditory input to one ear between target stimuli (75-msec signals) and much more frequent distractor stimuli (25-msec signals) when related, but not identical, stimuli were presented to the other ear. Which ear was relevant varied from one block of trials to the next. The frontal patients detected only 57% of the target stimuli, by comparison with 85% for the controls.[20]

The main part of this experiment was to examine the effect of frontal lesions on event-related evoked potentials and, in particular, on the negative potential occurring roughly 100 msec after stimulus onset, which is known to be modality-specific and influenced by the degree of attention (e.g. Hillyard & Picton, 1979). In normal subjects, it is much larger if the input channel on which the signal occurs is the relevant one. In frontal patients, this was not the case (Figure 14.4). These results were interpreted as a difficulty in focusing attention. Moreover, the frontal patients seemed to differ from normals primarily with respect to the response to the unattended channel. This increased response in the frontal group to the unattended ear was significantly greater for tones that were delivered contralaterally to the lesion than tones that were presented to the ipsilateral ear. The increased response to the irrelevant channel is evidence for increased distractibility.

A second supporting piece of evidence comes from an experiment of Salmaso and Denes (1982). In this study, subjects were presented with a very simple same–different discrimination task between simultaneously presented stimuli: letters in one condition, and lines of very different slope (e.g. horizontal vs. 45°) in the other. The stimulus pairs were exposed for 100 msec at the rapid rate of one pair every 2

---

19. This is particularly true of the second of the two procedures, so-called delayed matching-to-sample.
20. Technically, the control group was not adequate. It does not appear to have been matched to the patient group in any way. Moreover, while the mean age of the controls was 54, 8 of the 13 patients were over 60.

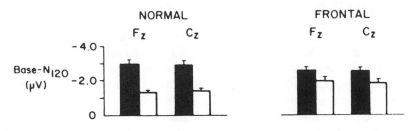

Figure 14.4. Mean amplitude of N120 component of the evoked response to attended (black) and unattended (white) stimuli with frontal patients and normal controls. Reprinted from Knight, Hillyard, Woods, and Neville (1981) by permission of Elsevier Science Publishers.

sec. Subjects had to respond to only the 20% of pairs that were in fact different. The subjects were 10 patients with frontal lobe lesions and 10 with more posterior lesions. The anterior patients missed nearly four times as many 'different' targets as the posterior ones (19% vs. 5%) and also produced more than twice as many false positive responses to the 'same' stimuli (13% vs. 6%). Both effects were significant. There were no significant effects of the hemisphere of lesion or of material. In view of the lack of effect of material, of the relative ease of the 'different' discrimination, and of the relative infrequency of targets, an interpretation of the difficulty of the frontal patients in terms of a disorder of attention was given by the authors.

A third relevant line of evidence comes from a study by Wilkins, Shallice, and McCarthy (1987). Patients were instructed to count trains of bleeps from 2 to 11, which were presented at a rate of one per second. The task is cognitively very simple, the only difficulty being in maintaining concentration because the task itself does not demand attention.[21] Thus errors were few. Two different sets of patients were tested. In the first set, 54% of the patients with lesions involving the right frontal lobe made at least one error, by comparison with 7% of the patients with right temporal lesions. In the second, smaller series, 4/6 (67%) of the right anterior patients made an error, and only 1/9 (11%) of the right posterior patients. The left hemisphere patients showed a similar trend, but the results were less clear-cut.

The experimental evidence is not, however, unequivocal. Stuss and Benson (1984) have argued that frontal lobe lesions do not necessarily produce attentional changes, even when patients have large lesions. Some of the studies they quoted are concerned with a lack of deficit on digit span, on which a momentary lapse of concentration would not necessarily be harmful. However, tasks like WAIS Digit Symbol, the Knox cubes – on which one must work out the number of cubes shown in a complex structure – and Serial Sevens – on which one has to count back in sevens – clearly require concentration. For all these tasks, Stuss et al. (1981) found no

---

21. Errors, when they occurred, were more frequent on very early trials, so this explanation may be oversimple.

difference between leucotomised and non-leucotomised schizophrenics. Many subjects with large frontal lesions performed like the non-operated patients. As Stuss and Benson pointed out, the effects of schizophrenia and frontal leucotomy on attention may have cancelled each other out. In addition, the tasks may be intrinsically interesting and so require less effort of will or be less dependent on instant-to-instant concentration. In general, the balance of the human neuropsychology evidence is in favour of the increased distractibility hypothesis, which fits with the animal literature. However, it is clear that none of the effects are as well established as the increased perseveration obtained in the Wisconsin Card-Sorting Test.

In general, the predictions made from the Supervisory System theory are supported. It is nevertheless possible to develop an explanation based solely on a failure of inhibition, as in the case of perseveration evidence. Concentration can be viewed as the ability to inhibit a response to an irrelevant stimulus that is potentially attention catching. Thus this class of phenomenon, too, cannot be used to differentiate the two theories. Tasks are needed that are more specifically tailored to the predictions of the model.

14.6 Problem Solving and Coping with Novel Situations

The primary function of the Supervisory System is that of producing a response to novelty that is planned rather than one that is routine or impulsive. The situations in which it is required are those where the routine triggering by the environment of the organism's battery of specialised thought or action schemata is insufficient to produce an appropriate response. Instead, some form of problem-solving behaviour, trying out hypotheses and learning from failed attempts, is required.

The problem-solving process of the normal subject typically involves a number of stages: The overall situation is assessed; an outline plan of attack is developed, refined, and revised if unsatisfactory aspects come to light; and any solution obtained is checked (see De Groot, 1965). Probably the first attempts to examine planning and problem solving quantitatively in frontal lobe patients used maze learning. Porteus had developed the idea that maze learning taps planning skills, and early in the history of quantitative neuropsychological investigations, he found that patients showed a loss on maze-learning ability after prefrontal leucotomies performed for psychiatric reasons (Porteus & Kepner, 1944); this finding was corroborated by later research (e.g. Mettler, 1952). Later research showed, though, that there was no *specific* frontal deficit (for a review, see Walsh, 1978). Patients with posterior lesions also had deficits. However, the frontal leucotomy patients who premorbidly had had psychotic symptoms showed few other cognitive deficits on quantitative tests, by comparison with their performance before their operation. In addition, because maze learning also has strong visuo-spatial aspects, the absence of a difference between frontal and posterior patient groups is most easily interpreted as arising from qualitatively different disorders leading to similar quantitative deficits in the two groups.

A very different approach was adopted by Klosowska (1976). Using the theoret-

Table 14.3. *Percentage of the different groups solving Klosowska's (1976) task with varying degrees of assistance*

Successful construction of action program	Frontal group	Posterior group	Normal subjects
Independently	26	56	74
With 1 act of assistance	28	36	} 26
With 2 acts of assistance	38	8	
Not at all	8	—	—

ical perspectives of Luria (1966) and Miller, Galanter, and Pribram (1960), she used a fairly complex and novel task that required the development of a plan in order to solve it. Subjects seated at a table were presented with (1) a tall burette attached to the table, in the bottom of which there was a cork, (2) a large receptacle, also attached to the table, that was filled with water and had a firmly fitting lid (the lid had no knob, but there was a 0.5-cm hole bored in it), (3) a metal cup with its bottom removed, (4) the bottom of the metal cup, (5) a metal hook 10 cm long, and (6) a small open bottle of gasoline. The problem was how the bottle of gasoline could be stoppered. This entails using the hook to open the lid of the receptacle, screwing the bottom of the cup back on, and pouring cupfuls of water into the burette so that the cork rises to the top.

Klosowska's subjects were 50 patients who had unilateral or bilateral frontal lobe damage arising from either trauma or tumour, and 25 patients with posterior lesions, from whom aphasic and agnosic patients had been excluded. All the patients were tested at least six months after surgery. The subjects had to give a verbal account of how they would accomplish the task. If the patient was unable to describe it, the experimenter would give a hint, such as removing the cover of the water receptacle with the hook and asking, 'Can you say now how to carry out this?' The results are shown in Table 14.3. They show a marked deficit in the frontal lobe group. In addition, 52% of the frontal lobe patients, compared with only 12% of the posterior patients, reported in a structured clinical interview that they were incapable of consistent realisation of a program of action when performing their vocational and household work.

It can be argued that in this study, the groups were not adequately matched. It remains possible that the exclusion of aphasic and agnosic patients from the posterior group meant that the lesions of the posterior group were on the whole smaller than those of the frontal group, who seem likely to have had large lesions, and hence that any generalised brain-damage effects would be less. However, the results are certainly strongly suggestive of a major frontal deficit on the task.

The solution to Klosowska's problem definitely appears to require planning, and, indeed, this was the rationale for her experiment. One type of planning task that has been much used in artificial-intelligence problem-solving simulations and in which both adult and child behaviour has been compared with that of computer

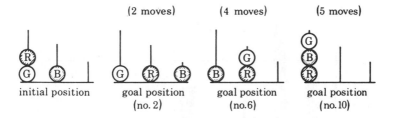

Figure 14.5. Three subproblems of the Tower of London test. The initial position is the same for all three. *R* stands for red; *G,* for green; *B,* for blue. Reprinted from Shallice (1982) by permission of the Royal Society.

programs is the Tower-of-Hanoi (see, e.g., Anzai & Simon, 1979). The Tower-of-Hanoi is not a task in which problem difficulty can be easily graded. This makes it an unsatisfactory test for psychometric purposes. McCarthy and I (see Shallice, 1982) therefore developed a related test in which difficulty can be graduated more easily. The patient must move from an initial position to a target position (Figure 14.5) in the smallest number of moves. In the simplest scoring system, the patient is allowed 1 min per problem, but must move from the initial to the target position without error. There was a significant left anterior deficit in our study.[22]

Indirect evidence that the deficit can be attributed to a planning difficulty arises if the results are compared with those of the same patients on Block Design, a task that is similar in many of the more basic processing subcomponents that it requires. Two left anterior patients scored below any normal subject on the 'Tower of London' test (25% and 42%), and yet did well on Block Design (scaled scores, 10 and 17),[23] while two right posterior patients showed the opposite pattern (Tower of London, 67%, Block Design, 5; and Tower of London, 84%; Block Design, 4). It would appear that performance on the Tower of London test has a major component that is a much less central part of Block Design. This seems likely to be planning.

An analogous deficit was not obtained in a later study, which investigated the possibility of detecting frontal impairments in patients whose brain damage could not be detected from the use of WAIS IQ (Shallice, Warrington, Watson, & Lewis, in preparation).[24] In this study, the left frontal group's performance was not impaired, by comparison with matched normal controls. Overall, the most plausible

22. The lesion groups were defined somewhat unusually. Each patient with a unilateral lesion was allocated to the anterior group if the lesion had its centre in the anterior part of the hemisphere *and* if the frontal lobe was involved. This had the effect of including most fronto-temporal and some fronto-parietal patients in the anterior group.
23. Scaled score 10 is the average adult score, and the range is 0 to 19.
24. Patients were included in the study only if WAIS IQ was no more than 10 points less than premorbid IQ, as estimated from the New Adult Reading Test (Nelson & O'Connell, 1978). Might the component impaired in the main study have something to do with language? After all, the impaired group had left hemisphere lesions. However, normal subjects do not appear to make use of verbalisation strategies when carrying out the task. Articulatory suppression has no effect on their performance.

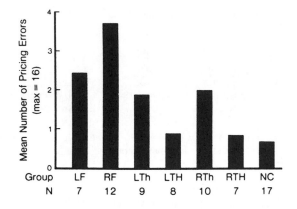

Figure 14.6. Mean number of extreme pricing errors in cognitive estimation by a number of subgroups (LF: left frontal; RF: right frontal; LTh: left temporal lobe with small hippocampal involvement; LTH: left temporal lobe with extensive hippocampal involvement; RTh and RTH: the right hemisphere equivalents of the previous two groups; NC: normal controls). Reprinted from Smith and Milner (1984); *Neuropsychologia* 22:701; by permission of Pergamon Journals, Ltd.

explanation is that the patient-selection process removed the patients with a planning deficit. However, it certainly must weaken the conclusions drawn from the previous study.

These studies concentrated on planning. A further task was concerned with two other aspects of dealing with a novel situation: thinking of a non-obvious approach, and checking the plausibility of a response. Shallice and Evans (1978) asked patients to give rough estimates for 15 mini-problems, such as 'How long is an average man's spine?' They were all questions that cannot, in general, be answered by simply consulting information already available in semantic memory. For some questions, a reasonable estimate can be simply obtained if an appropriate strategy is selected. For instance, one could answer the spine question by calculating [body − (head + legs)] or by imagining the length of a shirt. The difficulty lies in thinking of a means of using everyday information rather than in the mental operations required when the line of attack has been developed. Other questions, though, stressed more the ability to assess whether a guess is reasonable. So for a question like 'How fast do race horses gallop?' a response like 8 m.p.h. (13 km per hour) would be unreasonable; it is only twice as fast as a person's rapid walk. Similarly, 60 m.p.h. (97 km per hour) would be unreasonable; it is as fast as a car travels on a good road. So the space of possible answers can be narrowed. As the test concerned the inability to give a reasonable response, the measure of performance used was the number of bizarre responses made; the bizarreness of an answer was calculated on the basis of how extreme it was in terms of the distribution of responses that normal subjects make. Patients with frontal lobe lesions made significantly more such bizarre answers than patients with posterior lesions.

The procedure was simplified by Smith and Milner (1984). They showed sub-

Table 14.4. *Difference between the size of the P300 evoked response (in microvolts) measured at parietal and frontal skull sites in Knight's (1984) study (positive value means parietal greater).*

	Stimulus	
	Novel	Target
Frontals	3.5	4.6
Controls	−1.6	3.7

jects a series of toy objects – such as a trumpet, a cup, and a car – and asked subjects to estimate how much the real object would cost. Bizarre answers were considered as those that were more than 2 standard deviations from the normal mean. Subjects were patients who had had a unilateral excision for epilepsy and also normal controls. Patients with right frontal excisions produced more bizarre errors than did patients with right temporal or left temporal lesions (see Figure 14.6).

A very different type of demonstration of the difficulties that frontal lobe patients have in coping with novelty comes from a study by Knight (1984). Like his research discussed in section 14.5, this study used evoked potentials. The evoked responses of two groups of subjects were compared. One group consisted of 18 patients with unilateral lesions of varying aetiologies confined to the frontal lobe, according to CT scan results. The other was a control group of the same age as the patient group. Subjects had the simple task of pressing a button when they heard a tone of a particular frequency, which occurred on 9% of trials. They only very rarely missed these targets. The 'foil' stimuli, to which the subject did not have to give a response, occurred on over 80% of trials; they were tones of a higher frequency than the target tones (500 Hz). A well-known type of evoked response – the positive potential roughly 300 msec after stimulus onset (P300) – was generated for the target stimuli, but not for the foils. It was maximal over the parietal lobe. The P300 distribution produced by the frontal lobe group did not differ from that of the control group.

There were, however, an additional 9% of stimuli, about which the subjects had not been warned in the test instructions. These were recordings of the barking of a dog! In the control group, these novel stimuli generated a P300 distribution markedly different from that generated by the targets; in particular, it was larger over fronto-central regions of the brain than over the parietal lobes. However, in the frontal lobe group, the evoked response produced by the novel stimuli had the same parietal maximum as that obtained for the targets (Table 14.4). In addition, as the normal subjects habituated to the dog bark over trials, the amplitude of the P300 response to this stimulus declined to an asymptote, and it ceased to be primarily frontally located. The frontal patients, by contrast, showed no change in P300 amplitude over trials for this stimulus. Thus the special response to novel stimuli seems to be intimately related to the perseveration of the frontal cortex.

For the studies reviewed in this section, an explanation of the impaired performance of the frontal lobe patients in terms of a failure of inhibition of central sets has seemed increasingly inadequate. It might be possible to explain the failure to plan adequately or to estimate properly in terms of a failure to inhibit the initial line of thought that comes to mind. Knight's (1984) findings seem beyond even this recourse. Normal subjects do not appear to inhibit any response to the novel stimuli, but show a special type of response. The frontal response is not one of inadequate inhibition, but of a failure to show this novelty response.

On the whole, then, an impairment to the Supervisory System seems to give an adequate account of the findings on problem solving and responding to novelty. They are much more difficult to explain in terms of a lack of inhibition of central sets.

14.7   The Supervisory System: Is It Internally Equipotential or Modular?

If the Supervisory System exists, is it internally equipotential or internally modular? Considering its overall function, might it not correspond to Fodor's (1983) equipotential central system? After all, the Supervisory System is held to have access to all higher level schemata. There is, however, a contrasting position. Some artificial-intelligence theorists have assumed that planning systems that have a similar overall role in their programs to the Supervisory System are themselves modular. Figure 14.7 shows Sussman's (1975) model of the planning system that contains seven different processes and eight types of knowledge.

In fact, there is evidence that areas of the frontal lobes that are involved in tasks with a Supervisory System loading are not equipotential. The evidence for this point from studies on humans is not strong. In some studies, there has been a tendency to find greater deficits with left frontal than with right frontal lesions; in others, no such trend has been observed.[25] However, in animal experiments, where localisation can be much more adequately established, differences in lesion site within the frontal lobes have been shown to have an effect. Tasks that require suppression of prepotent response tendencies tend to be disrupted by lesions of the orbital and inferior convexity of the frontal lobe; the delayed-response type of deficits, however, occur with dorsolateral frontal lesions (for a review, see Fuster, 1980). In

25. Two other studies that show a specifically *left* frontal deficit required subjects to switch frequently between visually similar but conceptually opposite baselines for determining left and right in a figure (Semmes, Weinstein, Ghent, & Teuber, 1963; Butters, Soeldner, & Fedio, 1972), for instance by using front and back views randomly in a task of pointing to parts of the body. Here the similarity in the visual triggers will tend to lead to both the conflicting schemata being activated.

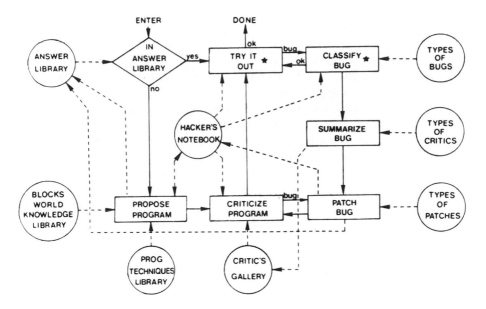

Figure 14.7. The sub-processes used in the programming part of the program HACKER, which learns from its mistakes. Reprinted from Sussman (1975), *A computational model of skill acquisition*, p. 22; © 1975 by Elsevier Science Publishing Co., Inc.

other words, an inability to deal with a prepotent response tendency and excessive distractibility arise from lesions in different areas of the frontal lobes.[26]

The Supervisory System does not therefore seem to be equivalent to Fodor's central system. It is not internally equipotential. However, if the Supervisory System is as complex in its internal structure as the planning component of Sussman's (1975) program, then it is entirely reasonable that two of its functions could be affected by damage to different subcomponents. Thus for Sussman's program, the ability to develop novel plans would be impaired if the Propose Program processes or the Program Techniques Library were damaged. Error correction would, by contrast, suffer if any of the Bug-related programs or their corresponding knowledge sources were affected. Thus the idea that the Supervisory System is internally modular is compatible with the physiological psychology evidence for dissociations among different supervisory functions within the frontal lobes. The idea is computationally plausible, too.

To assume that the Supervisory System is internally modular thus side-steps

26. This complicates the inference made earlier in the chapter. The claim was made earlier that the apparently conflicting pattern of deficits that is observed after frontal lesions – perseveration and distractibility – occurs as a result of an impairment of the same system but with different trigger-schema conditions. It has been corroborated if one considers the lesion site macroscopically, but not if one considers it microscopically. The inference procedure would be valid if the subsystems that are part of one functional system tended to be located near one another. I know of no solid evidence on whether or not this is the case.

apparent difficulties. However, to flesh out the possibility in an adequate fashion will almost certainly prove a most difficult undertaking. Any specific sub-process will presumably be characterisable only in highly abstract terms. Any impairment of such a subprocess is not likely to manifest itself simply in observable effects in behaviour. The functions of the frontal lobes seem set to remain one of neuropsychology's most intractable problems.

More positively, to characterise the functions of the frontal lobes as being concerned with the programming, regulation, and verification of behaviour, as Luria did, can be made more rigorous. It remains empirically plausible, too. From a cognitive science perspective, the way that the result of a frontal impairment can be viewed as leaving one system, contention scheduling, to operate inadequately modulated by a damaged Supervisory System supports the proposed three-level control structure for the regulation of subsystem operation: local attentional control system, contention scheduling, and the Supervisory System.

15   Amnesia: What Is Memory For?

15.1   The Amnesic Syndrome

Twenty-five years ago, human memory was a self-contained topic. It had its own laws, its own empirical paradigms, its chain of father figures leading back to Ebbinghaus. Yet in the past 15 years, memory research has been increasingly integrated with other areas of psychology. Short-term memory has almost hived off into perception and language. Semantic memory is now approached from the perspective of general models of cognition. Recently, links have been developed with attention (e.g. Hasher & Zacks, 1979). Before the mid-1970s, research on amnesia had much the same type of isolation as memory itself had had 15 years before. Admittedly, some ideas from the study of normal memory were beginning to be influential, such as 'levels of processing', and the phenomena being discussed were of much greater intrinsic interest than the interference paradigms of traditional memory research on normal subjects. Yet amnesia research was still very much a closed world, with debates couched in the conceptual terms of the 1950s. Moreover, there were fierce empirical disputes in the field about whether key results arose from artefacts.

Since the mid-1970s, there has been a great change. As was discussed in chapter 2, the disputes over replication have, to a considerable extent, been resolved. It is now widely accepted that many patients with severe memory disorders have additional damage to other processing systems, which can lead to the existence of observed associations between memory and non-memory disorders that may be functionally misleading. More positively, the dissociation approach is proving increasingly valuable; there is now ample evidence for the preservation of a number of aspects of long-term memory even in patients who are densely amnesic. Most positively of all, the gap that existed between studies of normal and abnormal memory has narrowed rapidly.

The change in amnesia research has been quantitative as well as qualitative. A flood of papers on research related to amnesia is now appearing. This chapter will make no attempt to provide a comprehensive review.[1] Instead, I will concentrate on the links between amnesia research and cognitive science.

---

1. Many specialist collections of papers exist – for example, Lynch, McGaugh, and Weinberger (1984). For review chapters, see Baddeley (1982a), Cermak (1982), Hirst (1982), Parkin (1984), Butters and Miliotis (1985), and Weiskrantz (1985).

Before considering the theoretical implications of the amnesic syndrome, it is necessary to outline more clearly its defining aspects and the differences in the way authors treat the concept. Amnesia can arise from a number of neurological causes. The Korsakoff state, which can be produced by alcoholism, has been the commonest aetiology of patients described in the neuropsychological literature, but the impairment can also arise from encephalitis, tumours, vascular disease (particularly of the posterior cerebral arteries), and Alzheimer's disease. In severe forms of the syndrome, patients may have no idea where they are, how old they are, what year it is, and who are the current political, sports, or cultural personalities. The patient may tell the same story 20 times in an hour, thinking it new on each telling. The clinician, who may have been seen fairly frequently before by the patient, can seem totally unfamiliar.

Adequate establishment of an amnesic deficit clearly requires that the patient exhibit severely impaired performance on standardised memory tests. The most widely adopted procedure has been the use of the Wechsler Memory Battery, a set of tests developed to assess memory performance in a parallel fashion to the way the WAIS IQ test assesses intelligence.[2] In addition to the gross memory impairment observed in a patient with a pure amnesia, performance on an IQ test should be at a level consonant with premorbid ability, and there should be no apparent deficits on perceptual, motor, or language tasks.

Severity of amnesia is measured by the difference between the WAIS IQ and the Memory Quotient (MQ), arrived at by an analogous calculation. When formal measures of severity of amnesia were compared across studies by Weiskrantz (1985), it became apparent that important differences in severity exist. Many investigations have continued to use groups of Korsakoff patients; in general, such studies appear to rely on a criterion for inclusion of a 20 to 30 point difference between IQ and MQ, where on both scales, 15 points equal 1 standard deviation (e.g. Butters & Cermak, 1980; Mayes, Meudell, & Neary, 1980; Winocur, Kinsbourne, & Moscovitch, 1981; Wetzel & Squire, 1982). However, single-case studies have involved patients with considerably more severe deficits – a difference of 35 to 50 points (e.g. Cermak, 1976; Heilman & Sypert, 1977). In addition, in certain group studies (e.g. Warrington & Weiskrantz, 1978, 1982), a more stringent criterion has been adopted – a recognition memory performance of 2 standard deviations below the age-corrected norm and with intelligence at its premorbid level.

This difference in severity of patients across studies can be of considerable importance. As an example, consider the way that grossly impaired performance on a recognition test can be used as a criterion measure for the inclusion of severely amnesic patients in some studies (e.g. Warrington & Weiskrantz, 1978, 1982). However, other investigators think that recognitioin is relatively spared in amnesia.

---

2. It is now widely agreed that the Wechsler Memory Battery does not provide a very adequate measure of amnesia. A number of its subtests (e.g. Digit Span) can be performed relatively well by amnesics because they tap processes other than the critical memory ones – for example, short-term memory skills that are not impaired in the amnesic syndrome (see Walsh, 1978; Hirst, 1982; Meudell & Mayes, 1982). Alternative standardised memory tests are therefore being developed (e.g. Warrington, 1984).

Indeed, Hirst (1982) has argued, 'Not only is recognition better than recall for amnesics but in many studies it rivalled the performance of controls' (p. 442) and Hirst et al. (1986) have drawn a number of theoretical conclusions from this empirical claim. Why should this discrepancy among studies occur? A simple explanation is that the 'recognition-sparing' phenomenon is, in essence, an artefact arising from a combination of two factors: the reduced task difficulty of recognition compared with recall, and the use of patients with a relatively mild disorder.[3]

In this chapter, a distinction will be made between 'severely' amnesic patients, who perform 2 standard deviations below their IQ on measured tests (or below MQ 70 if the IQ is not available), and 'mild' or 'moderate' amnesics, who have an IQ–MQ difference of between 20 and 30 points.

Might there be qualitative differences between amnesias as well as quantitative ones? Various authors have suggested that two forms of amnesia exist (e.g. Lhermitte & Signoret, 1972; Huppert & Piercy, 1978; Squire, 1981; for a contrary view, see Hirst, 1982). Three main criteria have been suggested. One is whether the rate of forgetting is or is not normal. This, however, requires that the memory of an amnesic subject can be matched to that of a normal subject by allowing the amnesic a much longer stimulus presentation in order to equate performance at first retrieval.[4] The second concerns the location of lesion, the medial temporal lobe and the hippocampus being contrasted with the diencephalon and, in particular, the mamillary bodies and nuclei in the thalamus. The third is the presence or absence of retrograde amnesia, whether events before the illness onset can be remembered. However, if all three criteria are applied, two clear sub-groups of patients do not emerge. More critically, after an exhaustive review of the issue, Weiskrantz (1985) concluded that no good evidence – anatomical or functional – exists for differentiating two forms of amnesia.[5]

---

3. See Figure 2.1 for examples of chance performance on recognition tests by amnesic patients. One interesting study, which gives a 'recognition sparing' result that cannot be explained away so easily, is that of Hirst et al. (1986). They employed a technique developed by Huppert and Piercy (1978) of matching amnesic patients and normal subjects on recognition performance by giving the amnesics a longer stimulus exposure duration – 8 sec for amnesics compared with 0.5 sec for normal subjects. In the Hirst et al. study, when recognition performance is matched between the two groups, the recall of the amnesic group is worse. There is, however, a problem with this procedure. The very rapid one stimulus per 0.5-sec presentation rate used with the normal group would be likely to lead to a large variance in trace strength across stimuli due to variability in attention and encoding. If this is the case, matching the groups on a low criterion (for recognition) would not ensure that the groups were matched on a higher one (for recall). The group with the larger variance would exceed a higher criterion more frequently. Thus a higher recall level would be expected in the control group than in the amnesics because recall would in general require higher 'trace strength'. In fact, the control group did show a higher difference in confidence between the correctly recognised items and the incorrectly recognised ones than did the Korsakoff patients, indicating a greater variance in the distribution of trace strengths across subjects in that group.
4. Whether this matching can be meaningfully achieved in severe amnesic patients has yet to be demonstrated (see Weiskrantz, 1985). The technique has problems similar to that discussed with respect to claims for 'spared recognition' (footnote 3).
5. Weiskrantz (1985) does not consider 'frontal amnesia'. It will be argued in section 15.9 that this is a qualitatively distinct disorder.

15.2   Amnesia and the Episodic–Semantic Distinction

The dissociations observed in amnesia can be even more dramatic than those between impaired memory and intact intelligence. The functions that can be spared
include some that are loosely describable as 'memory' ones. Short-term memory
storage, discussed in chapter 3, is one example. Also it is well known clinically that
knowledge of word meanings and even general knowledge can be preserved (see,
e.g., Lhermitte & Signoret, 1972). Quantitative evidence supports the earlier clinical claims. To give one example, a study by Meudell, Mayes, and Neary (1980)
involved four patients, each diagnosed as an alcoholic Korsakoff amnesic. Their
amnesia was quantitatively established with the Logical Memory subtest of the
Wechsler Memory Battery, which involves the remembering of a very short story,
used with a delay of 15 min between presentation and recall.[6] The amnesic patients
had a mean retention score of 0, in contrast to a score of 7.7 items (range 4.5 to 12)
for the matched control subjects. Yet the WAIS Vocabulary subtest scores of the
two groups were very comparable – 10.5 and 10.0 – indicating that the knowledge
of word meanings was as good in amnesics as in normal subjects. In addition, while
the amnesic patients were roughly 100 msec slower than the control subjects on
reaction-time tests, there was no interaction between the speed of making an identity judgement – searching for a specific word, say *baby*, – which requires no
knowledge of word meanings, and that of searching for a word in a given semantic
category, which does. Thus there appears to be no specific difficulty in accessing
semantic memory (see also Warrington & Weiskrantz, 1982).

The preservation of knowledge when autobiographical memory is grossly impaired is a dissocation that relates directly to a famous distinction in cognitive science between episodic and semantic memory, which was developed independently
of the neuropsychological evidence by Tulving (1972). Semantic memory, which
was discussed extensively in chapter 12, was viewed by Tulving as the organised
knowledge that one possesses about the meaning of words and other verbal symbols
and facts. It is natural to also include within it non-verbal knowledge, such as the
significance of objects or visual symbols. Episodic memory, by contrast, is autobiographical; following James (1890) and Reiff and Scheerer (1959), Tulving, in char-
acterising it, laid great stress on its role in the conscious experience of memory. In
Tulving's view, the two systems constitute two parallel and partly overlapping memory
systems. The correspondence between his conceptual framework and neuropsychological observations was sufficiently strong that very soon after the distinction
was made theoretically, amnesia became characterised as an impairment of episodic
memory, with semantic memory left intact (Kinsbourne & Wood, 1975; Warrington, 1975).

One simple consequence of Tulving's view is that if it were correct, it should be
possible to observe not only the dissociation between intact semantic and impaired

---

6. This is one of the more appropriate subtests of the Wechsler Memory Battery for obtaining a measure
   of memory impairment in amnesia, especially when used with a delay.

Table 15.1. *Episodic memory performance of EM*

	Memory score	
	Forced-choice paintings (recognition) (n = 50)	Delayed free recall
EM	44	2.6
Normal controls	40.6	3.3 ± 0.7
Amnesics	27.5	1.1 ± 0.6

From Coughlan and Warrington (1981); Baddeley and Warrington (1970);
Warrington (1975)

episodic memory found in amnesia, but also the complementary dissociation. Such a double dissociation has not been unequivocally established, but there are strong indications that it exists. Chapter 12 included an extensive discussion of patients with semantic memory impairments and, in particular, those with 'degraded store' deficits, whose knowledge of everyday words and objects is grossly blunted. Clinically, it is known that patients of the degraded store type need not be amnesic; two such patients were AB and EM, studied by Warrington (1975). These patients were well oriented in time and place, and their conversation was not repetitious. Obtaining an adequate measure of episodic memory capacities with such patients is, however, far from easy. Their loss of knowledge makes much of the stimulus material standardly used either unknown or poorly understood. Yet for any subject, long-term retention of a set of unknown units (e.g. nonsense syllables) is far inferior to that obtained when known units are used. It is therefore to be expected that on some long-term memory tasks, patients like EM and AB will perform poorly. For instance, EM and AB scored at roughly the same level as amnesic patients on Warrington's (1984) forced-choice memory test for words. Somewhat more surprisingly, they also performed at the amnesic level on a forced-choice recognition memory task for faces. However, on certain tests, EM, in particular, performed not only better than amnesic subjects, but even in the normal range (Table 15.1). This occurred on a forced-choice recognition test for paintings (where knowledge of basic units was less affected) and also on free recall of word lists when the words were selected so that EM knew them (see Coughlan & Warrington, 1981).

The existence of two seemingly complementary disorders – amnesia and a semantic memory syndrome – would provide strong support for the psychological importance of the distinction that Tulving (1972) drew. Indeed, even when theoretical criticisms were later made of the basic contrast between episodic and semantic memory, such was the explanatory power of its application to the amnesic syndrome that many of the critics paid it the indirect complement of retaining the basic division of long-term memory into two systems or processes; they produced alternative dichotomies. So now we have taxon and locale (O'Keefe & Nadel, 1978), 'horizontal' and 'vertical' associations (Wickelgren, 1979); integration or perceptual and elaboration or conceptual (Mandler, 1980), procedural and declarative (Cohen & Squire, 1980), semantic and cognitive (Moscovitch, 1982; Warrington & Weiskrantz, 1982), and memory and habit (Mishkin, Malamut, & Bachevalier, 1984).[7]

Why, though, should the semantic/episodic account of amnesia have receded in popularity? There have been certain problems for the approach in its account of normal memory (e.g. Anderson & Ross, 1980; McKoon, Ratliff, & Dell, 1986), but they are not clear-cut (Tulving, 1983, 1986). Other evidence unrelated to amnesia is rather favourable (e.g. Herrmann & Harwood, 1980; Jacoby & Dallas, 1981). There were, though, problems internal to the neuropsychology of memory.

There have been two major lines of criticism. The first is that the distinction is incomplete, that other memory systems exist apart from these two. The second is more serious, that the properties of the amnesic syndrome do not in fact square with what one would expect of a preserved semantic and an impaired episodic system.

15.3   Amnesia and Priming

The idea that there may be memory systems other than semantic memory and episodic memory is not particularly controversial if one adopts Tulving's rather restricted definition of semantic memory as concerned with facts, ideas, and concepts. The episodic/semantic distinction was never intended to be an exhaustive one that encompassed all possible forms of memory (Tulving, 1972, 1983). It is obvious that motor skills, say, are not in the semantic memory domain and are not concerned with conscious memories.

It was well established many years ago by Milner (1962) and Corkin (1968) that new motor skills can be learned by amnesics. It is now clear that this sparing of skill learning is not limited to motor skills only. For instance, Kinsbourne and Wood (1975) taught certain amnesics mathematical procedures that they had not known; Brooks and Baddeley (1976) taught such patients to solve particular jigsaw puzzles; and preserved reading of inverted script was shown by Cohen and Squire (1980). Moreover, in this last experiment, retention over a 13-week period was normal. This type of retention has been called by Cohen and Squire procedural memory. On the approach adopted in this book, it corresponds to the ability to develop new schemata. The normal retention of this sort of information presents no difficulty for the theory that amnesia is a deficit of episodic memory.

A more unexpected complication for the theory is that the amnesic patient can retain information within the verbal domain, too. Research on this topic forms a rapidly growing area (for a review, see Shimamura, 1986). It was originally stimulated by the finding that amnesic recall in a verbal-memory experiment is much

---

7. It should be noted that a double dissociation, particularly between memories that are not on an equivalent conceptual level, does not entail the existence of two functionally isolable subsystems (see chapter 11, particularly possibility 5). The explanation of the double dissociation might therefore be a more complicated one in terms of, say, damage to two processes within a common memory system, as argued by Rozin (1976) and Wickelgren (1979). This possibility is discussed again in footnote 21.

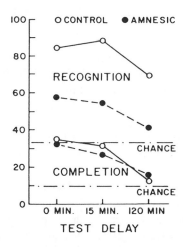

Figure 15.1. Performance of an amnesic group and a control group on a recognition and a completion task over different delay intervals between presentation and test. The upper curves and chance line refer to the recognition task; the lower ones, to the completion task. Reprinted from Graf, Squire, and Mandler (1984); *Journal of Experimental Psychology 10:*164; by permission of the American Psychological Association.

improved if recall is tested by presenting a cue that tightly constrains the response, such as the first three letters of the stimulus word – for example, *sco* for scorch (Warrington & Weiskrantz, 1970).

In the 1970s, there was a long debate about this finding. It was argued that this type of retrieval probe merely has the effect of allowing much weaker traces to be retrieved (e.g. Woods & Piercy, 1974; Mayes & Meudell, 1981). It has now been established that this 'weak-trace' explanation is insufficient. Performance of amnesics with this procedure can be at a level equal to that of controls and yet at neither ceiling nor floor (Warrington & Weiskrantz, 1978). In addition, on the weak-trace argument, amnesic performance should be equivalent to normal performance after a longer retention interval. However, Graf, Squire, and Mandler (1984) have shown that amnesic performance not only can be the same as normal performance, but also can show the same decline over time. The subjects in their experiment had two tasks: completion, a modification of the original Warrington and Weiskrantz (1970) first-three-letter cueing task, and recognition, to establish a dissociation with completion performance. In the retrieval phase of the completion task, subjects were told just that the three-letter cue began an English word and were asked to complete the word by guessing. No reference was made to the learning phase of the experiment. Despite the absence of a reference to memory in the instructions, performance on this task does have a genuine memory component, because it is influenced by the type of 'orienting task' used at input and because increased time between presentation and recall leads to a decline in performance. Performance on this task was equivalent for amnesic patients and controls (Figure 15.1). By contrast, the amnesics were inferior on their recognition performance, so it would seem that two qualitatively different processes are involved in the two tasks.[8]

The preserved performance of amnesic patients on the cueing or completion tasks occurs when memory instructions are not given. As the intention to recall appears to be irrelevant, it has been suggested that the completion effect may involve processes similar to those that occur in a paradigm much studied in normal subjects in recent years – repetition priming (see, e.g., Mandler, 1980; Warrington & Weiskrantz, 1982; Jacoby & Witherspoon, 1982). In the priming paradigm, words are presented in one situation and then presented again, say, 15 min later, in the context of another task (e.g. lexical decision); it is found that performance of the second task is speeded.[9]

Evidence that normal priming and cued amnesic retention are related comes from a number of sources. One is that the dissociation obtained in amnesia between recognition memory and completion/cueing has its parallel in the performance of normal subjects in priming tasks. Jacoby and Dallas (1981) showed that for normal subjects, a change in the orienting task used in the initial learning situation will alter the amount correctly retrieved when explicit recognition memory is required and yet can leave the degree of priming unaffected. Second, normal priming, like amnesic cueing, can occur when the subject has no conscious memory of the stimulus and when there is no intention to recall or remember; so Gipson (1986), in a detailed analysis of a number of priming experiments, was able to discard all instances in which the subject explicitly remembered having been presented with the initial prime, and still obtained typical priming facilitation.

The simplest explanation of these parallel phenomena in amnesics and normal subjects is that explicit recognition requires a subsystem different from that involved in completion or priming.[10] Might the system that acts as the basis for priming/completion in fact be semantic memory itself, as suggested by Warrington and Weiskrantz (1978)? There is a strong modality-specific effect in priming (see Winnick & Daniel, 1970; Morton, 1979a), and a major component of priming is often thought to be at the word-form level (see Kempley & Morton, 1982; Monsell, 1985). However, Tulving's (1972) characterisation of semantic memory as a contrasting concept to episodic memory is sufficiently loose to be able to include within it the word-form systems as well as the specific semantic subsystems discussed in chapter 12.

The idea that preserved verbal retention in amnesia might be based on semantic

8. It might seem that the recognition performance of the amnesic group is not sufficiently bad; compare, for instance, Figure 14.1 with Figure 2.1, which shows amnesic performance on Warrington's (1984) forced-choice recognition task. However, in the present study there were two presentations of 20 items, in Warrington's (1984) procedure there was one presentation of 50. In addition, the amnesics appeared to be of only mild-to-moderate severity. For related demonstrations, see Jacoby and Witherspoon (1982) and Tulving, Schachter, and Stark (1982).
9. For a brief discussion of other aspects of priming, see chapter 7.
10. A number of other paradigms in which preserved learning has been obtained in amnesia (e.g. lexical decision and homophone spelling) are reviewed by Shimamura (1986). They do not raise any different conceptual issues.

memory, as so defined, receives support from another amnesic dissociation. Wechsler (1917) claimed that Korsakoff patients were able to reproduce habitually used associations almost as readily as normal individuals, but that less habitual associations were not so adequately reproduced. Warrington and Weiskrantz (1982) showed this effect quantitatively. In their experiment, amnesics performed at roughly 50% of the normal level in retaining paired associates for a very short delay when the stimulus–response relationship was very close (e.g. *walk–run*), but at only about 25% of that level if the association was slightly more distant (e.g. *city–country*). Priming of an existing association within semantic memory is a plausible way that a very close association might be retained, but this process would work less well for an even slightly more distant associate because the number of potentially competing associates of equivalent strength in semantic memory would rise rapidly.

15.4 The Retention of Old Memories in Amnesia

The year 1982 was the high point for the popularity of the impaired episodic memory position. The complication of preserved verbal retention in certain situations seemed to be strengthening the distinction between semantic and episodic memory because it had led to the extrapolation of amnesia phenomena to normal subjects and seemed to be well encompassed by allowing semantic memory a certain degree of modifiability. In fact, the phenomena just discussed can be explained by other related theories, such as Mandler's (1980) contrast between retaining the activation of already integrated units and 'elaboration', acquiring new combinations of elements. Since 1982, the account of amnesia in terms of impaired episodic memory has come under increasing attack from other directions. Two main criticisms have been waged against it: that it does not account well for how amnesics retrieve information laid down before the onset of their illness, and that it cannot account for the retention of new associations.[11]

The inability of the patient to remember events that occurred before the onset of the disease is one of the best known aspects of amnesia. Famous, too, is the venerable claim that the retrieval difficulty lessens the farther back in time the event occurred (Ribot, 1882). The first quantitative investigation of this topic was that of Sanders and Warrington (1971). They studied memory for events and for faces. They chose events that at the time they had occurred had been very widely discussed, even though they might well be referred to only very rarely in later years –

---

11. It has also been argued that normal and amnesic priming effects have different time courses. Claims have been made that they are shorter lived in normals (Schacter & Tulving, 1982) and also the opposite (Shimamura, 1986)! In fact, amnesic cueing effects have been recorded three months after initial testing (Warrington & Weiskrantz, 1968; Cohen & Squire, 1980). In normals, Jacoby and Dallas (1981) have found priming effects lasting 24 hours. Too little is known about the time course of either effect to say that they have different time courses. What, though, is apparent is that the duration is almost certainly too long for priming or amnesic cueing to represent merely the continuing, if declining, activation of a pre-existing part of semantic memory (see Jacoby, 1983a, 1983b). The mechanism must be more complex than that.

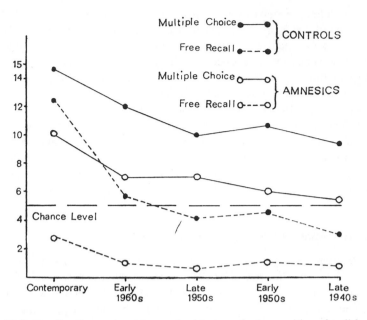

Figure 15.2. Results of amnesic and normal subjects on the 'recognition of well-known faces' test. Reprinted from Sanders and Warrington (1971); *Brain 94*:664; by permission of Oxford University Press.

an example would be a drama at sea, such as a famous shipwreck. The faces were of famous people who had disappeared from public view in a particular decade. With material selected in this way, a group of five amnesic patients performed at floor level for events as far back as they were tested (Figure 15.2).[12] Very lengthy retrograde amnesias were also obtained by Albert, Butters, and Levin (1979) for Korsakoff patients, although the degree of amnesia lessened for earlier memories (Figure 15.3). A very different pattern of results was, however, obtained from formal testing of certain other patients. These included HM, a famous bilateral temporal lobe surgery case (Marslen-Wilson & Teuber, 1975), a patient, NA, suffering from the effect of a sword thrust that had damaged, among other structures, the dorsomedial nucleus of the left thalamus (Squire & Slater, 1978; Cohen & Squire, 1981), and BY, a patient with a bilateral medial thalamic stroke (Winocur, Oxbury, Roberts, Agnetti, & Davis, 1985). All these patients seemed to have a retrograde amnesia limited to the last few months or, at most, few years before their brain injury.

A common way of resolving the difference in the findings has been to use the idea mentioned earlier that two types of amnesia exist. Thus Moscovitch (1982)

12. On recognition of famous faces, the patients performed at slightly above chance for contemporary faces but *not* for the older faces, an effect in the opposite direction from the preserved 'old memories' position.

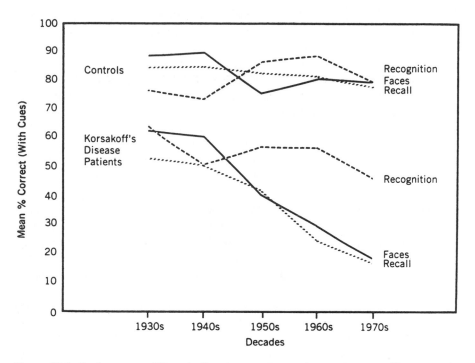

Figure 15.3. Performance of Korsakoff patients and normal controls on recalling memories of different ages. Note that duration of memory is plotted in the inverse way to Figure 15.2. Reprinted from Albert, Butters, and Levin (1979); Archives of Neurology 36:212; 1979, American Medical Association.

argued that patients whose memory difficulty arises from Korsakoff's psychosis do have a retrograde amnesia dating back to events many years before the onset of their illness. However, in his view amnesia arising from temporal lobe operations or encephalitis 'is primarily anterograde [i.e. post illness-onset], the retrograde [pre-onset] component being restricted to the period immediately preceding their trauma' (p. 354). These latter patients, he held, present difficulties for the theory of impaired episodic memory because 'contrary to the theory, not all episodic memory is equally affected – only those memories dating from the onset of the syndrome' (p. 358). Even the retrograde amnesia of the Korsakoff patients, he argued, presents a difficulty for the account of amnesia in terms of impaired episodic memory because it does not explain why there can be a distinct temporal gradient, later memories being the more affected. Others, such as Shimamura (1986), argue that any retrograde amnesia for public events or famous faces is difficult for this theory. Why, he pointed out, should such information not be in semantic memory?

The argument that different aetiologies produce forms of amnesia that differ in whether extensive retrograde amnesia is present or absent cannot be satisfactory. There are non-Korsakoff amnesics who have severe retrograde amnesias: for example, SS of Cermak and O'Connor (1983) and two of the five patients studied by

Sanders and Warrington (1971). Why, then, should there be such a large difference in the amount and temporal pattern of retrograde amnesia observed across different studies?[13] From Weiskrantz's (1985) review, it seems probable that the severity of the amnesia is a critical factor in this area too, although not enough comparable quantitative baseline information is available on the different patients.[14]

Another factor is how the testing of old memories was carried out. The picture is complicated by different investigators using different procedures to match the events or faces to be retrieved across time periods. Sanders and Warrington (1971), for instance, attempted to match for memorability at the time of occurrence, by using year-books that rank events. However, later investigators (e.g. Albert et al. 1979) have matched memories of different ages in how well normal subjects retrieve them at the time of testing.

There is a problem for this procedure. As Squire and Cohen (1982) have pointed out, quantitative matching at the time of testing does not ensure that the memories are qualitatively equivalent. Indeed, it is likely that there are crucial differences. Assume that memories for events and faces are laid down in both semantic and episodic memory. Bahrick (1984) has produced evidence that semantic memory traces can be very stable over long periods of time. If the semantic trace, while initially much weaker than the episodic one, declines more slowly – relatively speaking – then the following relation holds (see the Appendix to this chapter). If memories of different ages are matched for ease of recall at the time of testing, then the older memories will have the larger semantic component (Figure 15.4). In addition, Cermak (1984) has suggested that memories might be entirely episodic when originally laid down, but if repeated rehearsal or rearousal occurs, they would become increasingly a part of semantic memory. For some memories, then, the semantic memory component would actually grow with time.

With one or both of these effects operating, events of 1950 that controls remembered at, say, a 70% correct level would be much more likely to have been retrieved from semantic memory than those of 1986 remembered at the same level. Therefore, an amnesic lacking all episodic recall would perform much better on the 1950

13. The suggestion had been made by Cohen and Squire (1981) that brief retrograde amnesia is typically present whenever amnesia occurs, but that extensive remote memory impairment is a distinct difficulty arising from the presence of additional cognitive deficits. However, the purity of the amnesic disorder can hardly be a critical factor. SS had an IQ of 136. For a patient like SS, there was no insidious disease onset or additional cognitive deficits, which according to Cohen and Squire (1981), were the factors that might produce a severe remote memory deficit.

14. For example, patient BY (Winocur, Oxbury, Roberts, Agnetti, & Davis, 1985), who had no retrograde amnesia (RA) scored within the normal range on forced-choice recognition memory tests on which the two patients with lengthy RAs of Mair, Warrington, and Weiskrantz (1979) scored 2.7 standard deviations below the normal mean. Patient NA, who showed little RA, had only a very mild verbal memory deficit. His Wechsler MQ was 1.8 standard deviations below his IQ, and on Warrington's (1984) forced-choice words, he scored 40/50 (Squire & Shimamura, 1986), far better than her amnesics (see Figure 2.1). SS, who had a long RA, was 2.7 standard deviations below. Moreover, a more recent estimate is that HM does have a severe amnesia extending back at least 11 years prior to surgery (Corkin, 1984, quoted in Weiskrantz, 1985).

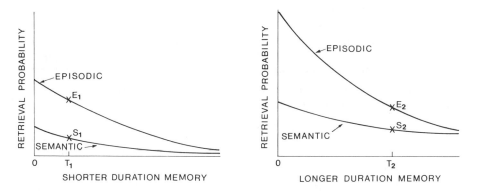

Figure 15.4. Relative contribution of the episodic and semantic traces for memories of different ages that are equally easily retrievable overall.

events than the 1986 ones, and so give the appearance of a retrograde amnesia limited in time. If, however, the events to be recalled are matched for memorability at the time they are experienced, as Sanders and Warrington (1971) did, no such effect would be expected, especially if the events were chosen so that they would not be rehearsed much after they were originally laid down. The way that different types of results occur when different matching procedures are used therefore supports the impaired episodic memory account that the very old memories retrieved by amnesics came from semantic memory.

An extensive study of retrograde amnesia in the very pure, highly intelligent post-encephalitic patient SS, studied by Cermak and O'Connor (1983; see also Cermak, 1976), provides further evidence for this position. When SS was tested using the formal procedures of Albert at al. (1979) the results suggested the existence of a temporal gradient. His amnesia appeared more severe for recent events than for older ones. However, Cermak and O'Connor also attempted to assess the patient's autobiographical memory; they found that 'SS was able to give accurate and often elaborate answers to the questions asked of him' (p. 230), which gave support to the possibility of his having an episodic memory of his early life. In addition, he was given a version of the procedure developed by Crovitz and Schiffman (1974) and Robinson (1976), in which the subject is asked to describe any memory experience that a word brings to mind. Cermak and O'Connor restricted SS to a particular time period for each word; for example, for *boat*, he had to produce a memory for the period between the ages of 20 and 30. They concluded, without giving any quantitative data, that 'it soon became apparent that he was not retrieving memories that could truly be considered as episodic. Instead his ''memories'' were of generalised events such as jobs he had held, not specific episodes for any one particular work experience' (p. 230). To account for SS's 'total inability to elaborate and specifically describe any single one of his past experiences' they concluded that he 'had *no* episodic memory for any events in his life, past or present. Recollections instead seemed to be drawn entirely from a personal pool of generalised knowledge about himself, i.e. his own semantic memory' (p. 230). The natural conclusion from their overall findings is that at least in this case, the apparent temporal gradient arises from the item-matching procedure used, as discussed earlier, and that retrieval is entirely from semantic memory.[15]

The idea that part of what one knows of oneself is obtained from a system closely related to semantic memory has recently received support in the normal memory literature. In a study by Conway (1987), positive responses to general autobiographical questions such as *'Do you often play football?'* were as fast as positive answers to matched semantic memory questions such as *'Is rugby a sport?'* and were equally speeded by a preceding semantically related prime – for example, *sport*. By contrast, Conway and Bekerian (1987) found no semantic priming for the elicitation of autobiographical memories with the Robinson technique when subjects recalled specific incidents. Instead, priming occurred if the trial was initiated with a prime of the appropriate lifetime period when the event occurred; this fits with episodic memory theory. It is only a short extrapolation to assume that important features of one's earlier life are organised in a fashion analogous to general autobiographical information and semantic information.

Thus the more detailed examination of temporal gradients obtained in tests of retrograde amnesia does not present grave difficulties for the impaired episodic memory account.[16] The different types of finding obtained by different investigators

15. A different conclusion was drawn from another study using the Robinson test with Korsakoff patients, that of Zola-Morgan, Cohen, and Squire (1983). Little information is, in fact, provided on the Korsakoff patients in their study, including whether they showed retroactive amnesia for public events. However, it would appear from the frequency of episodic memories rated 'good' that the patients had a much less severe amnesia than SS. The critical part of their study is that they found that when the memories generated are dated, the Korsakoff patients have older memories than the controls (30.4 vs. 20.1 years on average). They argued that this supports the temporal gradient theory. However, if the most recent memories (0–10 years) are excluded, the difference disappears. Hardly surprisingly, given their illness, the Korsakoff patients produced few (8%) recent memories, while the controls produced many (40%). Thus the effect can be explained by the time course of an alcoholic Korsakoff patient's illness and does not speak to the possible survival of early episodic memories.

16. Most of the retrograde amnesia studies discussed earlier, in addition to those using the Albert, Butters, and Levin test (1979), seem to have had a strong semantic memory component, and therefore to be irrelevant as far as Moscovitch's (1982) criticism of the impaired episodic memory account is concerned. In their study of the retrograde amnesia of HM, Marslen-Wilson and Teuber (1975) were not trying to select individuals who were famous only for a restricted period of time and then faded into obscurity. Their targets were very famous, for instance, including nine presidents. Much of the information that HM retained could well have been retrieved from semantic memory.

As far as NA was concerned, in the recognition of public events procedure used by Cohen and Squire (1981), he scored at over 70% on events in the 1940s, a decade in which he was between −2 and 8 and so not likely to have been attending much to public events; in the recognition of famous faces test (Squire & Cohen, 1982), he scored at 80% for the 1930s, before he was born! Thus semantic memory is also obviously involved in their test procedures. By contrast, Warrington and Sanders (1971) used intelligent schoolchildren as a means of roughly assessing the contribution that general semantic memory might be playing in answering their questions. Their schoolchildren performed poorly, which supports an episodic memory locus for their test.

and the way they may be influenced by whatever matching procedures they employed means that there is not a very solid data-base on which to theorise. However, it remains plausible that intact retention of earlier memories arises because they are represented *qualitatively* differently from the more recent events that cannot be retrieved.

On this analysis, though, there remain two theoretical puzzles. To account for Sanders and Warrington's (1971) results, much knowledge of public events and the faces of those who once were famous must be in episodic memory. Why should it not continue to remain in semantic memory, when other types of information, such as the vocabulary of a foreign language, can do so even when unused for a long time (Bahrick, 1984)? Why also should such information be part of episodic memory when it may have no personal significance for the patient (see, e.g., Moscovitch, 1982; Shimamura, 1986)? I will return to these questions later.

15.5 The Acquisition of New Memories

The issue of whether amnesics are able to acquire new information has been used both to support and to reject the impaired episodic memory position. Wood, Ebert, and Kinsbourne (1982) reported a post-encephalitic girl who they claimed, without presenting any quantitative evidence, to be densely amnesic and yet whose attainment of academic skills at school has kept pace with the level to be expected from her age. This they held to be unambiguous evidence for the dissociation between episodic and semantic memory.

A contrasting conclusion was drawn by Graf and Schachter (1985), who investigated whether the learning of novel associations could be used to prime performance in a word-completion test. Pairs of unrelated words (e.g. *window – reason*) were presented, and subjects were told to relate them by placing them in a sentence. Later, a word-completion test was presented, together with the same cue (e.g. *window – REA___*) and the instruction to read the initial stimulus and complete the second with the first word that came to mind. In a control condition, the three letters were presented with a word different from its original cue (e.g. *mold – REA___*). Amnesic patients produced the target-word response (*reason*) for about 30% of the same cue pairs, but in less than 20% of cases for different cue pairs. Yet on a conventional cued recall procedure demanding explicit recall of the second word without any word-fragment cues being available, amnesics could not remember any of the responses. This indicates that the association *window – REASON* had been formed, but was accessible only if indirectly tested by completion.

Graf and Schacter's interpretation was in line with a position articulated by Schachter and Tulving (1982):

As shown by many studies, semantic memory is a highly structured and organised system of interrelated facts and concepts (e.g. Collins & Loftus, 1975). It is not yet clear how new information becomes embedded in this complex structure, but common sense and experimental findings suggest that the acquisition of stable structures of new knowledge proceeds gradually, developing slowly over time (e.g. Homa, Rhoads, & Chambliss, 1979; Hull, 1920). It does not seem likely that the information retained by amnesics . . . could have become instantaneously integrated into the existing structures of semantic memory. (p. 44)

This is hardly a decisive argument against the impaired episodic memory position. More critically, the patients with whom Graf and Schachter (1985) obtained their effect were in the 'mild-to-moderate' amnesic range. More recently, they failed to replicate the finding on a more amnesic group whom they considered to be 'severely amnesic', but by the criteria given earlier, would still be in the mild-to-moderate range (Schacter & Graf, 1986). Given that the mild-to-moderate patients retain some reduced ability to form and use episodic traces, it would appear that the original result does not produce a critical problem for the impaired episodic memory account.

15.6 Developments of the Impaired Episodic Memory Account

The theory that amnesia arises from a specific impairment of the episodic memory system is only one of a large number of theories of amnesia that have been developed over the past 15 years.[17] I have concentrated on it because it is simple, gives a striking account of some surprising facts about amnesia, and uses a conceptual basis that also supports flourishing experimental studies within normal psychology.[18] It therefore provides a good example of the conceptual interaction of neuropsychology with cognitive psychology.

The distinction between impaired episodic and intact semantic memory gives a useful account of a number of aspects of the amnesic syndrome: the preserved knowledge, the relation with priming phenomena, the demonstration of retention in the absence of conscious remembering, the prolonged retrograde amnesias, and the ability to retain paired associates that are semantically closely related when more distant ones are not accessible. However, there are still major conceptual problems to be resolved on this approach. In my view, the principal ones are:

1. How the long duration of the priming and amnesic cueing completion phenomena, supposedly within semantic memory, is to be explained.
2. How episodic retrieval can be more effective than semantic retrieval for remote public-event-type memories in normal subjects.
3. How new information is laid down in semantic memory.
4. What the relation is between semantic and episodic memory.

The conclusions of the last three sections are as easily explained on some rival two-process theories as on the impaired episodic memory account. Consider, for instance, Mandler's (1979, 1980) approach that amnesic patients retain the ability to judge the familiarity of preexisting units. What they have lost are retrieval and elaboration processes based on inter-unit associations. This accounts well for the relation with normal priming – a temporary increase in familiarity – and, if anything, better for the loss of memories of old events and faces in amnesics. Intra-

17. Reviews of the other theories are presented by Baddeley (1982a) and Hirst (1982).
18. Another theory that has been widely applied both to normal subjects and in amnesia research – levels-of-processing theory – is now looking very sickly, both with respect to normal studies (e.g. Baddeley, 1978) and in its application to amnesia (e.g. Mayes, Meudell, & Neary, 1980) (see chapter 2).

unit bonds can be held to weaken with time generally, so that for old memories that are not rehearsed, the specific retrieval mechanisms become required and these are just what amnesics have lost.

There is, however, one further finding that puts additional constraints on theorising. It is conceptually of a different type from the ones just discussed. Indeed, its premise is one that ultra-cognitive neuropsychologists would view as of dubious validity (chapter 9)! In very few cases has there been a post-mortem examination of the brain of a pure amnesic.[19] In two such cases, EA_2 and HJ, a post-mortem took place (Mair, Warrington, & Weiskrantz, 1979). EA_2, in particular, was a severe pure amnesic who had an IQ after his illness that remained at its estimated premorbid level, no difficulties on short-term memory tasks, but very severe deficits on long-term memory tests of the episodic type. Both patients had two small subcortical lesions, to the mamillary bodies and in part of the medial thalamus; with the possible exception of a small and presumably irrelevant cerebellar lesion, there was no other sign of nerve-cell loss.[20] These two loci fit with sites frequently associated with amnesia in Korsakoff patients (e.g. Brierley, 1977). Mair et al. concluded that

it seems reasonable to consider the relatively restricted locus as forming a link in a circuit necessary for long-term memory rather than as constituting the repository of stored items as such, or even the single output of a store. The mamillary bodies are a narrow funnel through which connections from the mid-brain as well as the temporal lobe neocortex and limbic system gain access to the frontal lobes. (p. 779)

In other words it is most plausible that the classic locus for amnesia in humans produces a disconnection. These authors suggested that the existence of two lesions may interrupt two parallel pathways, hence making the 'disconnection more complete and the amnesic phenomena more profound and enduring' (p. 779).[21] A consequence would be that damage is not to an episodic store.

Given the many positive features of the impaired episodic memory account, it is not surprising that the systems held to be disconnected, according to Warrington and Weiskrantz (1982), have much in common with semantic and episodic memory. One, indeed, they assume to be semantic memory conceived of very much along the same general lines as in Tulving's (1972) account. They localise it in posterior cortical regions. The other system, which they situate in the frontal lobes, is what they term a 'mediational memory system, in which memoranda can be

19. For a general discussion of this issue in amnesia, see Markowitsch (1984).
20. A cerebellar lesion would be expected to affect motor movements, not memory.
21. That there are two parallel links fits with a related theory put forward by Mishkin (1982) to explain findings from the animal literature. Additional support for this disconnection position has come from a recent study by Von Cramon, Hebel, and Schuri (1985). They examined, from an anatomical perspective, all cases where an amnesic disorder had been claimed after a lesion to the thalamus. It was found that the common lesion sites were to two fibre tracts, one connecting the mamillary bodies to the thalamus and the other connecting the amygdala to it. One corollary of the disconnection findings is that any explanation of the double dissociation between amnesia and semantic memory impairment in terms of local resource dimensions (chapter 11, possibility 5) is made implausible.

manipulated, inter-related, and stored in a continually changing record of events' (p. 242) – in other words, an episodic memory that can be actively upgraded. The idea that amnesia involves the loss of more active memory processes – not too well captured by the label 'episodic' – is present in the accounts of three other theorists. For Cutting (1978), amnesia arises from the loss of active cognitive strategies. Baddeley (1982a), while viewing it as specifically a retrieval disorder, argued that its cause is a deficit of evaluative memory or in the process of recollection. Johnson (1983) has also claimed that a disruption in the part of memory necessary for the occurrence and later retrieval of reflective activity is responsible.

Rather than examine in detail any particular theories other than the impaired episodic memory account, I will use an alternative approach. This is to begin with a model of the cognitive system and then to ask what function would be served by a detailed memory of what happened in individual events, the capacity that amnesics principally lack. This will lead by a different route to a position related to this last set of theories.

15.7   'E-Mop' Theory

In chapter 14, a general model of cognitive functioning was developed in which to situate frontal lobe functioning. Change due to experience can take many forms according to this model: new modules may be developed, new entries can be added within modules, particular entries may be primed, new schemata can be created, and new triggers can be attached to them. All these changes are concerned with the refinement of the routine operation of the system.

There is, however, a type of memory required for effective functioning that differs from any of the above. This is the memory needed by the Supervisory System. What would happen if no existing routine thought or action schema were adequate to achieve a particular goal or, indeed, if none were strongly triggered by the present combination of goals and events? A person may be able to draw on knowledge of what happened in an analogous situation. For instance, I was recently asked how long it takes to drive from London to a place in the North of England. This is a route that I do not travel sufficiently often to know the answer by heart. However, I had recently driven it. The simple procedure I employed was to use my knowledge of the start and finish time on that particular occasion, and then compensate for any peculiarities of the traffic on that day. This is an example of the process of being reminded of a somewhat similar event, which Schank (1982) pointed out is an especially useful starting-point when confronting a novel situation. In this process the memory of a specific event is drawn on.

Another memory requirement of the Supervisory System is when a plan is being developed. Revising a provisional plan in the light of experience requires a detailed record of what happened when the attempt was made to implement it. Without a detailed record, one cannot efficiently correct an error. Take someone trying to improve the cooking of a dish that has not turned out just as was hoped or a climber trying a different way of tackling a stretch of rock on which he or she has just failed. They need to know why they tried what they did and what happened at each

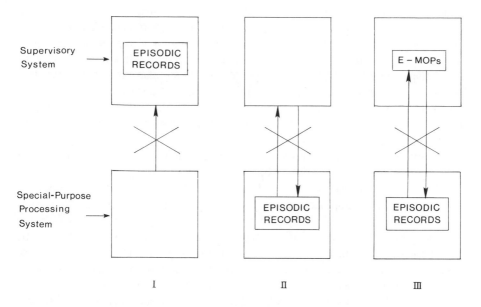

Figure 15.5. Three alternatives for the relation between episodic records and the Supervisory and processing systems (see text).

stage of the attempt. Finally, if a particular strategy does work, the critical aspects that have been provisionally retained until the outcome is known have to be stored for later use.

Certain planning programs record all their attempts to solve a problem – for example, Sussman's (1975) program HACKER. This program can operate in two modes. In CAREFUL mode, when planning, it keeps in a memory called CHRON-TEXT, a detailed chronological record of its attempts and the changing state of the world, and does a lot of cross-checking. Once the solution has been obtained, the program no longer operates in CAREFUL mode when executing the solution; it then keeps no information in CHRONTEXT unless something unexpected happens.

The types of theoretical consideration just outlined can be incorporated into the model presented in chapter 14. Two assumptions need to be made. The first is that the autobiographical record of the organism's previous environments, activities, plans, and intentions has the primary function of acting as raw material for the Supervisory System when it is directing some non-routine activity. The second is that the main way by which this material is accessed is indeed through transmission of information to the Supervisory System. If access to this material by the Supervisory System is what is lost in amnesia, then one has a position related to those advocated by Mandler (1980), by Baddeley (1982a), and by Warrington and Weiskrantz (1982). The Supervisory System is disconnected from the processing systems.

A set of alternative variants on this overall approach is possible (Figure 15.5). The first is to assume that the human equivalent of Sussman's CHRONTEXT is located in the frontal lobes. The theory then becomes similar to that of Warrington and Weiskrantz. However, a second possibility is that CHRONTEXT exists physically in the subsystems that provide its inputs. Engram formation, in Tulving's (1983) sense, has to occur when memories are formed, and this must involve the integrating of aspects of the cognitive processing taking place at a given time. It is by no means clear that such engrams require a separate subsystem for storage (see, e.g., Rumelhart & McClelland, 1985). Indeed, because an engram may well utilise the outputs of many processing systems, it would probably be computationally more parsimonious for the engram to involve associations between module outputs; these associations might then be reversed so that they can participate in on-line processing (see, e.g., Jacoby, 1983a, 1983b; Allport, 1985).

There is a third alternative. Some of the bundle of features that form the engram, to use the conceptual approach of Bower (1967), could be stored in the Supervisory System, while the rest of the bundle could be stored by associations within the standard processing systems. The specially stored aspects of the engram would be those necessary for effective integration of the memory into the overall structure of a person's life history. These would correspond to what Kolodner (1985) and Schank (1982) have called E-MOPs – episodic memory organisation packets.[22]

On these last two positions, the critical difference between episodic and semantic memory tasks lies not so much in the subsystems where the information is stored, as in Tulving's (1983) later formulation, or in the type of information required, as in Jacoby's (1983a, 1983b) approach, but in the retrieval procedure used, which is in accord with Mandler's (1980) position. Episodic memory tasks would utilise specialised retrieval procedures directable by only the Supervisory System; semantic memory tasks would involve accessing the relevant information through the operation of the schemata that control routine processing. Only the former would be impaired in classical amnesia, as a result of the Supervisory System being disconnected from the processing systems.

To provide a theory of amnesia rather than a computational speculation, it is useful to consider how such an approach would deal with the problems faced by the impaired episodic memory position. The five advantages listed in section 15.6 are retained by all the alternative versions of the present theory. The preservation of knowledge, the relation with priming phenomena, the possibility for information to be retained in the absence of conscious remembering, and the ability to retain paired associates that are closely related semantically follow from the position that the 'routine' processing systems – those underlying semantic memory – remain intact.[23] The existence of prolonged retrograde amnesias results, as in the basic Warrington and Weiskrantz theory, from the disconnection impairing non-routine retrieval.

22. An 'E-MOP' (episodic-MOP) characterises a particular event in terms of the general-purpose MOPs active at the time *and* the differences from the prototype that are operative in that specific situation. Thus a specific memory is abstractly indexed by the general units that are organising activity at the time.
23. The issue of awareness will be discussed in chapter 16.

The five primary disadvantages of the impaired episodic memory position are simply overcome on the second and, particularly, on the third of the alternatives. It is obviously no longer a problem why amnesia can arise from an anatomical disconnection. The assumption that lower level 'episodic' information is laid down in the same subsystems that carry out on-line semantic processing means that it is no problem that priming and amnesic completion phenomena can have a long time course. Nor is there a difficulty about how new information can be laid down in semantic memory. The problem of the confused conceptual relation between semantic and episodic memory is obviously dissolved.

More complex is the issue of why amnesia should involve an impairment in the retrieval of events that are not part of the current frame of reference or of faces that were in the news long ago. This, though, is an example of the grey area lying between episodic memory and semantic memory, which is more easily discussed after the process of memory retrieval has been more tightly specified. Specifying the retrieval process in more detail has an additional major advantage. It can help to provide an account of a different type of memory disorder – that which arises from frontal lobe lesions.

15.8 The Norman–Bobrow Theory

What sort of information would the Supervisory System require of a specific memory of events? Take a concrete example. You arrive home one day to find a damp patch on a wall or ceiling. Why has it happened? If this sort of event occurs fairly often from the same cause, then the event will be easily structured by a single MOP. If not, many types of event might be relevant: recent high wind or heavy rain, the recent work by plumbers on the central-heating system, an occasion sometime before when your upstairs neighbour's washing machine flooded. How does a useful memory come to mind?

One set of ideas related to this issue is Norman and Bobrow's (1979) original, if rather loose, speculations. Memories are stored in individual 'records'. In fact, their 'records' are not all that different from Bower's (1967) 'feature bundles', Tulving's (1976) 'unique episodic traces', and so on. What is interesting about the approach of Norman and Bobrow is what they say about how records are accessed and what happens after access. More classical theories of memory, such as that of Tulving (1967, 1983), stress the importance of retrieval cues, typically representations of stimuli, in accessing the memory trace. Norman and Bobrow, however, emphasise the importance of a description of the information required. They give the example of a subject trying to remember the names of high-school class-mates (see Williams & Hollan, 1981) and trying to produce as precise a description as possible. This proves to be an extended process:

Subject: I was imagining the whole room and I was imagining the instruments set up and I'm trying to remember the name of this guy – who used to do art, and he was in my 10th grade art class, which would also bring a whole lot of people too – first on that (lots of banging and tapping) What's his name now? Let's see – (whistle) I'm trying to – remember his name, at his house was the first time I ever heard a Jefferson Airplane album. Umm, plays the bass guitar. Really strungout-looking dude, uh, wow. (p. 112)

It should be noted that the formulation of a description of what record is being sought need not occur in as explicit a manner as in the example given by Norman and Bobrow. For instance, consider the example given in the section 15.7 of my being asked how long it would take to drive from London to a region in the North of England. The memory of the recent occasion on which I had driven the journey came spontaneously to mind. It was not preceded by any thought, such as 'Have I recently driven there?' It would seem that faced with a non-routine problem, the search carried out by the Supervisory System for promising lines of attack – of which one has no conscious knowledge – includes the formulation of the descriptions of memory records that would be relevant if they existed.

Norman and Bobrow do not theorise about how the record is actually retrieved when the description has been specified. What they do claim is that this is not the end of the memory process; they suggest that retrieval of a candidate record is followed by a process of verification. They give another example from the study of Williams and Hollan (1981):

Subject: I was just looking at the wheel of, of that chair, and I was thinking of Wheeler – Linda Wheeler? That name, I don't know if that was in my – Linda Wheeler, that name – Now there's a name that doesn't have a face that goes with it. I'm not even sure that – No! That's not in high school. That's here. That's here in college. Scratch that. That was Lynn Wheeler. She was a roommate of one of the friends I have here on campus. (p. 112)

The whole process of remembering is thus viewed by Norman and Bobrow as a series of cycles of specifying description, matching with records, and verifying retrieval candidate memories. This approach fits well with the position that the primary function of episodic memory is providing the Supervisory System with an additional means of tackling non-routine problems.[24] On the model developed in section 15.7, the articulation of descriptions and the process of verification would be controlled by the frontally located Supervisory System. The records would contain the schemata selected in contention scheduling, together with their triggering conditions; they would therefore be located primarily in the posterior processing systems, but some 'headings' might be frontally situated. The memory theory is now sufficiently developed to situate 'frontal lobe amnesia'.

15.9 Frontal Lobe Amnesia

It has long been known that patients with frontal lobe lesions can have memory difficulties. Thus Hécaen (1964), in a series of 131 patients with frontal lobe tu-

---

24. Norman and Bobrow's (1979) model is broadly compatible with the idea that memories are accessed through abstract descriptions. Indeed, a version of the model – that of Morton, Hammersley, and Bekerian (1985) – explicitly assumes that records are accessed via 'headings'. Such 'headings', like 'E-MOPs', could be frontally located.

mours, said that 20% of his patients had an isolated memory disorder.[25] Moreover, in a number of experimental group studies, it has been shown that frontal patients perform poorly on memory tasks. Petrides and Milner's (1982) study, discussed in chapter 14, is a good example. Another is a study by Corsi (see Milner, 1971), showing a specific frontal difficulty in recency discrimination.

It is, however, unclear in these studies whether the deficit is of the organisation of material for memorisation rather than in its storage or retrieval. Memory difficulties of patients with frontal lobe lesions can arise from organisational problems, as one would expect from the nature of frontal lobe functions. Thus Signoret and Lhermitte (1976) described two patients with anterior communicating artery lesions who were unable to learn verbal paired associates. Following 5 presentations of 6 pairs, they retained only 1 pair after 10 min. On average, normal subjects retained 5.2 pairs. If, however, the patients were given an organisational structure – either by each stimulus pair being presented in a sentence frame (e.g. 'The *beggar* carries the *cupboard*') or by being instructed to imagine a picture of the relevant pair – their performance improved greatly; they retained 5 pairs, on average.[26]

There are, however, aspects of the memory disorders of some frontal patients that are hard to explain in terms of a general organisational problem in encoding material. Thus Smith and Milner (see Milner, Petrides, & Smith, 1985) found that patients who had had a frontal lobectomy had more difficulty on a frequency discrimination task than did other subjects. In one version of the task, patients were shown a series of designs and had to decide whether they were composed entirely of straight lines or curved lines or were mixed. Each design occurred one, three, five, seven, or nine times. Afterwards, they were asked to assess how many times the design had occurred. The frontal lobe patients showed a significant lack of sensitivity to actual frequency at the higher end of the range, when compared with temporal lobe patients or normal controls (Figure 15.6). The authors argued that the task requires an orderly search to be made through memory, and that this process may be the source of the difficulty seen in patients with frontal lesions. Damage to the description and verification stages of Norman and Bobrow's (1979) theory would produce just these types of difficulty. Can one obtain more direct evidence that this theory is a useful way of analysing frontal lobe memory disorders?

In a study by Grafman (1985) with Vietnam veterans with penetrating brain injuries, it was noted that the frontal lobe group produced significantly more confabulations on delayed story recall. Confabulation used to be considered a general property of the amnesic syndrome, or at least a frequently observed component. Nowadays, though, it is thought of as fairly unusual in the context of pure amnesia (e.g. Zola-Morgan, Cohen, & Squire, 1983). However, some patients do show it to a very marked degree. The most frequent causes are strokes that affect the anterior communicating artery, which result in lesions of the medial parts of the frontal

25. Little psychometric information is provided about what is counted as a memory disturbance in this study.
26. It is stated, although no results are given, that an amnesic subject with a hippocampal lesion showed no such effect.

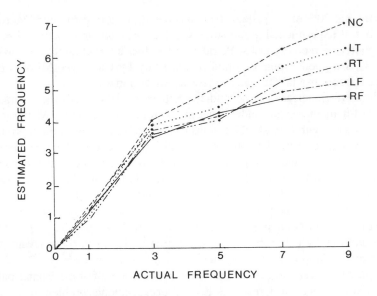

Figure 15.6. Mean estimated frequency of occurrence of designs as related to actual frequency in an investigation by Smith and Milner; the frontal lobe groups perform like normal controls on recognition (NC: normal controls; LT: left temporals; LF: left frontals; RT and RF: the right hemisphere equivalents of the previous two groups). Reprinted from Milner, Petrides, and Smith (1985) by permission of Springer.

lobes (e.g. Logue, Durward, Pratt, Piercy, & Nixon, 1968; Luria, 1976; Stuss, Alexander, Lieberman, & Levine, 1978; Kapur & Coughlan, 1980; Damasio, Graff-Radford, Eslinger, Damasio, & Kassell, 1985), and head injury (e.g. Baddeley & Wilson, 1986).

In such patients, confabulations can be almost instantaneoulsy produced, and yet be grossly inaccurate. Thus RJ, a head injury patient of Baddeley and Wilson (1986), produced a large number of gross confabulations both in memory testing and in everyday-life situations. For instance, in the Robinson test (section 15.4), where the subject has to give a specific memory elicited by a word, his response to the word *letter* was, 'I sent a letter to my great aunt in South Wales when my younger brother was killed saying just that.' He gave the date of his brother's death (eight years before), how he had heard of it (by telephone), and how it had happened. RJ does have a brother, but he is still alive.

Confabulations are sometimes thought to represent the patient's attempt to cope with task demands or to hide his or her memory deficiency in social situations. Baddeley and Wilson argued convincingly that this was not the case for their patient RJ. He gave many examples of acting on the basis of his confabulations, even when there was no social pressure. For example, on one occasion, he was discovered standing on the lavatory seat attempting to reach the ceiling. He said he was attempting to find his baggage, which was stored in the loft above. He refused to move until it was demonstrated to him that there was no loft.

A possible explanation of such confabulation that is made plausible by the way it can occur in senile dementia is that it is just one manifestation of generalised intellectual deterioration and an inability to concentrate or think straight in any situation. To be of theoretical interest as a specific impairment of memory, it needs to be shown that in general the patient is capable of organised thought. One study in which this was done was that of Kapur and Coughlan (1980). Their patient, SB, had had a haemorrhage of the anterior communicating artery three months before. He produced frequent confabulations in everyday life and clinical interviews. For instance, he claimed to have fictitious business appointments, frequently dressed for dinner as though guests were coming, and attempted to take tea outside to someone who had stopped working for him years before. His full-scale WAIS IQ of 112 was close to the estimated premorbid level. Moreover, he performed at normal level (45/50) on Warrington's (1984) forced-choice memory tests; he did have memory difficulties on some tasks, being, for instance, totally unable to remember a short story after an hour. He also showed some impairment on two frontal lobe tasks, the Wisconsin Card-Sorting and the Cognitive Estimation tests (chapter 14).

If it is granted that the impairment in these patients is one of memory and not a general disorder of concentration, is there any evidence that the problem is one of retrieval rather than storage? Evidence for this conclusion can be obtained from the study of an anterior communicating artery patient, RW (Derouesné, Beauvois, & Shallice, 1985). RW, a former manager, scored well on some IQ tests (e.g. Progressive Matrices, IQ 118) and showed no aphasic, motor, or perceptual difficulties on formal testing. Apart from poor performance on verbal fluency and some slowness on the Trail-Making test (Armitage, 1946) – a test that involves drawing a route through a labelled sequence of points – he performed reasonably well on tests of frontal lobe function.[27] He had no apparent failure of concentration; thus he was able to hold six digits for 1 min correctly on 8/10 trials.

On memory tests, his performance varied greatly. On some – the forced choice recognition tests of Warrington (1984) – he was at an amnesic level of performance: faces 32/50; words 34/50. On others – such as free recall – he was within the normal range but not high within it. On one – the Paired Associate Learning subtest of the Wechsler Memory Scale, a test on which amnesic patients hardly score at all on the more difficult items – he performed above the mean of controls. One aspect of his performance on memory tests was relatively consistent. On most tests, he produced very significantly more confabulations than did normal controls.

The interpretation given by the authors was that RW was unable to distinguish between associations elicited by stimuli and memories. So on another version of the

---

27. The major exception was word fluency (Milner, 1964), on which his performance was very poor. In this test, which is very sensitive to left frontal damage, the subject must generate as many words as possible beginning with a particular first letter over a 1- to 2-min period.

Warrington (1984) forced-choice recognition test for faces, in which he scored 3 standard deviations below normal, he claimed to be confident about his incorrect response on 15/20 errors. Further supporting evidence occurred in an experiment on the retention of short stories. The experiment involved memory for four stories. In two of them, he was questioned after each sentence was presented in order to check that he could repeat the sentence. At retrieval, two of the stories were recalled without prompts. In the other two, he was asked a series of specific questions. Over the experiment as a whole, he scored within the normal range on the amount recalled. However, he produced four times as many erroneous responses as normal controls. Moreover, if one eliminates vague descriptions (e.g. *dog* for *poodle*) and co-ordinate errors, RW produced 30 times as many of the other errors – confabulations – as controls. Moreover, unlike controls, RW made such erroneous responses considerably more frequently when he was asked questions than when he was asked just to recall unprompted. This suggests that the provision of any stimulus that leads to an irrelevant association was the major cause of his difficulties.

Similar confabulations occurred in real-life recall, and they could at times be traced to related events. Thus when asked to recall what had happened two afternoons before, he correctly recalled many details of a visit he had made with friends to his local town, including, for instance, who had eaten what pizza; this is something that a classical amnesic would never achieve. However, a striking event – the trying on of a feather boa (by his wife) – was transposed in time and place. It had actually taken place in his home on the intervening day, but he included it as an event on the critical afternoon. He said it had taken place in a shop in the town, which in fact he had not even entered that afternoon, although his wife had been there. Similarly, he conflated dramatic events that had happened three years apart in an account of his life.

An impairment at the verification stage in Norman and Bobrow's (1979) model seems to account well for RW's difficulty. Where, as in the retention of a paired associate, little strain is placed on the verification process, he can perform well; in this respect, his disorder differs markedly from that of classical amnesics. Derouesné et al. (1985) argued that, by contrast, if stimuli are present that elicit an irrelevant association, RW is incapable of selecting appropriately which of the responses retrieved is the valid one.

Frontal amnesia, then, appears to be an impairment of that part of the Supervisory System concerned with formulating the description of any memories that might be required and of verifying that any candidate memories that have been retrieved are relevant. Classical amnesia, by contrast, would arise from an interruption of the flow of memory information from the processing systems to the Supervisory System. On this theory, the contrast between semantic and episodic memory is replaced by a related one. The new contrast is between information accessible by the operation of some routine schema operating directly on the processing systems (the semantic memory system) and that which requires the formulation of a description by the Supervisory System and verification of any record retrieved.

This theory of classical and frontal amnesia has one additional advantage. It helps understand why there should be a grey area between episodic and semantic memory, and how amnesics behave when presented with tests that tap this domain. Intact retrieval should occur in amnesia when information can be obtained from processing systems by the use of well-learned schemata. This facility would normally take a fair degree of practice to set up. Such schemata would not be available to retrieve certain information that would not typically be thought of as 'episodic'. For instance, one of Norman and Bobrow's best examples of the description and verification process in action concerns a student trying to remember a programming language command he had learned in a previous session. This was an attempt to retrieve not a unique event, but a poorly learned one.

Of more direct relevance to the phenomena discussed earlier in the chapter, an event that was striking long ago but has since disappeared from general view will not be a part of any standard semantic memory retrieval routine, so it, too, will require the description and verification procedure controlled by the Supervisory System. Thus the failure of classical amnesic patients to retrieve events and faces that they knew well long before becomes understandable.

If the study of memory disorders is considered more generally, one again sees a parallel between the phenomena uncovered in neuropsychological studies and those obtained in later experiments on normal subjects – in this case, on priming. Certain striking properties of amnesia fit well with a phenomenologically based theory of normal memory function, that concerned with the distinction between episodic and semantic memory systems. The properties of classical amnesia and of frontal amnesia can now be seen to fit even better with a theory of memory derived from computationally plausible assumptions.

15.10 Appendix

Let the probability that an event can be retrieved from episodic memory be $ae(t)$, where a is its initial strength and t is the length of time it has been in memory. Let the probability that it can be retrieved from semantic memory be $as(t)$, where $s(t)$, like $e(t)$, is a monotonically decreasing function. Initially, $e(0)$ will be greater than $s(0)$. If, however, the episodic trace declines more rapidly in time, then

$$s(T_2)/s(T_1) > e(T_2)/e(T_1)$$
$$\text{where } T_2 > T_1$$

Therefore, if the probabilities of the two events being retrieved from semantic and episodic memory are S_1 and E_1, and S_2 and E_2, respectively,

then $S_2/E_2 > S_1/E_1$ . . . (1),

as: $$\frac{a_2 s(T_2)}{a_2 e(T_2)} > \frac{a_1 s(T_1)}{a_1 e(T_1)}$$

If the probabilities of retrieval from semantic and episodic memory are independent and two events of different age have an equal overall probability, P, of being retrieved, then:

$$S_1 + E_1 - S_1 E_1 = P = S_2 + E_2 - S_2 E_2 \text{ where } 1 > P > S, E > 0.$$

So

$$S_1 = (P - E_1)/(1 - E_1) \text{ and } S_2 = (P - E_2)/(1 - E_2) \qquad \ldots (2)$$

From (2)

$$\text{if } S_2 \leqslant S_1 \text{ then } (P - E_2) \cdot (1 - E_1) \leqslant (P - E_1) \cdot (1 - E_2).$$

That is,

$$E_1 \cdot (1 - P) \leqslant E_2 \cdot (1 - P) \text{ and } E_1 \leqslant E_2.$$

Thus

$$S_1/E_1 \geqslant S_2/E_2, \text{ which is in conflict with (1) above.}$$

Hence by exclusion $S_2 > S_1$.[28]

28. I should like to thank Ian Nimmo-Smith for his criticisms of an earlier version of this argument.

16   Modularity and Consciousness

16.1   The Relevance of Modelling Consciousness

There is an even more severe conceptual difficulty for the modular view of mind than how it can operate efficiently. The efficiency problem can at least be posed in a 'mechanistic' framework closely related to the framework in which 'modularity' itself is expressed. A more complex issue is why the human cognitive-processing system, which is apparently modular, should have the property of being conscious, unlike most modular systems – for example, present-day complex machines.

The obvious strategy within a modular approach is to identify some aspects of the operation of some particular module – say, its input – as conscious experience. However, one is then faced with the question of what could be so special about the processing in that module as to give its input such exceptional status. No real progress appears to have been made. One appears merely to be taking the first step on the road to infinite regress.

The situation is worse than it appears. Not only is there no apparent line of attack on how and why a modular system might be conscious, but an explanation of consciousness within the conceptual framework of modularity would probably need to be 'functionalist' (Putnam, 1960). In other words, consciousness would correspond to some 'system-level' property (i.e. information-processing characteristic), of the brain and not to some aspect of its material constituents. In wait for any explanation of this form that might be produced, there already lie the prepared tank traps of philosophical criticism. Attempting to refute a functionalist explanation is at present a popular enterprise for philosophers (e.g. Block, 1980; Searle, 1980).[1]

---

1. The most critical issue is how functionalism accounts for so-called qualia, or 'raw-feels' – that is, the *redness* of red, the experience of pain and, so on. I prefer to think of the relationship between information processing explanations and accounts of experience as analogous to the relation between two different maps of the *same* part of the world; neither map need be totally deducible from the other, but there will be many correspondences (see Shallice, 1972). In my view, the best strategy as far as the philosophical problems are concerned is to assume, hopefully, that any paradoxes represent an intellectual eddy that can be safely neglected, if *positive* evidence for a functionalist position can be obtained. There are precedents for such intellectually psychopathic behaviour. Darwin, in his theorising on evolution, was quite at a loss to account for the similarity among the flora of South America, Africa, and Australia, which should, on the theory, mean that the three regions were close together. The phenomenon became comprehensible only with the development of the theory of continental drift.

There is a simple and basically behaviourist response to these types of conceptual difficulty. Worry about consciousness has historically been a snare and a delusion in psychology. What, it might be asked, is so special about the system-level of explanation of human thought that it needs to incorporate consciousness? After all, a number of philosophical positions on consciousness are in conflict with the idea that consciousness has any particular relation to an information-processing level of explanation of cognition. Consciousness has been conceived of as a property of non-material entities, as in classical dualism, of more molecular constituents of the brain, such as matter itself, and also of persons (e.g. Strawson, 1959), all in conflict with any priority for an information-processing explanation. Why should cognitive psychology and neuropsychology not progress as nicely as, say, neurophysiology without being concerned about consciousness?

The obvious response is that consciousness exists. Historically, there have been other phenomena as basic and obvious that in their time have been as inexplicable as the existence of consciousness or were explained in a way antithetical to modern scientific thought. Life is an obvious example, but planetary motions or fire would be others. It seems ahistorical to assume that consciousness is some freak phenomenon totally resistant to a scientific account. Yet for such an explanation to be achieved, the existence of awareness must be interpretable in terms of some scientific level of explanation of human cognition or of the more basic processes that are required for it to operate. No progress has been made in linking consciousness with concepts relevant to these more basic processes, those of physics, biology, or physiology.[2] The conceptual framework that cognitive psychology offers is tantalisingly different. The names of its subject areas – memory, attention, perception, and so on – come from terms denoting mental states. In its practice, cognitive psychology even requires that subjects understand such terms in order to carry out the instructions of experiments, and it uses procedures that require subjects to comment on their mental states (see, e.g., Ericcson & Simon, 1985).

The most convincing concrete support for the need to understand consciousness in system terms would be provided by the existence of unexpected phenomena within the domain of system-level explanations of human cognition that are best describable in terms of consciousness. Consciousness would then become part of the scientific phenomena requiring explanation and not just a philosophical luxury. In fact, two of the neuropsychological phenomena that have created general interest in recent years – blindsight and the split-brain – have been compelling for this very

2. Indeed, one might almost say that consciousness viewed from the perspective of those levels of explanation is becoming more paradoxical! Thus Libet, Wright, Feinstein, and Pearl (1979) and Libet, Gleason, Wright, and Pearl (1983) have discovered counterintuitive phenomena concerning correlations between evoked potential recordings and reported experience. This led them to the paradoxical conclusion that the subjective timing of experiences is 'retroactively antedated'. (For criticisms of this claim, see Bisiach, in press.) For discussion of the more general issue of whether the existence of consciousness should be interpretable in terms of a scientific conceptual framework, see the articles in Marcel and Bisiach (in press), which take conflicting positions.

reason.[3] They will be considered in the following sections, together with lesser known neuropsychological phenomena relating to knowledge without awareness.

This argument has an Achilles heel. It can be reversed. Bisiach (in press) has recently claimed that there are neuropsychological phenomena that show the limitations of consciousness as a scientific concept. These phenomena have led him to argue that 'we may have to learn to live together with the idea that some of the questions set by commisurotomy [the split-brain operation], blind-sight, unilateral neglect of space etc. will remain forever unanswerable.' His arguments will be considered in section 16.5.

16.2 Blindsight

One of the most commonplace observations in neurology is the existence of a scotoma, a loss of visual capacity over a certain region of the visual field. It is known that it can arise from lesions to the striate cortex (area 17) (Holmes, 1918; Teuber, Battersby, & Bender, 1960). In its most extreme form, the patient has *no* visual experience of anything in that area of the field; in other cases, the patient can be aware of stimuli, but only when they move or flicker (Riddoch, 1917). One of the most interesting developments in modern neuropsychology has been the discovery of an unexpected potential in some patients for the visual processing of stimuli presented in a scotoma.

The initial investigation was made by Pöppel, Held, and Frost (1973). They studied four patients, each of whom had a visual-field defect involving at least one quadrant of the visual field. The patients were tested along an axis in one of the quadrants in which they were totally blind. A brief flash was presented, together with a tone. When the patients heard the tone, their task was to move their eyes to the position in the visual field where they guessed the flash had been presented. The patients could make a voluntary eye movement in the general direction of a stimulus projected into the scotoma, even though they denied seeing the stimulus. All four subjects showed a slight tendency to move the eyes farther when the flash was presented 25° eccentrically than when it was presented 10° eccentrically. Pöppel et al. present a statistical analysis to support their main finding, but it is based on combining results across subjects in a rather arbitrary fashion. Although the correspondence between stimulus and response positions was above chance, there was only a weak correlation in three of the four patients.

A more extensive study of an individual patient, DB, was made the following year by Weiskrantz, Warrington, Sanders, and Marshall (1974). As blindsight is a condition that does not manifest itself in an identical way in different patients, it is worth considering one prototypic patient in more detail. DB is by general consent the prototypic patient.

DB had had an arteriovenous malformation in the right occipital pole removed

---

3. For related phenomena in cognitive psychology, see Marcel (1983a, 1983b) and Groeger (1984, 1986).

at the age of 26. The initial experiments on his blindsight were conducted in the year following the operation. At the time they were carried out, he had no visual experience in the left visual field, except for a crescent of preserved vision at the periphery of the upper quadrant. All experiments at that time were performed on the horizontal meridian in order to remain in the entirely blind part of the field.

The procedure adopted by Pöppel et al. (1973) was also used with DB. In locating a light turned on in different positions in his blind field by means of a voluntary eye movement, DB showed only a non-significant trend towards matching his eye movement to the light position. However, when the response of making a voluntary eye movement was replaced by one of the reaching to the position of the light with a finger, he was remarkably accurate (see Figure 16.1).[4] In addition, DB could discriminate a long horizontal from a long vertical line exposed in the lower quadrant of the blind half-field at over 97% accuracy, even for an exposure duration of less than 100 msec. Any unreliability of fixation is not therefore a relevant factor. DB could also discriminate a circle from a cross at 90% accuracy. Moreover, he showed an acuity threshold using gratings in his blind half-field that was no more than double that obtained in his normal sighted field.

When the stimulus crossed the border of his scotoma, he was very reliable about reporting it. Otherwise, throughout these experiments, DB reported having no visual experience. When repeatedly pressed, he said at times that he had a 'feeling' about a stimulus pointing in a particular direction or that it was 'smooth' (the circle) or 'jagged' (the cross). He repeatedly, though, stressed that he had no sensation of seeing and that he was always guessing.

Since these experiments were done, a number of related studies have been carried out (e.g. Perenin & Jeannerod, 1978; Barbur, Ruddock, & Waterfield, 1980; Zihl, 1980).[5] None of the patients reported in these studies is as clear a case of blindsight as DB. These authors do, though, agree on two conclusions. The first is that there are patients who can use visual information for a number of purposes, such as reaching to a point, without any visual experience being available to guide the act. Second, it is believed that these functions depend not on information transmitted from the retina via the lateral geniculate to the visual cortex, but on information transmitted by other pathways, probably including one that involves a subcortical structure – the superior colliculus.

In a critical review article, Campion, Latto, and Smith (1983) have challenged both these conclusions. They have argued that all the phenomena claimed for blind-

---

4. This was so for all but the smallest diameter (23`) light spot used.
5. The patients reported in the studies are often collectively referred to as having 'blindsight'. However, the tests that have been carried out by the different authors vary considerably, and the patients themselves are also rather heterogeneous. Thus the patients of Perenin and Jeannerod (1978) had had a whole hemisphere removed at operation, while DB had most of his right hemisphere including poststriate visual regions intact. This heterogeneity means that it is premature to treat their visual impairments as exemplars of the same underlying functional syndrome. The argument will therefore primarily be based on DB, with other patients referred to in a secondary fashion.

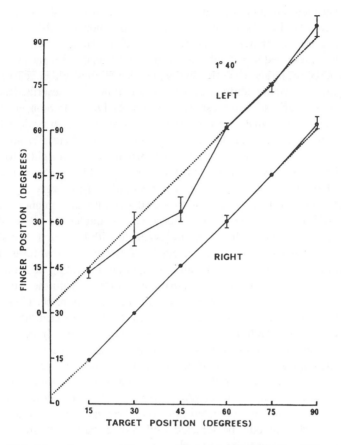

Figure 16.1. Mean finger-reaching responses to stimuli flashed to different positions in the sighted (right) and blind (left) half-fields of DB. The left results are plotted against the upper of the two scales. Reprinted from Weiskrantz, Warrington, Sanders, and Marshall (1974); *Brain 97*:714; by permission of Oxford University Press.

sight can be attributed to one or other of two processes. The first is that light from the target might have spread to portions of the retina unrelated to the scotoma as a result of reflection off structures external to the eye or off ones within the eye, such as the retina itself (the 'scattering' hypothesis). The second is that there may be spared, if abnormally functioning, tissue within the cortical region mediating visual analysis of the area of the field covered by the scotoma (the 'residual striate vision' hypothesis). In addition, they argued that the phenomenological accounts given by the patients are inconsistent and irrelevant.

Light scattering within the eye is a far from negligible phenomenon (see, e.g., Bartley, 1941). The weight that Campion et al. gave to this effect as an explanation of blindsight is based on two types of experiments they carried out on normal subjects.[6] One experiment attempted to mimic the reaching results shown in Figure 16.1 using the blind field of a simulated hemianopia in a normal subject. Both the left eye and the right visual field of the right eye of the subject were occluded. Targets were then presented to the subject's right visual field. This meant that the subject could not see the targets directly, so that any detection would have to depend on scattered light. Localisation ability under these conditions was described as 'very accurate', but it is clearly less impressive than that of DB. Campion et al. also reported experiments on normal subjects on the detection of stimuli projected onto the blind spot using this as an analogue of a scotoma. They held that any intact capacity in this situation must also depend on the use of scattered light. However, as Barbur and Ruddock (1983) pointed out, there are great differences in degree of scatter between the blind-spot situation, in which stimuli must be very close to the intact field, and those in which stimuli are projected well into an hemianopic field.[7]

A variety of additional arguments have been given to counter the scattered-light claims.[8] Two particularly compelling ones are available with DB. First, Weiskrantz (1986) pointed out that DB was able to detect *black* stimuli on a white ground – for instance, in the X versus O discrimination – and that the testing of acuity used a grating with light intensity modulated sinusoidally. Indeed, with the latter technique, acuity could be *better* in part of the blind field than in more peripheral parts of the sighted field, although this was never the case for form discrimination. It is very hard to see how these findings could be explained by scattered light.

A second procedure devised by Weiskrantz (in press) used the fact that a stimulus projected onto the blind spot in the *blind* field would not produce a neural response to light. However, light would be reflected to other parts of the retina. Therefore, if DB were using scattered light, he should have been able to detect the stimulus. DB could not detect a stimulus projected onto the blind spot in the blind field at above chance level when it could be detected well in other parts of the field defect. DB's blindsight would appear to be a real phenomenon.

The other line of criticism made by Campion et al. (1983) remains more prob-

6. Campion, Latto, and Smith (1983) also carried out two experiments on three hemianopic patients. However, the results, even given their assumptions, did not clearly support their position that 'blindsight' results are artefacts.
7. These differences are not just quantitative. Light from stimuli projected onto the blind spot can be detected, whichever way it scatters. When a patient has a hemianopia, only scatter towards the intact field is relevant. The findings of experiments on stimuli projected onto the blind spot are to be treated cautiously, especially if accurate measurement of fixation is not made. Thus Bartley (1941) found that in this situation, 'a great variety of results . . . occurred, and that by deliberately shifting slightly from the original good fixation in which the direct illumination undoubtedly fell within the bounds of the optic disc [i.e. the blind spot], the variety of results reported by different observers will be repeated' (p. 106). In the experiments conducted by Campion et al. (1983), deviations of fixation of 1°, sufficient to bring the stimulus to the edge of the sighted field for two of the three subjects, could not be reliably detected by the procedure adopted to check fixation position.
8. Barbur, Ruddock, and Waterfield (1980) attempted to calculate the amount of scattering of light from the blind to the sighted field that would be needed to produce the 'blindsight' results they obtained from a hemianopic patient, G. They deduced that the stimulus light would need to scatter 15 times its own energy into the sighted field to be detected, which is obviously impossible.

lematic. They claimed that there is no strong evidence that the blindsight phenomenon can be attributed to the operation of subsystems not involved in conscious perception. Thus they point out that over time, DB's scotoma reduced in size (see Weiskrantz, 1980) and that parts of the field previously used for blindsight testing functioned normally later. This, they argued, suggests recovery of function of parts of the visual cortex and hence is compatible with blindsight having been mediated earlier by the visual cortex operating in a damaged but not totally impaired fashion.

What this account fails to explain is the close match between what DB can and, more critically, cannot do and how monkeys perform after striate cortex lesions. DB, in particular, could not perform above chance on any pattern-discrimination test that could not be mediated by a simple sensory cue, such as orientation (Weiskrantz, in press). Thus he could not carry out the simple discrimination of a square from a rectangle discussed in the context of the pseudo-agnosias in chapter 8. Moreover, the functions that have been shown to return in the monkey after visual cortex lesions, although not to the same level as before the operation – spatial localisation, orientation detection, spatial frequency discrimination, and very simple shape discrimination (see Pasik & Pasik, 1982) – are those that can be carried out by DB in a scotoma (see Weiskrantz, 1980). Overall, the idea that 'blindsight' depends on a processing route that involves structures other than the visual cortex seems most plausible.

Finally, how do these behavioural and anatomical issues relate to questions of awareness? Campion et al. (1983) advocated the standard behaviourist position that as there is no way of verifying the fidelity of the report of personal experiences, reports of phenomenal experience should not be a part of scientific psychology. The inappropriateness of using reports of experience as scientific evidence was, they claimed, shown by the way that the reports given by blindsight patients in test sessions are very heterogenous.

The reports given by these patients, when light is presented to their impaired field, do differ. They appear to fall into three classes. DB, for instance, showed a variation in what he experienced within his scotoma (Warrington, personal communication). In one part, which he called the 'dead' part of his field, he never had any form of experience. His responses were complete guesses. A second type of experience, that mentioned earlier, occurred in another part of the blind field. When pressed, he admitted some form of awareness of the stimulus, but it was not described as a *visual* awareness. Thus he reported feelings like a 'feeling of smoothness' for the O in the X versus O discrimination. Similarly, two of Zihl's (1980) subjects reported that they could 'feel' the correspondence between target and eye position.

It is noteworthy that in the scattered-light experiments performed by Campion et al. (1983) on the blind spot of normal subjects, the subjective reports were not of these two types. Subjects reported instead some form of *visual* experience. A 'halo of light' was perceived, and the experience of the light 'waxed and waned'. Reports of visual experience do also occur with blindsight subjects; such reports constitute the third type of experience described by the patients. Often, they arise when intense light sources like flash bulbs are used (e.g. Perenin & Jeannerod, 1978), where light scatter might indeed be producing the experience. Occasionally, visual experiences can occur in these patients with lower intensity stimuli. For instance, DB's scotoma reduced in size in the years after he was initially tested, and within the reduced scotoma, he now acknowledged *seeing* something under certain condition – namely, when moving stimuli were used.

It is now clear that the difference in visual experience between normal subjects and blindsight patients is not an absolute one. Nor is it predictable under what conditions any given subject will have a visual experience (see Weiskrantz, 1980), although moving stimuli and, particularly, the beginning or end of movement seem to be the most likely conditions to produce it. Yet good performance on tasks that use visual input in the absence of *visual* experience occurs reliably across tasks and across blindsight patients. It is not reported in scattered-light experiments in normal subjects. The heterogeneity of experiential reports of blindsight patients is therefore no grounds for ignoring their most surprising characteristic. The absence of *visual* experience when a response can be made to a visually presented stimulus is a phenomenon that requires explanation.[9]

It is clear that blindsight is not an artefact. Certain types of judgements or actions can be based on input processes that differ from those involved in normal object identification. Most critically for the argument of this chapter, these judgements are not associated with a visual experience.

Our everyday intuition is that a reaching action requires an awareness of what one is trying to touch or grasp. The study of blindsight shows that this is not necessarily so. Moreover, this unexpected fact about awareness is tightly linked to one about processing systems; the absence of visual awareness seems to occur when the standard input to the visual cortex is not available. It seems anomalous to ban such phenomena concerned with awareness from science, while the rest of the patient's behaviour is admitted. If one does attempt to link accounts of awareness and scientific conceptual systems, a functionalist framework – a system-level one – provides a natural starting place for a phenomenon of this sort. In the case of blindsight, it seems most plausible that information transmitted from the input is failing to arrive at some higher level subsystem, but the subsystems to which it can arrive are sufficient to effect appropriate reaching behaviour. It is simple to assume that it is the failure of the input to arrive at these higher level subsystems that is responsible for the patient's lack of visual awareness of the stimulus (Figure 16.2).

16.3   Knowledge Without Awareness

An issue that has been vigorously debated over the past 30 years in cognitive psychology is whether semantic processes can take place for stimuli of which the subject does not become aware. During the 1950s, there was great interest in whether

9. To argue that the phenomenon is only analogous to effects that occur in normal subjects with near-threshold stimuli only substitutes one experiential phenomenon that requires explanation for another. The two situations are probably qualitatively different.

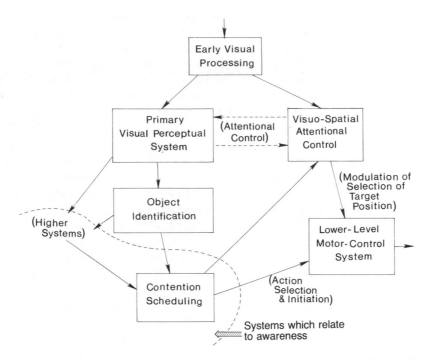

Figure 16.2. Functionalist model of subsystems involved in reaching to objects detected by normal or blindsight vision. It is presupposed that the visuo-spatial attentional control system (chapter 13) is also linked to the system controlling the direction of action. (If this figure is related to Figure 13.5, Contention Scheduling replaces the General Attentional Control System of that figure.) Object Identification refers to the processing undertaken by visual semantic memory systems (chapter 12).

it was more difficult to recognize a taboo word than a control word – so-called perceptual defence. By the 1960s, workers in the field had split into two non-communicating camps. One group believed that the effects are artefacts (e.g. Eriksen, 1960). The other argued that the effects are real (e.g. Dixon, 1971) and arise from subconscious identification of the taboo word before it can be consciously identified. During the 1970s, new paradigms were developed. The most popular were concerned with whether there could be any effect on the processing of a subsequent word from the rapid presentation of a word that was followed virtually immediately by a pattern mask, so that the subject had no awareness of it. The most widely supported position is that the masked word can facilitate recognition of an associate that follows it (e.g. Marcel, 1983a, 1983b). However, again, as with perceptual defence, critics have attacked the phenomenon on methodological grounds, claiming it to be an artefact (see, e.g., Holender, 1986; see also Cheesman & Merikle, 1985).

Can neuropsychology shed any light on the controversy? Recently, Tranel and Damasio (1985) reported a study of autonomic responses (galvanic skin response, or GSR) in two patients who did not recognize the stimuli presented to them. The patients were 'prosopagnosics'; in other words, they had a specific difficulty in recognising faces.[10] Tranel and Damasio investigated the GSRs to faces that would have been familiar to the patients if they had not been prosopagnosic. The faces of three types of people were used in the study: family members of the patients, famous people, and hospital personnel who under normal circumstances the patients would have learned to recognize while in hospital. These faces were interspersed with unknown faces and shown one at a time to the patients at intervals of 20 sec. The GSR response was recorded. Afterwards, they were shown the faces again and had to rate them for familiarity under a scale of 1 (familiar) to 5 (unfamiliar). Subject 1 recognised no faces and yet showed a significantly higher GSR reading to those that, but for her prosopagnosia, would have been familiar. Subject 2 failed to recognise only the faces of people she had met since her illness. However, for these faces, she, too, showed a significantly greater GSR than for faces of people she had not met.

A closely related study was carried out by Bauer (1984). De Haan, Young, and Newcombe (in press) have shown analogous effects using entirely psychological procedures. They found that semantic-category judgements about printed names showed interference from distracting faces in a different category in a prosopagnosic patient who could not explicitly identify the faces.

Tranel and Damasio (1985) explained their findings in terms of a four-stage theory of face perception:

1. Early visual processes.
2. Matching the face to a template; the function of this stage is similar to the perceptual-classification stage of Warrington and Taylor (1978) or the pictogens of Seymour (1979) in object perception (see chapter 8).
3. The activating of multi-modal associations.
4. Read-out of the evoked associations, which permits a conscious experience of familiarity and verbal report or non-verbal matching of the stimulus.

They held that the impairment lies in stage 3, and on their account, awareness of whose face it is requires stage 3 so the impairment leads to a loss of awareness. Stages 1 and 2 were held to be relatively intact in their patient, so that the GSR response can be triggered. They were not specific about how it is triggered, but Bauer (1984) argued that this is because GSR activation requires a different route from stage 2 onwards. This is a parallel account to that given for blindsight (see

10. For a review of this syndrome, see Damasio, Yamada, Damasio, Corbett, and McKee (1980) and Bauer and Rubens (1985). In one case, the impairment occurred from bilateral occipital lobe strokes; in the other, from herpes simplex encephalitis. It is stated that patient 1 was normal on tests of language, intellect, and visual perception. For patient 2, it is rather obscurely stated that 'language abilities are intact and her visual perception is compatible with normal recognition of faces learned before the onset of her illness' (Tranel & Damasio, 1985, p. 1454). Unfortunately, no quantitative data are given on these points. However, it does not seem too likely that other deficits unrelated to the prosopagnosia influence the results.

Figure 16.2). Awareness depends on input reaching certain higher level systems, and some other responses are based on a diverging processing route.

All these findings on prosopagnosia have a family resemblance to the semantic access phenomena discussed in chapter 12. Thus in semantic access dyslexia, the patient has no explicit knowledge of what the stimulus is and yet can make certain correct semantic decisions about it. An account that has been given for these phenomena is that the preserved function requires a weaker or more noisy input reaching critical systems than does explicit identification; explicit identification requires inhibition of competing possibilities as well as activation of the representation of the stimulus itself (Shallice & Saffran, 1986; see also Shallice & McGill, 1978). A similar explanation could be given for the prosopagnosia phenomenon. Reduced activation at Tranel and Damasio's (1985) Stage 3 would be sufficient to produce a GSR response, but insufficient for conscious identification of the stimulus. Whichever interpretation is accepted, the phenomenon itself offers a neuropsychological parallel to experiments on normal subjects that are held to show unconscious semantic priming (e.g. Marcel, 1983a, 1983b; Cheeseman & Merikle, 1985). Moreover, both of the two explanations are basically system-level ones. They fit well with a functionalist perspective.

16.4 The Split-Brain Patient and Dual Consciousness

One of the most widely known neuropsychological syndromes is that of the split-brain patient. It is the condition produced by a rarely carried out operation in which the corpus callosum and the anterior commissure – the fibre tracts that link the hemispheres – are sectioned for the relief of intractable epilepsy (see, e.g., Gazzaniga & Le Doux, 1978). This syndrome has become famous because its implications seem so dramatic. The operation was widely interpreted in the 1960s and 1970s as resulting in two relatively normal hemispheres being present in the same skull but each disconnected from the other. It was generally believed that by using appropriate input and output processes, one could study the operation of the normal right hemisphere in isolation from its partner. Moreover, it was widely believed that the operation resulted in two conscious entities being present within the same body.

The first of these beliefs no longer seems plausible according to Gazzaniga (1983a), the investigator with probably the greatest experience of these patients. By 1983, at least four series of split-brain patients had been described. In the original series, studied by Akelaitis and his colleagues (see Geschwind, 1965), no remarkable behavioural problems or capacities were noted. The second series of 11 patients, that of Bogen and Vogel (1962) – the California series – was dramatically different. At least two patients, NG and LB, showed evidence of considerable language ability in their right hemispheres, a finding at variance with earlier views of right hemisphere function. It therefore became widely believed that the normal right hemisphere has considerable language capacities.[11]

---

11. See chapters 5 and 10, for further discussion of this issue.

Evidence for the existence of language abilities in the right hemisphere had been obtained in a variety of ways. The most elegant and reliable procedure used a device developed by Zaidel (1975), which occludes one-half of the visual field while allowing prolonged viewing of the display with the other half-field. The Peabody test – a word–picture matching test – was carried out with the word presented auditorily and the four pictures presented to the patient's left visual field and so to the right hemisphere. NG had a raw score of 82 and LB, of 103 (Zaidel, 1976). These scores indicate that the right hemispheres of these patients had comprehension skills equivalent to those of children of mental ages of 11 and 16.

The other two series, though, show that these results are not typical of split-brain patients. A later East Coast series, carried out by Wilson, consisted of 28 patients, and an additional patient has been operated on by Rayport in the Midwest (see Gazzaniga, 1983a). Of these 29 patients, Gazzaniga stated that only 3 (PS_2, VP, and JW) show clear evidence of language processing in the right hemisphere. He concluded that right hemisphere language in split-brain patients can be attributed in almost every case to left hemisphere brain damage occurring at an early age, at which time language capacities can transfer better to the right hemisphere.

This was disputed by Zaidel (1983b), who argued that LB and NG are not atypical as far as the California series is concerned. He said that 'all of these patients have by now shown evidence of right hemisphere language' (p. 544), but quoted no specific findings. Gazzaniga (1983b) assumed that Zaidel was referring to the six most studied patients in the California series. He retorted sceptically, 'We look forward to examining the data finally acquired from patients in whom the existence of right hemisphere language resisted empirical demonstration for over 15 years' (p. 548). If someone who worked extensively with both the major series of split-brain patients – the California one in the 1960s and the East Coast one in the 1970s and 1980s – considers that right hemisphere language is a rare abnormality in such patients and objective evidence is not available to disprove him, then the safest conclusion is to accept the conservative position. This implies that the most widely studied split-brain patients can tell us little about the capacities of the normal right hemisphere.

The split-brain syndrome bears on a second issue. Indeed, it is for this second reason that the syndrome has been so widely discussed. The anatomical separation of the two hemispheres has been held to result in the presence of two conscious entities in the same body (Sperry, 1968, 1984). As far as the wider implications of this claim are concerned, it is not critical whether the right hemisphere cognitive systems in the most widely studied split-brain patients are or are not normal. For there is no reason to assume that before their operation, such patients differed from normal subjects in how unitary was their experience of the world.

What evidence, though, is there that the 'right hemisphere' of a split-brain patient like NG is conscious? As the right hemisphere of the classical split-brain patients produces no language, no evidence can be obtained through report about whether it experiences the world. The standard argument is to list a set of capacities for the right hemisphere and to infer from them that the right hemisphere must be aware. So Sperry (1984) stated:

The mental performance of this hemisphere after commissurotomy has been found repeatedly to be superior and dominant to that of the speaking hemisphere in a series of nonverbal, largely spatial tests. . . . Examples include the copying of designs, reading faces [*sic*], fitting forms into molds, discrimination and recall of nondescript tactual and visual forms, spatial transformations and transpositions, judging whole circle size from a small arc, grouping series of different sized and shaped blocks into categories, perceiving whole plane forms from a collection of parts and intuitive apprehension of geometrical properties. (p. 666)[12]

He concluded that 'after watching repeatedly the superior performance of the right hemisphere in tests like the above, one finds it most difficult to think of this half of the brain as being only an automaton lacking in conscious awareness' (p. 666).

This is undoubtedly the natural assumption of those who work with split-brain patients, but one can hardly take what observers assume as a strong form of evidence. An observer, watching a mute blindsight patient reaching towards a spot of light would, for instance, if ignorant of the literature, assume that the patient could see the light. The work discussed in section 16.3 and that on action lapses in normals indicate that our intuitive assumptions of what cognitive processing is possible without awareness is not solidly based. Does this mean that one can hold a position like that advocated by Eccles (1965) and MacKay (1966b) that the right hemisphere in split-brain subjects is some form of non-conscious automaton?

Consider, as one example, the study of Zaidel, Zaidel, and Sperry (1981) on the performance of the right and left hemispheres of two classic split-brain patients, NG and LB, on a standardly used non-verbal reasoning test – Progressive Matrices. The test was carried out using the device developed by Zaidel (1975). The task was done first with the left visual field and left hand, to assess the capacity of the right hemisphere. A week later, it was performed with the right visual field and right hand, to assess the capacities of the left hemisphere. Finally, a week after that, it was carried out with free vision. Both patients did as well or nearly as well with their right hemisphere as with their left (Table 16.1). Indeed, with his right hemisphere, LB scored at a level equivalent to an 11-year-old child. To perform correctly on this test, the relation between two items has to be abstracted and then extrapolated so as to infer the third item in a progression; finally, the result must be matched to one of a set of possible answers. The processes involved are far more demanding than, say, those used in picture–word matching in the number of components, the level of abstraction, and the involvement of more than the operation of a routine schema. If this level of performance could be obtained unconsciously, then it would be really difficult to argue that consciousness is not an epiphenome-

---

12. Sperry (1984) continues at this point, 'the literature is still scattered but see reviews' (p. 666), and then gives five references, four of which are to reviews of the older split-brain literature of the 1960s. In fact, descriptions of methodologically adequate quantitative experiments are very rare in the split-brain literature until the 1970s.

Table 16.1. *Mental-age equivalents of performance on Progressive Matrices of two split-brain patients given input to right visual field, to left visual field, and bilaterally*

	Input		
	Right field	Left field	Bilateral
NG	7.9	7.9	8.2
LB	>14	11.3	>14

From Zaidel, Zaidel, and Sperry (1981)

non. Given that it is not, it is therefore very likely, if not unequivocally established, that the split-brain right hemisphere is aware.

If one does accept that the split-brain right hemisphere can be conscious, then this has created much difficulty for some philosophical positions.[13] Thus the philosopher Nagel (1971) has argued, referring to split-brain patients,

If we decide that they definitely had two minds, then it would be problematical why we didn't conclude on anatomical grounds that everyone has two minds, but that we don't notice it except in these odd cases because most pairs of minds in a single body run in perfect parallel due to the direct communication between the hemispheres which provide their anatomical base. (p. 409)

This, he pointed out, would be a *reductio ad absurdum* position because the unitariness of mind derives directly from our own experience. Another philosopher – Puccetti (1973) – has grasped the nettle and claimed that normal subjects are indeed two distinct conscious entities. On Puccetti's approach, the left hemisphere self is unaware of the other and so considers mind to be unitary. The right hemisphere self, however, 'has known the true state of affairs from a very tender age. It has

13. One way of avoiding the difficulties is to adopt a suggestion of Kinsbourne (1974b), that a function of the corpus callosum is to maintain the activation level of both hemispheres at reasonable levels. Without it, he argued, only one hemisphere, at most, can be reasonably activated by mid-brain structures. It seems unlikely that this is always true. It would not, for instance, seem possible on this account to explain 'cross-cueing', where one hemisphere detects the inner response of the other. For instance, Gordon (1974) described, but did not document, a split-brain patient who could name a picture of a common object flashed to the right hemisphere, 'The patient's eyes rove about until he sees some square shape or cubic object. As he stares the left hemisphere picks up the cue and guesses "box" ' (p. 145). Another phenomenon that would present difficulties is the perception of chimeric figures: two half-faces joined down the middle so that a different half-face is presented to each visual field and analysed by each hemisphere. If the patient has to point with the left hand to a match of one half-face (the left visual one) or to give the name of the other verbally, then the subject can perform either task and can do so fairly accurately, even though the task that has to be performed is not known until after the stimulus is presented (Levy, Trevarthen, & Sperry, 1972). Both half-faces must therefore have been registered in their respective hemispheres.

known this because beginning at age two or three it heard speech emanating from the common body' (Puccetti, 1981, p. 97).

That two fairly self-contained processing systems inhabit the same body in normal people is a common, but quite unjustified, extrapolation from split-brain research. In the normal person, processing in the two hemispheres is frequently complementary. As earlier chapters should have demonstrated, the different processes involved in simple tasks like reading a word in script or recognising a picture taken from an unusual angle or copying a drawing can involve different hemispheres. Any conscious experience limited to one hemisphere would be quite unlike the one we have.

A system-level, or functionalist, approach to consciousness provides a very simple answer to these philosophical puzzles. As Kinsbourne (1974a) pointed out, the conceptual difficulties over split-brain conscious experience are not basically different from those arising from any other major disconnection syndrome or from what normal subjects experience over short intervals of time when carrying out two fairly demanding tasks simultaneously.[14] If consciousness is some, as yet unspecified, property of the system-level organisation of cognition, then the split-brain operation has the effect of creating two separate, if peculiarly functioning, systems where originally the subsystems operated as a co-ordinated whole.

To flesh out this argument, one would need to specify what these system-level properties might be so that it is clear why before the separation, they apply to one system and after the operation, to two. Before discussing this issue, it is necessary to consider certain views on consciousness that derive directly from neuropsychological research. The first – that of Le Doux, Wilson, and Gazzaniga (1979) derives directly from split-brain research, particularly from work with three East Coast patients with some capacity both to comprehend and to produce language in both hemispheres (see Gazzaniga, Holtzman, Deck, & Lee, 1985).

Le Doux, Wilson, and Gazzaniga were interested in responses made by the left hemisphere to a stimulus presented to the left visual field and so to the right hemisphere. In the test situation used, two stimuli were presented simultaneously, one to each visual field. The subject's task was to select those two pictures out of an array of eight that were semantically related to the two stimuli presented. One picture had to be selected with either hand. Thus if a snow scene was presented to the right visual field and a chicken claw to the left, the left hand is supposed to choose a shovel and the right hand, a chicken. Split-brain patients PS$_2$ and VP are said to be able to perform this task.

Of particular relevance to Le Doux, Wilson, and Gazzaniga's theory is what the left hemisphere said about responses presumed to be generated by the right hemisphere. When in the example just given PS$_2$ was asked what he saw, he replied, 'I saw a claw and I picked the chicken and you have to clean out the chicken shed

14. For a discussion of the phenomenology of carrying out two demanding tasks simultaneously, see Spelke, Hirst, and Neisser (1976).

with a shovel.' From examples such as this, Gazzaniga and Le Doux (1978) have developed the following 'metaphor':

Our sense of subjective awareness arises out of our dominant left hemisphere's unrelenting need to explain actions taken from any one of a multiplicity of mental systems that dwell within us. . . . These systems, which coexist with the language system, are not necessarily in touch with language processes prior to a behavior. Once actions are taken, the left, observing these behaviors, constructs a story as to the meaning, and this in turn becomes part of the language system's understanding of the person. (Gazzaniga, 1983a, p. 536)

The argument is inadequate. Assume that the evidence obtained by Gazzaniga and Le Doux does indeed support the idea that if an action is produced and the left hemisphere systems responsible for language production have no information about the causal antecedents of the action, then a rationalisation will tend to be produced to account for the action. To generalise from the split-brain patient to the normal subject, one has to assume that for the normal subject, too, there is usually no information about the causal antecedents of an action available to the cognitive system. The idea that one acted from an 'intention' would need to be a delusion.

To make this position plausible, the normal cognitive system must contain some functional analogue of the disconnection of the split-brain system or some other means by which part of the overall system might operate independently of the rest to produce actions that have causes 'unknown' to the rest of the system. Gazzaniga offers no evidence that this is generally the case or that 'a cognitive system that strives for consistency and order in the buzzing chaos of behaviors that are constantly being produced by the total organism' (p. 536) is indeed what is responsible for our sense of subjective awareness. For he does not show that a 'buzzing chaos of behaviors' is an appropriate way to characterise human action. Indeed, it is a classical position about consciousness (James, 1890) that it is the product of a mechanism that has come about in evolution to prevent just such a 'buzzing chaos' from existing. The behavior of split-brain patients can be a misleading guide to normal function in more ways than one!

16.5 Bisiach's Critique

The three types of phenomena discussed so far in this chapter are paradoxical from a lay view of consciousness. They are, though, easily explicable on functionalist theories of consciousness. Two other types of neuropsychological observation – also paradoxical to the lay perspective – have been used by Bisiach (1985) to argue more subtly against attempting to explain conscious experience in scientific terms.

Bisiach begins his argument with an aspect of unilateral neglect that was not discussed in chapter 13 – the patient's denial of any deficit. Denial of deficit, anosagnosia, can also occur for other syndromes, such as cortical blindness or aphasia. It is far from universal in the syndromes in which neglect is observed, but when it occurs, it can be dramatic. Take, for instance, the hemiplegic patient described by Bisiach, Meregalli, and Berti (1985):

E (Holding one of his fingers in the patient's right visual field) 'Seize my finger with your left hand.' . . . 'Well? Can't you move your left hand at all?'

P . . . 'Just give me time to proceed from thought to action.'

E 'Why don't you need time to proceed from thought to action when you use your right hand? Maybe you *can't* move your left hand?'

P 'I can move it perfectly. Only, there are sometimes illogical reactions in behavior; some positive and some negative. . . .'

E (Placing the patient's left hand between his own hands) 'Whose hands are these?'

P 'Your hands.'

E 'How many of them?'

P 'Three.'

E 'Ever seen a man with *three* hands?'

P 'A hand is the extremity of an arm. Since you have three arms you must have three hands.' (Bisiach, Meregalli, & Berti, 1985; unpublished)

Bisiach, Luzzatti, and Perani (1979) have argued that dementia is not a sufficient explanation for such denial of symptoms. It would not account, they say, for phenomena like the classic one of Anton (1899), where the patient denied being cortically blind even though she was vividly aware of much milder dysphasic difficulties. Instead, Bisiach and his colleagues argue that all *expectations* concerning the damaged function can be lost as a result of relatively local damage as well as the perceptual processing itself.

Why else would the evidence of other senses have so little effect? Bisiach and Berti (in press) say,

In severe cases, any effort to beset the patient and force him to admit and critically evaluate his pathological conditions is doomed to failure; either the patient eludes the problem altogether, or he cuts short and shelters his cognitive disorder by arguments of which a confrontation would be in vain. . . . This seems to entail that consciousness is *inherent* in the representational activity of these analog structures, both as referring to the monitoring of these activities and as referring to their control . . . no further mechanisms for consciousness seem to exist, either in the form of a unitised hierarchically superimposed component of the cognitive machinery or emerging from the whole of cognitive activities of the brain.

Here Bisiach and Berti are attacking the idea of consciousness as an all-seeking homunculus. The critique of functionalist theories of consciousness is taken further in Bisiach (in press), where he uses some observations of Bisiach, Berti, and Vallar (1985). In the experiment described in this study, subjects were asked to respond manually to the red or green colour of a 200-msec light flash presented to the left or right half-field. The subjects had four panels to press, two for each side (Figure 16.3). On any trial, two would light up on different sides – one red and one green – and the subject had to press the lighted panel of the same colour as the flash.

In his interpretation of the results, Bisiach (in press) discussed the observations made on a patient, FS, who had an extensive right frontal lesion. Of particular interest were the responses FS made when the flash was to the right half-field, which projects to the undamaged left hemisphere. In a preliminary experiment in which he just had to name the colour, FS was completely accurate with this stimulus in this situation. This was also the case in the main experiment, when FS had to

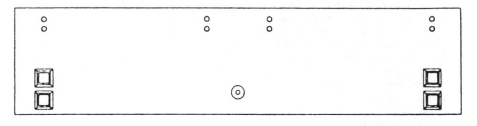

Figure 16.3. The apparatus used with patient FS. There are pairs of lights (one red, one green) at four positions in the upper half of the apparatus. The stimulus flash was the illumination of one of these eight lights. The response was to press one of the four response panels in the lower half, two of which lighted up on a trial. Subjects always used their unimpaired hand (i.e. the one ipsilateral to the lesion). Reprinted from Bisiach, Berti, and Vallar (1985); *Attention and Performance 11*:240; by permission of Erlbaum.

respond to the colour by pressing one of the right-side keys. If, however, the response to the right-field stimulus had to be with a left-side key, FS made no response on 8 out of 16 trials. More critically, on several occasions, he spontaneously stated that no stimulus had occurred.

Bisiach (in press) considered the possibility that FS did not become aware of the stimulus until he made a response, but argued that this suggestion is implausible because we are normally aware of many stimuli to which we make no response. So he continued that it seems more sensible to hold that 'denial of supra-threshold stimuli . . . would be better interpreted as an inhibitory effect of the action made which suppresses or overrides any experience of the stimulus after its fleeting appearance in consciousness, and prevents recovery of episodic memory of it'.

Given the other anosagnosia phenomena he had investigated, denial is a natural explanation for Bisiach of why his right frontal patient FS said that no stimulus had occurred on some of the trials on which he failed to respond.[15] The purpose of Bisiach's argument is not, though, to establish a denial explanation. The conclusion he draws 'is that in trying to explain neuropsychological disorders we cannot turn from the Spinozian "inner perspective" of the mental events lived by our subjects to the functionalist level'.[16] Instead, he believes that we should be concerned with the information-processing properties that allow such processes as reflection or intersubjective communication to occur, but not with their relation to 'inner experiences', 'raw feels', or the like.

Bisiach's argument that it makes little sense to speculate on the inner experience

15. In favour of an explanation of this type is the way that right frontal patients are the group most likely to confabulate (see the discussion of frontal amnesia in chapter 15) and to produce an association of ideas rather than an appropriate response.
16. Bisiach's (in press) arguments are concerned with the irrelevance for science of the nature of a subject's phenomenal experience; he does not, however, reject the use of phenomenal reports. His is basically a 'double aspect' theory of mind.

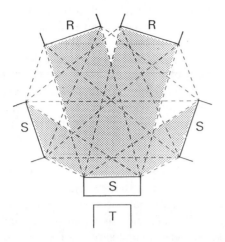

Figure 16.4. A purposefully tendentious and highly simplified model of the organisation of the cognitive system developed to illustrate a theoretical argument about consciousness. *T* are sensory transducers, *S*, higher level sensory processes, *R*, response organisation systems. From Bisiach, Meregalli, and Berti (1985).

of a patient like FS seems apt. Indeed, in the spirit of his argument, one might even say that 'inner experience' is not an appropriate phrase to use of FS's state during the episodes that he discussed. However, it is not valid to extrapolate and assume that all phenomenal experience is irrelevant for science or that it is invalid to attempt to explain an abstraction based on it – consciousness – in scientific terms.

As far as the reporting of phenomenal experience is concerned, it is useful for science only if its subject has concepts that, at least roughly, capture it and when the complex mechanisms of abstraction, categorisation, memory, and language required to articulate it are intact. These mechanisms function effectively in many psychological experiments on normal subjects (see Ericcson & Simon, 1984). They can be presumed to be intact in, say, blindsight patients and in Tranel and Damasio's (1985) prosopagnosic patient. They may well, however, be impaired in FS. Thus Bisiach's argument about FS could be valid, and the phenomenal experience of other subjects still be of value for science.

This defence does not, however, help as far as Bisiach's deeper objections about anosagnosia are concerned. Denial phenomena have led Bisiach, Meregalli, and Berti (1985) to propose the following 'purposefully tendentious' model (Figure 16.4). In the model, the T components are sensory transducers, the S are multi-level sensory processors that carry out both perceptual and representational activities, and the R are response systems. The essence of the model is its modularity, the relative segregation of S-R paths, and the absence of a superordinate general-purpose module for detecting and controlling failures in the system. Neglect arises on this view because a certain level of operation of S is responsible not only for the processing of the stimulus, but also expectations concerning it. Such a model provides no reasonable correspondence for consciousness, for there is no element that controls and no unitariness in its processing.

How, then, can anosagnosic denial be explained? The position developed by Bisiach and his colleagues is that the locus of the impairment is close to that of the sensory processors themselves. To make this type of position more concrete, it is useful to consider a phenomenon discovered by Gregory (personal communication). He constructed a self-luminant outline cube. It is possible to invert the cube as one would a Neckar cube so that in the dark what appears to be its near face is actually the far one. Gregory then asks the subject to rotate the cube. The visual and kin-aesthetic cues are now in conflict because they suggest that the cube is rotating in diametrically opposed ways. Either one observes a strange visual distortion of the cube or, alternatively, the object remains a cube but one's wrist feels as though it were breaking. The power of 'unconscious inference' is so great that one or the other percept, which would otherwise be clear, cannot survive. The outputs of the two perceptual modules – visual and tactile – have to produce representations of the world, which are consistent.

An analogous explanation can be given for denial in anosagnosia. If the mechanisms that mediate perceptual 'unconscious inference' are intact, but part of the perceptual subsystems – because they are damaged – give a grossly distorted reading, the preceptual-inference system has to resolve the discrepancy. Knowledge is no help. In Gregory's example, one knows that one is seeing a real cube inverted like a Neckar cube, but one still feels one's wrist breaking. So for Bisiach, Meregalli, and Berti's patient, it may be that the knowledge that the doctor attempts to induce in the patient cannot shift the operation of the 'unconscious inference' mechanism. Its output continues to register the position of the arm as elsewhere than in the doctor's hands.

How do these positions on anosagnosic denial relate to the theoretical perspective being advanced in this book? On the surface, the model seems diametrically opposed to the conceptual framework of contention-scheduling and Supervisory Systems, developed in chapters 13 and 14. Yet the opposition is more apparent than real. The distributed processing that characterises the model of Bisiach and his colleagues, is, in fact, present in the schemata that are selected in contention scheduling and in the modules on which they are implemented.

The denial phenomenon, itself, is compatible with the idea that perceptual subsystems, including spatial representations, are 'impenetrable' – to use Pylyshyn's (1980) term – to higher systems. It does not, however, rule out the possibility that a general-purpose Supervisory System exists, especially one that activates *schemata* not modules. The way that schemata utilise modules would not be known to the Supervisory System; it does not need to know because if one schema is activated, any incompatible one will be automatically inhibited. So why should the Supervisory System be in a position to know what is happening to modules when they are damaged? As the use of Helmholtz's views on unconscious inference should make clear, the position being developed is entirely compatible with consciousness corresponding to the operation of some higher level processing system that has access only to the outputs of the perceptual system.

16.6 Conclusion

Neuropsychological research is not, then, in conflict with the need to explain consciousness scientifically. It is entirely compatible with a functionalist solution of the body–mind dilemma. Over the past 15 years, a wide variety of theories for an information-processing correspondence for consciousness have been offered by cognitive psychologists. It has been identified with the operation of a high-level processing system, as in my early idea that it corresponded to the input that selects which action-system (action or thought schema) is dominant and sets its goal for that particular operation (Shallice, 1972).[17] Related positions are Posner and Klein's (1973) view that it corresponds to a limited-capacity processing system and Johnson-Laird's (1983) suggestion that it corresponds to the operating system of a computer. It has been identified with a system analogous to the Supervisory System by MacKay (1966a), Luria (1969), Marshall and Morton (1978), and Mandler (1975, 1985). It has been held to correspond to the contents of a short-term store by Atkinson and Shiffrin (1971), the input to the speech system by Dennett (1969), the contents of a globally distributed data-base by Baars (1983), the recovery of synthesised percepts by Marcel (1983b), and the functions carried out by the hippocampus by O'Keefe (1985)!

It is natural to view these as competing hypotheses, although their very variety suggests that little progress is being made. One could, however, ask whether neuropsychological research can help to choose between them. At present, it seems to offer relatively little in this respect. From a neuropsychological perspective, it can, for instance, be argued that short-term stores are various and specific and lowly in function, and so their contents are not satisfactory candidates for a correspondence with consciousness. One can point out that no syndrome has yet been characterised as damage to a globally distributed data-base. Yet this still leaves many alternatives. However, to a considerable extent, it can contribute little because the theories themselves are too vaguely specified and so difficult to falsify.

I will take a different tack. The arguments of the last few chapters support two basic assumptions. First – and here there are echoes of Fodor's (1983) position – there are many subsystems with internal mechanisms and even outputs that are 'unknown' to higher systems. Second – and here there is a resemblance to Bisiach's view – it seems likely there is no single higher-level system that directly controls the operation of the lower level modules. There are a variety of higher level systems, and *control* is too strong a term to describe their relation to lower level sub-

---

17. This would correspond to the most activated thought and action schema, to use the terminology of earlier chapters.

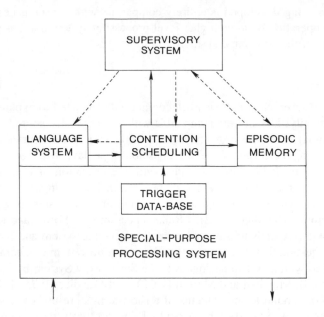

Figure 16.5. The four subsystems or processes hypothesised to have a relation with aware-ness (those extensively interconnected by arrows). Solid arrows represent obligatory trans-mission operations; dashed arrows are optional (i.e. under the control of the Supervisory System).

systems. The higher level systems influence the activation of schemata, each of which, in its specific way, will, if selected, determine which modules will be op-erative and modulate their activities. On the present approach, these control systems include contention scheduling, the Supervisory System, episodic memory process-ing, and the language system.

My position is to reject a common denominator in the theories listed earlier, the attempt to identify any particular subsystem – or, better, its output or some other aspect of its processing – with consciousness. Instead, I would argue that another aspect of the operation of our information-processing system holds the key. The processes of willed action, of reflection, of remembering, and of speaking about something do not involve identical subsystems or even the same control system, but it is normal for these control systems to operate in an integrated way. The output of episodic memory, say, feeds the Supervisory System, which feeds the language system or contention scheduling; alternatively, the activities of contention schedul-ing are fed to episodic memory and the Supervisory System (Figure 16.5). Consider the information that is successively represented, in different forms, in different control systems in such a process. By comparison with the other types of informa-tion being processed at the same time in various special-purpose modules, this in-formation would be both much more widely accessible and especially important for present and future activities. If the organism also has sufficient powers of abstraction to attempt to categorise its internal states, the distinction between the two types of information would be a key aspect of the concepts that it employs to understand itself. The conscious/non-conscious contrast would correspond to the distinction between the two types of information.[18]

If the process that corresponds to having a conscious experience is one that necessarily involves more than one control system, then it is apparent why each of two theorists could take a different control system and produce a plausible argument about why the properties of conscious experience map with what is happening in the particular control system that he or she chose. Also, there will be rare occasions in normal subjects or frequent occasions in rare patients when the control systems operate in an uncoordinated fashion. Patient FS of Bisiach, Berti, and Vallar (1985) may well be an example. In these cases, the adjective *conscious* could not be unambiguously applied. For instance, it might happen that the language system could, say, be controlled by the Supervisory System, but a strong input to episodic memory could be coming from contention scheduling. The person would then be unable to remember what had been said because of what else was being done. On such occasions, there would be no clear answer to the question of whether one is conscious of what one was saying or doing. As an example, in the course of an action-lapse, the operations of contention scheduling and the Supervisory System are in conflict. It would not be appropriate to say of people in this situation either that they are conscious of how they are acting or that they are not.[19]

Whatever the merit of this particular approach to consciousness, neuropsychology's most fundamental contribution to our understanding of human cognition, however, is to provide by far the strongest evidence for its modular basis. The conception of the organisation of the cognitive system as composed of specialised subsystems in turn offers few openings for a concept like consciousness. Yet neuropsychology, with a phenomenon like blindsight, seems to require that consciousness be included within science. Neuropsychological research thus poses a deep conceptual problem in an acute fashion.

The discussion in this chapter has strayed increasingly far from the more solid aspects of cognitive neuropsychological research. In a way, though, these issues concerning consciousness are typical of modern cognitive neuropsychology. The phenomena that have been uncovered are stunningly counterintuitive, challenging many of our most standard assumptions about the mechanisms underlying cogni-

18. This is a descendant of William James's (1890) idea that consciousness is an organ, added for the sake of steering a nervous system too complex to handle itself.
19. There are various surprising consequences of this position. For instance, one cannot determine a precise time at which a conscious experience occurs; thus paradoxes like those described by Libet et al. (1983) (footnote 2) would be dissolved. Also, if one considers an organism that has a rudimentary form of contention scheduling but no other control systems, it would be inappropriate to say *either* that it had consciousness or that it did not have it. One of the requirements for consciousness – the existence of a scheduling control system – would be present, but the other requirement – that the information that 'dominated' that system was represented in other control systems – would not hold. The arguments presented in this section are given in more detail in Shallice (in press).

tion. Thirty years ago, except for certain seemingly outdated schools of neurologists, the modular view of the cognitive system that cognitive neuropsychology offers would have seemed as implausible as that provided by Gall. The answers that have been given for the variety of phenomena discovered and documented over many aspects of perception, language, memory, and cognition may not survive. The range of conceptual problems that these phenomena pose will, however, remain. When they can be adequately answered, psychology will have become a science.

References

Ach, N. (1905). *Ueber die Willenstatigheit und das Denken.* Göttingen: Vardenhoek.

Ackley, D. H., Hinton, G. E., & Sejnowski, T. J. (1985). A learning algorithm for Boltzmann Machines. *Cognitive Science, 9,* 147–169.

Ajax, E., Schenkenberg, T., & Kosteljanetz, M. (1977). Alexia without agraphia and the inferior splenium. *Neurology, 27,* 685–688.

Alajouanine, T., Lhermitte, F., & Ribaucourt-Ducarne, B. De (1960). Les alexies agnosiques et aphasiques. In T. Alajouanine (Ed.), *Les Grandes Activités de lobe occipital.* Paris: Masson.

Albert, M. L. (1979). Alexia. In K. M. Heilman & E. Valenstein (Eds.), *Clinical neuropsychology.* New York: Oxford University Press.

Albert, M. L., Reches, A., & Silverberg, R. (1975). Associative visual agnosia without alexia. *Neurology, 25,* 322–326.

Albert, M. L., Yamadori, A., Gardner, H., & Howes, D. (1973). Comprehension in alexia. *Brain, 96,* 317–328.

Albert, M. S., Butters, N., & Levin, J. (1979). Temporal gradients in the retrograde amnesia of patients with alcoholic Korsakoff's disease. *Archives of Neurology, 36,* 211–216.

Allport, D. A. (1977). On knowing the meaning of words we are unable to report: The effects of visual masking. In S. Dornic (Ed.), *Attention and performance* (Vol. 6). Hillsdale, N.J.: Erlbaum.

Allport, D. A. (1979). Word recognition in reading. In P. A. Kolers, M. E. Wrolstad, & H. Bouma (Eds.), *Processing of visible language* (Vol. 1). New York: Plenum Press.

Allport, D. A. (1980). Attention and performance. In G. L. Claxton (Ed.), *New directions in cognitive psychology.* London: Routledge.

Allport, D. A. (1984). Auditory–verbal short-term memory and conduction aphasia. In H. Bouma & D. G. Bouwhuis (Eds.), *Attention and performance X: Control of language processes.* Hillsdale, N.J.: Erlbaum.

Allport, D. A. (1985). Distributed memory, modular systems and dysphasia. In S. K. Newman & R. Epstein (Eds.), *Current perspectives in dysphasia.* Edinburgh: Churchill Livingstone.

Allport, D. A., Antonis, B., & Reynolds, P. (1972). On the division of attention: A disproof of the single channel hypothesis. *Quarterly Journal of Experimental Psychology, 24,* 225–235.

Allport, D. A., & Funnell, E. (1981). Components of the mental lexicon. *Philosophical Transactions of the Royal Society of London B, 295,* 397–410.

Anderson, J. A., & Mozer, M. C. (1981). Categorization and selective neurons. In G. E. Hinton & J. A. Anderson (Eds.), *Parallel models of associative memory.* Hillsdale, N.J.: Erlbaum.

Anderson, J. A., Silverstein, J. W., Ritz, S. A., & Jones, R. S. (1977). Distinctive features, categorical perception, and probability learning: Some applications of a neural model. *Psychological Review, 84,* 413–451.

Anderson, J. R. (1976). *Language, memory and thought.* Hillsdale, N.J.: Erlbaum.

Anderson, J. R. (1980). *Cognitive psychology and its implications.* San Francisco: Freeman.

Anderson, J. R. (1983). *The architecture of cognition.* Cambridge, Mass.: Harvard University Press.

Anderson, J. R., & Ross, B. H. (1980). Evidence against a semantic–episodic distinction. *Journal of Experimental Psychology: Human Learning and Memory, 6,* 441–465.

405

Anton, G. (1899). Ueber die Selbstwahrnemung der Herderkrankungen des Gehirns durch den Kranken bei Rindenblindheit und Rindentaubheit. *Archiv für Psychiatrie und Nervenkrankheiten, 32*, 86–127.

Anzai, Y., & Simon, H. (1979). The theory of learning by doing. *Psychological Review, 86*, 124–140.

Arbib, M. A., & Caplan, D. (1979). Neurolinguistics must be computational. *Behavioral and Brain Sciences, 2*, 449–483.

Armitage, S. G. (1946). An analysis of certain psychological tests used for the evaluation of brain injury. *Psychological Monographs, 60* (277).

Arrigoni, G., & De Renzi, E. (1964). Constructional apraxia and hemisphere locus of lesion. *Cortex, 1*, 170–197.

Assal, G., Buttet, J., & Jolivet, R. (1981). Dissociations in aphasia: A case report. *Brain and Language, 13*, 223–240.

Assal, G., & Regli, F. (1980). Syndrome de disconnection visuo-verbale et visuo-gestuelle. *Revue Neurologique, 136*, 365–376.

Atkinson, R. C., & Shiffrin, R. M. (1968). Human memory: A proposed system and its control processes. In K. W. Spence & J. T. Spence (Eds.), *The psychology of learning and motivation: Advances in research and theory* (Vol. 2). New York: Academic Press.

Atkinson, R. C., & Shiffrin, R. M. (1971). The control of short-term memory. *Scientific American, 224*, 82–90.

Audley, R. J., & Jonckheere, A. R. (1956). The statistical analysis of the learning process: II. Stochastic processes and learning behaviour. *British Journal of Statistical Psychology, 9*, 87–94.

Baars, B. J. (1983). Conscious contents provide the nervous system with coherent global information. In R. J. Davidson, G. E. Schwartz, & D. Shapiro (Eds.), *Consciousness and self-regulation* (Vol. 3). New York: Plenum Press.

Baddeley, A. D. (1966). Short-term memory for word sequences as a function of acoustic, semantic and formal similarity. *Quarterly Journal of Experimental Psychology, 18*, 362–365.

Baddeley, A. D. (1968). How does acoustic similarity influence short-term memory? *Quarterly Journal of Experimental Psychology, 20*, 249–264.

Baddeley, A. D. (1970). Estimating the short-term component in free recall. *British Journal of Psychology, 61*, 13–15.

Baddeley, A. D. (1976). *The psychology of memory*. New York: Basic Books.

Baddeley, A. D. (1978). The trouble with levels: A re-examination of Craik and Lockhart's framework for memory research. *Psychological Review, 85*, 139–152.

Baddeley, A. D. (1982a). Amnesia: A minimal model and an interpretation. In L. S. Cermak (Ed.), *Human memory and amnesia*. Hillsdale, N.J.: Erlbaum.

Baddeley, A. D. (1982b). Implications of neuropsychological evidence for theories of normal memory. *Philosophical Transactions of the Royal Society of London B, 298*, 59–72.

Baddeley, A. D. (1986). *Working memory*. Oxford: Clarendon Press.

Baddeley, A. D., & Hitch, G. (1974). Working memory. In G. H. Bower (Ed.), *The psychology of learning and motivation* (Vol. 8). New York: Academic Press.

Baddeley, A. D., & Hitch, G. (1977). Recency re-examined. In S. Dornic (Ed.), *Attention and performance* (Vol. 6). Hillsdale, N.J.: Erlbaum.

Baddeley, A. D., & Lieberman, K. (1980). Spatial working memory. In R. S. Nickerson (Ed.), *Attention and performance*. (Vol. 8). Hillsdale, N.J.: Erlbaum.

Baddeley, A. D., Thomson, N., & Buchanan, M. (1975). Word length and the structure of short-term memory. *Journal of Verbal Learning and Verbal Behavior, 15*, 575–589.

Baddeley, A. D., & Warrington, E. K. (1970). Amnesia and the distinction between long- and short-term memory. *Journal of Verbal Learning and Verbal Behavior, 9*, 176–189.

Baddeley, A. D. & Wilson, B. (1986). Amnesia, autobiographical memory and confabulation. In D. Rubin (Ed.), *Autobiographical memory*. Cambridge: Cambridge University Press.

Badecker, W., & Caramazza, A. (1985). On considerations of method and theory governing the use of clinical categories in neurolinguistics and cognitive neuropsychology. *Cognition, 20*, 97–125.

Bahrick, H. P. (1984). Semantic memory content in permastore: Fifty years of memory for Spanish learned in school. *Journal of Experimental Psychology: General, 113*, 1–29.

Baker, R. C., & Smith, P. T. (1976). A psycholinguistic study of English stress assignment rules. *Language and Speech, 19*, 9–27.

Balint, R. (1909). Die Seelenhahmung des 'Schauens', optische Ataxie, raumliche Storung der Aufmerksamkheit. *Monatschrift für Psychologie und Neurologie, 25*, 51–81.

Barbur, J. L., & Ruddock, K. H. (1983). The analysis of scattered light effects in hemianopic and normal vision. *Behavioral and Brain Sciences, 6*, 448–449.

Barbur, J. L., Ruddock, K. H., & Waterfield, V. A. (1980). Human visual response in the absence of the geniculo-calcarine projection. *Brain, 103*, 905–928.

Barnard, P. J., Hammond, N. V., MacLean, A., & Morton, J. (1982). Learning and remembering interactive commands in a text-editing task. *Behaviour and Information Technology, 1*, 347–358.

Baron, J. (1977). Mechanisms for pronouncing printed words: Use and acquisition. In D. A. Laberge & S. J. Samuels (Eds.), *Basic processes in reading: Perception and communication*. Hillsdale, N.J.: Erlbaum.

Baron, J., & Strawson, C. (1976). Use of orthographic and word-specific knowledge in reading words aloud. *Journal of Experimental Psychology: Human Performance and Perception, 2*, 386–393.

Barry, C. (1984). Consistency and semantic errors in a deep dyslexic patient. In R. N. Malatesha & H. J. Whitaker (Eds.), *Dyslexia: A global issue*. The Hague: Martinus Nijhoff.

Bartlett, F. C. (1932). *Remembering: A study in experimental and social psychology*. Cambridge: Cambridge University Press.

Bartley, S. H. (1941). *Vision*. New York: Van Nostrand.

Basso, A., & Capitani, E. (1985). Spared musical abilities in a conductor with global aphasia and ideomotor apraxia. *Journal of Neurology, Neurosurgery and Psychiatry, 48*, 407–412.

Basso, A., Capitani, E., Laiacona, M., & Luzzatti, C. (1980). Factors influencing type and severity of aphasia. *Cortex, 16*, 631–636.

Basso, A., Capitani, E., & Moraschini, S. (1982). Sex differences in recovery from aphasia. *Cortex, 18*, 469–475.

Basso, A., Spinnler, H., Vallar, G., & Zanobia, E. (1982). Left hemisphere damage and selective impairment of auditory–verbal short-term memory. *Neuropsychologia, 20*, 263–274.

Basso, A., Taborelli, A., & Vignolo, L. A. (1978). Dissociated disorders of speaking and writing in aphasia. *Journal of Neurology, Neurosurgery and Psychiatry, 41*, 556–563.

Bastian, H. C. (1869). On the various forms of loss of speech in cerebral disease. *British and Foreign Medical-Chirurgical Review 43*, 209–236, 470–492.

Bastian, H. C. (1898). *Aphasia and other speech defects*. London: Lewis.

Battersby, W. S., Bender, M. B., Pollack, M., & Kahn, R. L. (1956). Unilateral 'spatial agnosia' ('inattention') in patients with cerebral lesions. *Brain, 79*, 68–93.

Bauer, R. H., & Fuster, J. M. (1976). Delayed-matching and delayed-response deficit from cooling dorsolateral prefrontal cortex in monkeys. *Journal of Comparative and Physiological Psychology, 90*, 293–302.

Bauer, R. H., & Fuster, J. M. (1978). The effect of ambient illumination on delayed-matching and delayed-response deficits from cooling dorsolateral prefrontal cortex. *Behavioral Biology, 22*, 60–66.

Bauer, R. M. (1984). Autonomic recognition of names and faces in prosopagnosia: A neuropsychological application of the guilty knowledge test. *Neuropsychologia, 22*, 457–469.

Bauer, R. M., & Rubens, A. B. (1985). Agnosia. In K. M. Heilman & E. Valenstein (Eds.), *Clinical neuropsychology* (2nd ed.). New York: Oxford University Press.

Baxter, D. M. (1982). *The development of a graded spelling test for adults*. Paper presented at the Fifth International Neuropsychological Society European Conference, Deauville, France.

Baxter, D. M., & Warrington, E. K. (1983). Neglect dysgraphia. *Journal of Neurology, Neurosurgery and Psychiatry, 46*, 1073–1078.

Baxter, D. M., & Warrington, E. K. (1985). Category-specific phonological dysgraphia. *Neuropsychologia, 23*, 653–666.

Baxter, D. M., & Warrington, E. K. (1986). Ideational agraphia: A single case study. *Journal of Neurology, Neurosurgery and Psychiatry, 49*, 369–374.

Baxter, D. M., & Warrington, E. K. (1987). Transcoding sound to spelling: Single or multiple sound unit correspondences. *Cortex, 23*, 11–28.

Bay, E. (1953). Disturbances of visual perception and their examination. *Brain, 76*, 515–551.

Bay, E. (1962). Aphasia and non-verbal disorders of language. *Brain, 85*, 411–426.

Beauvois, M.-F. (1982). Optic aphasia: A process of interaction between vision and language. *Philosophical Transactions of the Royal Society of London B, 298*, 35–47.

Beauvois, M.-F., & Derouesné, J. (1979). Phonological alexia: Three dissociations. *Journal of Neurology, Neurosurgery and Psychiatry, 42*, 1115–1124.

Beauvois, M.-F., & Derouesné, J. (1981). Lexical or orthographic agraphia. *Brain, 104*, 21–49.

Beauvois, M.-F., & Derouesné, J. (1982). Recherche en psychologie cognitive et rééducation: Quel rapports? In X. Seron (Ed.), *Rééduquer le cerveau*. Brussels: Mardaga.

Beauvois, M.-F., Derouesné, J., & Saillant, B. (1980). Syndromes neuropsychologiques et psychologie cognitif trois exemples: Aphasie tactile, alexie phonologique et agraphie lexicale. *Cahiers de Psychologie, 23*, 211–245.

Beauvois, M.-F., & Saillant, B. (1985). Optic aphasia for colours, and colour agnosia: A distinction between visual and visuo-verbal impairments in the processing of colours. *Cognitive Neuropsychology, 2*, 1–48.

Beauvois, M.-F., Saillant, B., Meininger, V., & Lhermitte, F. (1978). Bilateral tactile aphasia: A tacto-verbal dysfunction. *Brain, 101*, 381–401.

Bender, M. B., & Feldman, M. (1972). The so-called visual agnosias. *Brain, 95*, 173–186.

Bender, M. B., & Teuber, H. L. (1947). Phenomena of fluctuation, extinction and completion in visual perception. *Archives of Neurology and Psychiatry, 55*, 627–658.

Benson, D. F. (1967). Fluency in aphasia: Correlation with radioactive scan localisation. *Cortex, 3*, 373–394.

Benson, D. F., & Geschwind, N. (1969). The alexias. In P. J. Vinken & G. W. Bruyn (Eds.), *Handbook of clinical neurology* (Vol. 4). Amsterdam: North Holland.

Benson, D. F., Segarra, J., & Albert, M. L. (1974), Visual agnosia–prosopagnosia. *Archives of Neurology, 30*, 307–310.

Benson, D. F., Sheremata, W. A., Bouchard, R., Segarra, J. M., Price, D., & Geschwind, N. (1973). Conduction aphasia: A clinicopathological study. *Archives of Neurology, 28*, 339–346.

Benton, A. L. (1961). The fiction of the Gerstmann syndrome. *Journal of Neurology, Neurosurgery and Psychiatry, 24*, 176–181.

Benton, A. L. (1965). The problem of cerebral dominance. *Canadian Psychologist, 6*, 332–348.

Benton, A. L. (1977). Reflections on the Gerstmann syndrome. *Brain and Language, 4*, 45–62.

Bergson, H. (1896). *Matière et mémoire*. Paris: Alcan.

Berndt, R. S. (1987). Symptom co-occurrence and dissociation in the interpretation of agrammatism. In M. Coltheart, G. Sartori, & R. Job (Eds.), *The cognitive neuropsychology of language*. London: Erlbaum.

Berndt, R. S., & Caramazza, A. (1980). A redefinition of the syndrome of Broca's aphasia: Implications for a neuropsychological model of language. *Applied Linguistics, 1*, 225–278.

Bianchi, L. (1921). *La Mécanisme du cerveau et la fonction du lobes frontal*. Paris: Arnette.

Bianchi, L. (1922). *The mechanism of the brain and the function of the frontal lobes*. Edinburgh: Livingstone.

Binford, L. R. (1976). Forty-seven trips: A case study in the character of archaeological formation processes. In E. S. Hall (Ed.), *Contributions to anthropology: The interior peoples of northern Alaska: Archaeological survey of Canada* (Vol. 49). Ottawa: Ottawa National Museum of Man.

Bisiach, E. (in press). The (haunted) brain and consciousness. In A. J. Marcel & E. Bisiach (Eds.), *Consciousness in contemporary science*. Oxford: Oxford University Press.

Bisiach, E., & Berti, A. (in press). Dyschiria: An attempt at its systemic explanation. In M. Jeannerod

(Ed.), *Neurophysiological and neuropsychological aspects of spatial neglect.* Amsterdam: North Holland.

Bisiach, E., Berti, A., & Vallar, G. (1985). Analogical and logical disorders underlying unilateral neglect of space. In M. I. Posner & O. S. M. Marin (Eds.), *Attention and performance* (Vol. 11). Hillsdale, N.J.: Erlbaum.

Bisiach, E., Capitani, E., Luzzatti, C., & Perani, D. (1981). Brain and conscious representation of outside reality. *Neuropsychologia, 19,* 543–551.

Bisiach, E., & Luzzatti, C. (1978). Unilateral neglect of representational space. *Cortex, 14,* 129–133.

Bisiach, E., Luzzatti, C., & Perani, D. (1979). Unilateral neglect, representational schema and consciousness. *Brain, 102,* 609–618.

Bisiach, E., Meregalli, S., & Berti, A. (1985, June). *Mechanisms of production–control and belief–fixation in human visuospatial processing: Clinical evidence from hemispatial neglect.* Paper presented at the Eighth Symposium on Quantitative Analyses of Behavior. Cambridge, Mass.

Block, N. (1980). Troubles with functionalism. In N. Block (Ed.), *Readings in the philosophy of psychology* (Vol. 1). Cambridge, Mass.: Harvard University Press.

Blumstein, S. E., Cooper, W. E., Zurif, E. B., & Caramazza, A. (1977). The perception and production of voice-onset time in aphasia. *Neuropsychologia, 15,* 371–383.

Blumstein, S. E., Milberg, W., & Shrier, R. (1982). Semantic processing in aphasia: Evidence from an auditory lexical decision task. *Brain and Language, 17,* 301–315.

Bodamer, J. (1947). Die prosopagnosia. *Archiv fur Psychiatrie und Zeitschrift für Neurologie, 179,* 6–54.

Boden, M. (1977). *Artificial intelligence and natural man.* New York: Basic Books.

Bogen, J. E. (1985). The callosal syndromes. In K. M. Heilman & E. Valenstein (Eds.), *Clinical neuropsychology* (2nd ed.). New York: Oxford University Press.

Bogen, J. E., & Vogel, P. J. (1962). Cerebral commissurotomy in man. *Bulletin of the Los Angeles Neurological Society, 27,* 169–172.

Boller, F., & Grafman, J. (1983). Acalculia: Historical development and current significance. *Brain and Cognition, 2,* 205–223.

Bornstein, B. (1963). Prosopagnosia. In L. Halpern (Ed.), *Problems of dynamic neurology.* Jerusalem: Hadasseh Medical Organization.

Bower, G. H. (1967). A multicomponent view of the memory trace. In K. W. Spence & J. T. Spence (Eds.), *The psychology of learning and motivation: Advances in research and theory.* New York: Academic Press.

Brain, R. (1941). Visual disorientation with special reference to the lesions of the right cerebral hemisphere. *Brain, 64,* 244–272.

Brierley, J. B. (1977). The neuropathology of amnesic states. In C. W. M. Whitty & O. L. Zangwill (Eds.), *Amnesia* (2nd. ed.). London: Butterworth.

Broadbent, D. E. (1958). *Perception and communication.* London: Pergamon.

Broadbent, D. E. (1971). *Decision and stress.* London: Academic Press.

Broadbent, D. E. (1984). The Maltese cross: A new simplistic model for memory. *Behavioral and Brain Sciences, 7,* 55–94.

Broadbent, D. E., Vines, R., & Broadbent, M. (1978). Recency effects in memory, as a function of modality of intervening events. *Psychological Research, 40,* 5–13.

Broca, P. (1861). Remarques sur le siège de la faculté du langage articulé, suives d'une observation d'aphemie. *Bulletin et Mémoires de la Société anatomique de Paris, 2,* 330–357.

Brooks, D. N., & Baddeley, A. D. (1976). What can amnesic patients learn? *Neuropsychologia, 14,* 111–122.

Brown, J. S. (1981). Review of *Deep dyslexia, Brain and Language, 14,* 386–392.

Brown, W. P., & Ure, D. M. N. (1969). Five rated characteristics of 650 word association stimuli. *British Journal of Psychology, 60,* 223–250.

Brust, J., Shafer, S., Richter, R., & Bruun, B. (1976). Aphasia in acute stroke. *Stroke, 7,* 167–174.

Bryant, P., & Impey, L. (1986). The similarities between normal readers and developmental and acquired dyslexics. *Cognition, 24,* 121–137.

Bub, D., Cancelliere, A., & Kertesz, A. (1985). Whole-word and analytic translation of spelling-to-sound in a non-semantic reader. In K. E. Patterson, M. Coltheart, & J. C. Marshall (Eds.), *Surface dyslexia*. London: Erlbaum.

Bub, D., & Kertesz, A. (1982a). Evidence for lexicographic processing in a patient with preserved written over oral single word naming. *Brain, 105*, 697–717.

Bub, D., & Kertesz, A. (1982b). Deep agraphia. *Brain and Language, 17*, 146–165.

Buckingham, H. W. (1979). Linguistic aspects of lexical retrieval in the posterior fluent aphasias. In H. Whitaker & H. A. Whitaker (Eds.), *Studies in neurolinguistics* (Vol. 4). New York: Academic Press.

Buckingham, H. W., & Kertesz, A. (1976). *Neologistic jargon aphasia*. Amsterdam: Swets & Zeitlinger.

Butters, N., & Cermak, L. S. (1974). Some comments on Warrington and Baddeley's report of normal short-term memory in amnesic patients. *Neuropsychologia, 12*, 283–285.

Butters, N., & Cermak, L. S. (1975). Some analyses of amnesic syndromes in brain-damaged patients. In R. Isaacson & K. Pribram (Eds.), *The hippocampus* (Vol. 2). New York: Plenum Press.

Butters, N., & Cermak, L. S. (1976). Neuropsychological studies of alcoholic Korsakoff patients. In G. Goldstein & C. Neuringer (Eds.), *Empirical studies of alcoholism*. Cambridge, Mass.: Ballinger.

Butters, N., & Cermak, L. S. (1980). *Alcoholic Korsakoff's syndrome: An information-processing approach to amnesia*. New York: Academic Press.

Butters, N., & Miliotis, P. (1985). Amnesic disorders. In K. M. Heilman & E. Valenstein (Eds.), *Clinical neuropsychology* (2nd ed.). New York: Oxford University Press.

Butters, N., Soeldner, C., & Fedio, P. (1972). Comparison of parietal and frontal lobe spatial deficits in man: Extrapersonal vs personal (egocentric) space. *Perceptual and Motor Skills, 34*, 27–34.

Butterworth, B. (1979). Hesitation and the production of verbal paraphasias and neologisms in jargon aphasia. *Brain and Language, 8*, 133–161.

Butterworth, B. (1980). Some constraints on models of language production. In B. Butterworth (Ed.), *Language production* (Vol. 1). London: Academic Press.

Butterworth, B., Campbell, R., & Howard, D. (1986). The uses of short-term memory: A case study. *Quarterly Journal of Experimental Psychology, 38A*, 705–738.

Campbell, R. (1983). Writing non-words to dictation. *Brain and Language, 19*, 153–178.

Campion, R. L., Latto, R., & Smith, Y. M. (1983). In blindsight an effect of scattered light, spared cortex and near-threshold vision. *Behavioral and Brain Sciences, 6*, 423–486.

Canavan, A. G. M., Janota, I., & Schurr, P. H. (1985). Luria's frontal lobe syndrome: Psychological and anatomical considerations. *Journal of Neurology, Neurosurgery and Psychiatry, 48*, 1049–1053.

Caplan, D. (1981). On the cerebral localisation of linguistic functions: Logical and empirical issues surrounding deficit analysis and functional localisation. *Brain and Language, 14*, 120–137.

Caplan, D., Vanier, M., & Baker, C. (1986). A case study of reproduction conduction aphasia: II. Sentence comprehension. *Cognitive Neuropsychology, 3*, 129–146.

Caramazza, A. (1984). The logic of neuropsychological research and the problem of patient classification in aphasia. *Brain and Language, 21*, 9–20.

Caramazza, A. (1986). On drawing inferences about the structure of normal cognitive systems from the analysis of patterns of impaired performance: The case for single-patient studies. *Brain and Cognition, 5*, 41–66.

Caramazza, A., Basili, A. G., Koller, J. J., & Berndt, R. J. (1981). An investigation of repetition and language processing in a case of conduction aphasia. *Brain and Language, 14*, 235–271.

Caramazza, A., & Berndt, R. S. (1978). Semantic and syntactic processes in aphasia: A review of the literature. *Psychological Bulletin, 85*, 898–918.

Caramazza, A., Berndt, R. S., & Basili, A. G. (1983). The selective impairment of phonological processing: A case study. *Brain and Language, 18*, 128–174.

Caramazza, A. Berndt, R. S., & Hart, K. J. (1981). 'Agrammatic' reading. In F. L. Pirozzolo & M. C. Wittrock, (Eds.), *Neuropsychological and cognitive processes in reading*. New York: Academic Press.

Caramazza, A., & McCloskey, M. (in press). Number system processing: evidence from dyscalculia. In N. Cohen, M. Schwartz, & M. Moscovitch (Eds.), *Advances in cognitive neuropsychology*. New York: Guilford Press.

Caramazza, A., Miceli, G., & Villa, G. (1986). The role of the (output) phonological buffer in reading, writing and repetition. *Cognitive Neuropsychology, 3,* 37–76.

Caramazza, A., Miceli, G., Villa, G., & Romani, C. (1987). The role of the graphemic buffer in spelling: Evidence from a case of acquired dysgraphia. *Cognition, 26,* 59–85.

Caramazza, A., & Zurif, E. B. (1976). Dissociation of algorithmic and heuristic processes in language comprehension: Evidence from aphasia. *Brain and Language, 3,* 572–582.

Cermak, L. S. (1976). The encoding capacity of a patient with amnesia due to encephalitis. *Neuropsychologia, 14,* 311–326.

Cermak, L. S. (Ed.). (1982). *Human memory and amnesia,* Hillsdale, N.J.: Erlbaum.

Cermak, L. S. (1984). The episodic/semantic distinction in amnesia. In N. Butters & L. R. Squire (Eds.), *The neuropsychology of memory*. New York: Guilford Press.

Cermak, L. S., & Butters, N. (1972). The role of interference and encoding in the short-term memory deficits of Korsakoff patients. *Neuropsychologia, 10,* 89–95.

Cermak, L. S., & O'Connor, M. (1983). The anterograde and retrograde retrieval ability of a patient with amnesia due to encephalitis. *Neuropsychologia, 21,* 213–234.

Charcot, J. M. (1884). *Differenti forme d'afasia*. Milan: Vallardi.

Charniak, E., & McDermott, D. (1985). *Introduction to artificial intelligence*. Reading, Mass.: Addison-Wesley.

Chase, W. G., & Clark, H. H. (1972). Mental operations in the comparison of sentences and pictures. In L. Gregg (Ed.), *Cognition in learning and memory*. New York: Wiley.

Chedru, F., & Geschwind, N. (1972). Writing disturbances in acute confusional states. *Neuropsychologia, 10,* 343–353.

Cheesman, J., & Merikle, P. M. (1985). Word recognition and consciousness. In D. Besner, T. G. Waller, & G. E. MacKinnon (Eds.), *Reading research: Advances in theory and practice* (Vol. 5). New York: Academic Press.

Chomsky, N. (1980). Rules and representations. *Behavioral and Brain Sciences, 3,* 1–61.

Chorover, S. L., & Cole, M. (1966). Delayed alternation performance in patients with cerebral lesions. *Neuropsychologia, 4,* 1–7.

Cicerone, K. D., Lazar, R. M., & Shapiro, W. R. (1983). Effects of frontal lobe lesions on hypothesis sampling during concept formation. *Neuropsychologia, 21,* 513–524.

Claparede, E. (1911). Reconnaissance et moitié. *Archives de Psychologie, 11,* 79–90.

Clark, H. H., & Clark, E. V. (1977). *Psychology and language*. New York: Harcourt Brace Jovanovich.

Cohen, N. J. & Squire, L. R. (1980). Preserved learning and retention of pattern-analysing skill in amnesia: Dissociation of 'knowing how' and 'knowing that.' *Science, 210,* 207–209.

Cohen, N. J., & Squire, L. R. (1981). Retrograde amnesia and remote memory impairment. *Neuropsychologia, 19,* 337–356.

Cole, M., Schutta, H. S., & Warrington, E. K. (1962). Visual disorientation in homonymous half-fields. *Neurology, 12,* 257–263.

Colle, H., & Welsh, A. (1976). Acoustic masking in primary memory. *Journal of Verbal Learning and Verbal Behavior, 15,* 17–32.

Collins, A. M. & Loftus, E. F. (1975). A spreading-activation theory of semantic processing. *Psychological Review, 82,* 407–428.

Collins, A. M. & Quillian, M. R. (1969). Retrieval time from semantic memory. *Journal of Verbal Learning and Verbal Behavior, 8,* 240–247.

Coltheart, M. (1978). Lexical access in simple reading tasks. In G. Underwood (Ed.), *Strategies of information processing*. London: Academic Press.

Coltheart, M. (1980a). Deep dyslexia: A review of the syndrome. In M. Coltheart, K. E. Patterson, & J. C. Marshall (Eds.), *Deep dyslexia*. London: Routledge.

Coltheart, M. (1980b). Deep dyslexia: A right-hemisphere hypothesis. In M. Coltheart, K. E. Patterson, & J. C. Marshall (Eds.), *Deep dyslexia*. London: Routledge.

Coltheart, M. (1980c). The semantic error: Types and theories. In M. Coltheart, K. E. Patterson, & J. C. Marshall (Eds.), *Deep dyslexia*. London: Routledge.

Coltheart, M. (1981). Disorders of reading and their implications for models of normal reading. *Visible Language, 15*, 245–286.

Coltheart, M. (1982). The psycholinguistic analysis of acquired dyslexias: Some illustrations. *Philosophical Transactions of the Royal Society of London B, 298*, 151–164.

Coltheart, M. (1983). The right hemisphere and disorders of reading. In A. Young (Ed.), *Functions of the right cerebral hemisphere*. London: Academic Press.

Coltheart, M. (1985). Cognitive neuropsychology and the study of reading. In M. I. Posner & O. S. M. Marin (Eds.), *Attention and performance*. (Vol. 11). Hillsdale, N.J.: Erlbaum.

Coltheart, M., Besner, D., Jonasson, J. T., & Davelaar, E. (1979). Phonological encoding in the lexical decision task. *Quarterly Journal of Experimental Psychology, 31*, 489–507.

Coltheart, M., Masterson, J., Byng, S., Prior, M., & Riddoch, J. (1983). Surface dyslexia. *Quarterly Journal of Experimental Psychology, 35A*, 469–495.

Coltheart, M., Patterson, K., & Marshall, J. C. (Eds.). (1980). *Deep dyslexia*. London: Routledge.

Conrad, K. (1932). Versuch einer psychologisches Analyse des Parietalsyndroms. *Monatschrift für Psychiatrie und Neurologie, 84*, 28–97.

Conrad, R. (1964). Acoustic confusion in immediate memory. *British Journal of Psychology, 55*, 75–84.

Conway, M. A. (1987) Verifying autobiographical facts. *Cognition, 26*, 39–58.

Conway, M. A., & Bekerian, D. A. (1987) Organization in autobiographical memory. *Memory and Cognition, 15*, 119–132.

Corkin, S. (1968). Acquisition of motor skill after bilateral medial temporal-lobe excision. *Neuropsychologia, 6*, 225–265.

Coslett, H. B., & Saffran, E. M. (in press). Evidence for preserved reading in 'pure alexia.' *Brain*.

Costa, L., & Vaughan, H. (1962). Performance of patients with lateralised cerebral lesions: I. Verbal and perceptual tests. *Journal of Nervous and Mental Diseases, 134*, 162–168.

Costello, A. de L., & Warrington, E. K. (1987). Dissociation of visuo-spatial neglect and neglect dyslexia. *Journal of Neurology, Neurosurgery and Psychiatry, 50*, 1110–1116.

Coughlan, A. K., & Warrington, E. K. (1978). Word-comprehension and word-retrieval in patients with localised cerebral lesions. *Brain, 101*, 163–185.

Coughlan, A. K. & Warrington, E. K. (1981). The impairment of verbal semantic memory: A single case study. *Journal of Neurology, Neurosurgery and Psychiatry, 44*, 1079–1083.

Cowey, A. (1982). Sensory and non-sensory visual disorders in man and monkey. *Philosophical Transactions of Royal Society of London B, 298*, 3–13.

Cowey, A. (1985). Aspects of cortical organisation related to selective attention and selective impairments of visual perception: A tutorial review. In M. I. Posner & O. S. M. Marin (Eds.), *Attention and performance* (Vol. 11). Hillsdale, N.J.: Erlbaum.

Craik, F. I. M. (1968a). Two components in free recall. *Journal of Verbal Learning and Verbal Behavior, 7*, 996–1004.

Craik, F. I. M. (1968b). Types of error in free recall. *Psychonomic Science, 10*, 353–354.

Craik, F. I. M., & Lockhart, R. S. (1972). Levels of processing: A framework for memory research. *Journal of Verbal Learning and Verbal Behavior, 11*, 671–684.

Craik, F. I. M., & Watkins, M. J. (1973). The role of rehearsal in short-term memory. *Journal of Verbal Learning and Verbal Behavior, 12*, 599–607.

Crick, F. (1984). Function of the thalamic reticular complex: The searchlight hypothesis. *Proceedings of the National Academy of Sciences, 81*, 4585–4590.

Critchley, M. (1965). Acquired anomalies of colour. *Brain, 88*, 711–724.

Crompton, A. (1982). Syllables and segments in speech production. In A. Cutler (Ed.), *Slips of the tongue and language production*. Berlin: Mouton.

Crossman, E. R. F. W. (1961). Information and serial order in human memory. In C. Cherry (Ed.), *Information theory*. London: Butterworth.

Crovitz, H. F., & Schiffman, H. (1974). Frequency of episodic memories as a function of their age. *Bulletin of the Psychonomic Society, 4*, 517–518.

Crowder, R. G. (1979). Similarity and order in memory. In G. H. Bower (Ed.), *The psychology of learning and motivation* (Vol. 13). New York: Academic Press.

Crowder, R. G. (1982a). General forgetting theory and the locus of amnesia. In L. S. Cermak (Ed.), *Human memory and amnesia*. Hillsdale, N.J.: Erlbaum.

Crowder, R. G. (1982b). The demise of short-term memory. *Acta Psychologica, 50,* 291–323.

Cutler, A. (1981). Making up materials is a confounded nuisance, or: Will we be able to run any psycholinguistic experiments at all in 1990? *Cognition, 10,* 65–70.

Cutting, J. (1978). A cognitive approach to Korsakoff's syndrome. *Cortex, 14,* 485–495.

Czopf, J. (1972). Uber die Rolle der nicht dominanten Hemisphäere in der Restitution der Sprache der Aphasischen. *Archiv fur Psychiatrie und Nervenkrankheiten, 216,* 162–171.

Damasio, A. R. (1985). The frontal lobes. In K. M. Heilman & E. Valenstein (Eds.), *Clinical neuropsychology* (2nd ed.). New York: Oxford University Press.

Damasio, A. R., Damasio, H., & Van Hoesen, G. W. (1982). Prosopagnosia: Anatomic basis and behavioural mechanisms. *Neurology, 32,* 331–341.

Damasio, A. R., Graff-Radford, N. R., Eslinger, P. J., Damasio, H., & Kassell, N. (1985). Amnesia following basal forebrain lesions. *Archives of Neurology, 42,* 263–271.

Damasio, A. R., & Van Hoesen, G. W. (1983). Emotional disturbances associated with focal lesions of the frontal lobe. In K. Heilman & P. Satz (Eds.), *The neuropsychology of human emotion: Recent advances.* New York: Guilford Press.

Damasio, A. R., Yamada, T., Damasio, H., Corbett, J., & McKee, J. (1980). Central achromatopsia: Behavioral, anatomic and physiological aspects. *Neurology, 30,* 1064–1071.

Damasio, H., & Damasio, A. R. (1980). The anatomical basis of conduction aphasia. *Brain, 103,* 337–350.

Davidoff, J., & Wilson, B. (1985). A case of visual agnosia showing a disorder of presemantic visual classification. *Cortex, 21,* 121–134.

Day, J. L. (1979). Visual half-field recognition as a function of syntactic class and imageability. *Neuropsychologia, 17,* 515–519.

De Bleser, R. (1987). From agrammatism to paragrammatism: German aphasiological traditions and grammatical disturbances. *Cognitive Neuropsychology, 4,* 187–256.

De Groot, A. D. (1965). *Thought and choice in chess.* The Hague: Mouton.

De Haan, E. H. F., Young, A., & Newcombe, A. (in press). Face recognition without awareness. *Cognitive Neuropsychology.*

Dejerine, J. (1891). Sur en case de cécité verbale avec agraphie, suivi d'autopsie. *Compte rendu des séances de la societé de biologie, 3,* 197–201.

Dejerine, J. (1892). Contribution à l'étude anatomoclinique et clinique des differentes variétés de cécité verbale. *Mémoires de la Société de Biologie, 4,* 61–90.

Deloche, G., Andreewsky, E., & Desi, M. (1981). Lexical meaning: A case report, some striking phenomena, theoretical implications. *Cortex, 17,* 147–152.

Deloche, G., Andreewsky, E., & Desi, M. (1982). Surface dyslexia: A case report and some theoretical implications to reading models. *Brain and Language, 15,* 21–31.

Deloche, G., & Seron, X. (Eds). (in press). *Mathematical disabilities: A cognitive neuropsychological perspective.* Hillsdale, N.J.: Erlbaum..

Denes, G., Ballellio, S. Volterra, V., & Pellegrini, A. (1986) Oral and written language in a case of childhood phonemic deafness. *Brain and Language, 29,* 252–267.

Denes, G., Ciplotti, L., & Semenza, C. (1987). How does a phonological dyslexic read words she has never seen? *Cognitive Neuropsychology, 4,* 11–31.

Denes, G., & Semenza, C. (1975). Auditory modality-specific anomia: evidence from a case of pure word deafness. *Cortex, 11,* 401–411.

Dennett, D. C. (1969). *Content and consciousness.* London: Routledge.

Dennis, M. (1976). Dissociated naming and locating of body parts after left anterior temporal lobe resection: An experimental case study. *Brain and Language, 3,* 147–163.

De Renzi, E. (1982). *Disorders of space exploration and cognition.* Chichester: Wiley.

De Renzi, E., Faglioni, P., & Ferrari, P. (1980). The influence of sex and age on the incidence and type of aphasia. *Cortex, 16,* 627–630.

De Renzi, E., Faglioni, P., & Scotti, G. (1970). Hemispheric contribution to exploration of space through the visual and tactile modality. *Cortex, 6,* 191–203.

De Renzi, E., Scotti, G., & Spinnler, H. (1969). Perceptual and associative disorders of visual recognition. Relationship to the side of the cerebral lesion. *Neurology, 19,* 634–642.

De Renzi, E., & Spinnler, H. (1966). Visual recognition in patients with unilateral cerebral disease. *Journal of Nervous and Mental Disorders, 142,* 513–525.

De Renzi, E., & Spinnler, H. (1967) Impaired performance on color tasks in patients with hemispheric damage. *Cortex, 3,* 194–216.

De Renzi, E., & Vignolo, L. A. (1962). The Token Test: A sensitive test to detect receptive disturbances in aphasics. *Brain, 85,* 665–678.

Derouesné, J., & Beauvois, M.-F. (1979). Phonological processing in reading: Data from alexia. *Journal of Neurology, Neurosurgery and Psychiatry, 42,* 1125–1132.

Derouesné, J., & Beauvois, M.-F. (1985). The 'phonemic' stage in the non-lexical reading process: Evidence from a case of phonological alexia. In K. E. Patterson, M. Coltheart, & J. C. Marshall (Eds.), *Surface dyslexia.* London: Erlbaum.

Derouesné, J., Beauvois, M.-F., & Shallice, T. (1985). Confabulation following anterior arterial surgery. *Journal of Clinical and Experimental Neuropsychology, 7,* 175.

Derouesné, J., Seron, X., & Lhermitte, F. (1975). Rééducation de patients atteints de lésions frontales. *Revue Neurologique, 131,* 677–689.

Deutsch, J., & Detusch, D. (1963). Attention: Some theoretical considerations. *Psychological Review, 70,* 80–90.

Dixon, N. F. (1971). *Subliminal perception: The nature of a controversy.* London: McGraw-Hill.

Dixon, N. F. (1981). *Preconscious processing.* Chichester: Wiley.

Dodd, B. (1980). The spelling abilities of profoundly pre-lingually deaf children. In U. Frith (Ed.), *Cognitive processes in spelling.* London: Academic Press.

Drachman, D. A., & Arbit, J. (1966). Memory and the hippocampal complex II. *Archives of Neurology, 15,* 52–61.

Drewe, E. A. (1974). The effect of type and area of brain lesion on Wisconsin Card Sorting Test performance. *Cortex, 10,* 159–170.

Dricker, J., Butters, N., Berman, G., Samuels, I., & Carey, S. (1978). The recognition and encoding of faces by alcoholic Korsakoff and right hemisphere patients. *Neuropsychologia, 16,* 683–692.

Dubois, J. (1977). L'agraphie des aphasiques sensoriels: Les troubles a la dictée des mots et des logatomes. *Langage, 47,* 81–119.

Dubois, J., Hécaen, H., Angelergues, R., Maufras Du Chatelier, A., & Marcie, P. (1964). Étude neurolinguistique de l'aphasie du conduction. *Neuropsychologia, 2,* 9–44.

Duncan, J. (1980). The locus of interference in the perception of simultaneous stimuli. *Psychological Review, 87,* 272–300.

Duncan, J. (1984). Selective attention and the organization of visual information. *Journal of Experimental Psychology: General, 113,* 501–517.

Duncan, J. (1986). Disorganization of behaviour after frontal lobe damage. *Cognitive Neuropsychology, 3,* 271–290.

Duncan, J. (1987). Attention and reading: Wholes and parts in shape recognition. In M. Coltheart (Ed.), *Attention and performance* (Vol. 12). London: Erlbaum.

Dunn, L. M. (1965). *Manual for the Peabody Picture Vocabulary Test.* Circle Pines, Minn.: American Guidance Service Inc.

Eccles, J. C. (1965). *The brain and the unity of conscious experience.* The 19th Arthur Stanley Eddington Memorial Lecture. Cambridge: Cambridge University Press.

Efron, R. (1968). What is perception? In R. S. Cohen & M. Wartofsky (Eds.), *Boston studies in the philosophy of science* (Vol. 4). New York: Humanities Press.

Egeth, H. (1977). Attention and preattention. In G. H. Bower (Ed.), *The psychology of learning and motivation* (Vol. 11). New York: Academic Press.

Ellis, A. W. (1979a). Speech production and short-term memory. In J. Morton & J. C. Marshall (Eds.), *Psycholinguistics series: Vol. 2. Structures and processes.* London: Elek.

Ellis, A. W. (1979b). Slips of the pen. *Visible Language, 13,* 265–282.

Ellis, A. W. (1982a). Spelling and writing (and reading and speaking). In A. W. Ellis (Ed.), *Normality and pathology in cognitive function.* London: Academic Press.

Ellis, A. W. (1982b). Modality-specific priming of auditory word recognition. *Current Psychological Research, 2,* 123–128.

Ellis, A. W. (1987). Intimations of modelarity, or, the modularity of mind: Doing cognitive neuropsychology without syndromes. In M. Coltheart, G. Sartori, & R. Job (Eds.), *The cognitive neuropsychology of language.* London: Erlbaum.

Ellis, A. W., Flude, B. M., & Young, A. W. (1987). 'Neglect dyslexia' and the early visual processing of letters in words and nonwords. *Cognitive Neuropsychology, 4,* 439–464.

Ellis, A. W., Miller, D., & Sin, G. (1983). Wernicke's aphasia and normal language processing: A case study in cognitive neuropsychology. *Cognition, 15,* 111–144.

Ellis, H. D., & Shepherd, J. W. (1974). Recognition of abstract and concrete words presented in left and right visual fields. *Journal of Experimental Psychology, 103,* 1035–1036.

Ericsson, K. A., & Simon, H. A (1985). *Protocol analysis: Verbal reports as data.* Cambridge, Mass.: MIT Press.

Eriksen, C. W. (1960). Discrimination and learning without awareness. *Psychological Review, 67,* 279–300.

Eslinjer, P. J., & Damasio, A. R. (1985). Severe disturbance of higher cognition after bilateral frontal ablation: Patient EVR. *Neurology, 35,* 1731–1741.

Fahlman, S. E. (1974). A planning system for robot construction tasks. *Artificial Intelligence, 5,* 1–49.

Fay, D., & Cutler, A. (1977). Malapropisms and the structure of the mental lexicon. *Linguistic Inquiry, 8,* 505–520.

Feuchtwanger, E. (1923). Die Funktionen des Stirnhirns, ihre Pathologie und Psychologie. In O. Foerster & K. Williams (Eds.), *Monographien aus dem Gesamtgebiete der Neurologie und Psychiatrie.* Berlin: Springer.

Feyerabend, P. (1975). *Against method: Outline of an anarchist theory of knowledge.* London: New Left Books.

Finger, S., & Stein, D. G. (1982). *Brain damage and recovery.* New York: Academic Press.

Fodor, J. A. (1983). *The modularity of mind.* Cambridge, Mass.: MIT Press.

Fodor, J. A. (1985). Multiple book review of *The modularity of mind. Behavioral and Brain Sciences, 8,* 1–42.

Fodor, J. A., Bever, T. C., & Garrett, M. F. (1974). *The psychology of language.* New York: McGraw-Hill.

Forster, K. I. (1976). Accessing the mental lexicon. In R. J. Wales & E. C. T. Walker (Eds.), *New approaches to the language mechanisms.* Amsterdam: North Holland.

Frankish, C. (1985). Modality-specific grouping effects in short-term memory. *Journal of Verbal Learning and Verbal Behavior, 24,* 200–209.

Freedman, J. L., & Loftus, E. F. (1971). Retrieval of words from long-term memory. *Journal of Verbal Learning and Verbal Behavior, 10,* 107–115.

Freud, S. (1891). *Zur Auffassung der Aphasien.* Vienna: Deuticke.

Freund, D. C. (1889). Uber optische Aphasie und Seelenblindheit. *Archiv für Psychiatrie und Nervenkrankheiten, 20,* 276–297.

Friedman, A., & Polson, M. C. (1981). Hemispheres as independent resource systems: Limited capacity processing and cerebral specialisation. *Journal of Experimental Psychology: Human Perception and Performance, 7,* 1031–1058.

Friedman, R. B. (1982). Mechanisms of reading and spelling in a case of alexia without agraphia. *Neuropsychologia, 20,* 533–545.

Friedman, R. B., & Alexander, M. P. (1984). Pictures, images, and pure alexia: A case study. *Cognitive Neuropsychology, 1,* 9–23.

Friedman, R. B., & Perlman, M. B. (1982). On the underlying causes of semantic paralexias in a patient with deep dyslexia. *Neuropsychologia, 20,* 559–568.

Freidrich, F. J., Glenn, C. & Marin, O. S. M. (1984). Interruption of phonological coding in conduction aphasia. *Brain and Language, 22,* 266–291.

Friedrich, F. J., Walker, J. A., & Posner, M. I. (1985). Effects of parietal lesions on visual matching: Implications for reading errors. *Cognitive Neuropsychology, 2,* 253–264.

Frith, U. (1980). Unexpected spelling problems. In U. Frith (Ed.), *Cognitive processes in spelling.* London: Academic Press.

Funnell, E. (1983). Phonological processing in reading: New evidence from acquired dyslexia. *British Journal of Psychology, 74,* 159–180.

Fuster, J. M. (1980). *The prefrontal cortex.* New York: Raven Press.

Gainotti, G., Messerli, P., & Tissot, R. (1972). Qualitative analysis of unilateral spatial neglect in relation to laterality of cerebral lesion. *Journal of Neurology, Neurosurgery and Psychiatry, 35,* 545–550.

Gardner, H., & Zurif, E. B. (1975). Bee but not be: Oral reading of single words in aphasia and alexia. *Neuropsychologia, 13,* 181–190.

Garrett, M. F. (1980). Levels of processing in sentence production. In B. Butterworth (Ed.), *Language production* (Vol. 1). London: Academic Press.

Gazzaniga, M. S. (1983a). Right hemisphere language following bisection: A 20-year perspective. *American Psychologist, 38,* 525–537.

Gazzaniga, M. S. (1983b) Reply to Levy and to Zaidel. *American Psychologist, 38,* 547–549.

Gazzaniga, M. S., Bogen, J. E., & Sperry, R. W. (1962). Some functional effects of sectioning the cerebral commisures in man. *Proceedings of the National Academy of Sciences, 48,* 1765–1769.

Gazzaniga, M. S., Holtzman, J. D., Deck, M. D. F., & Lee, B. C. P. (1985). MRI assessment of human callosal surgery with neuropsychological correlates. *Neurology, 35,* 1763–1766.

Gazzaniga, M. S., & Le Doux, J. E. (1978). *The integrated mind.* New York: Plenum Press.

Geiselman, R. E., Woodward, J. A., & Beatty, J. (1982). Individual differences in verbal memory performance: A test of alternative information processing models. *Journal of Experimental Psychology: General, 111,* 109–134.

Gelb, A., & Goldstein, K. (1920). *Psychologische analyser Hirnpathologischer Falle.* Leipzig: Bartke.

Gerstmann, J. (1930). Zur Symptomatologie der Hirnlaesionen im Ubergangsgebiet der unteren Parietal- und mittelerem Occipitalwindung. *Nervenarzt, 3,* 691–695.

Geschwind, N. (1965). Disconnection syndromes in animals and man. *Brain, 88,* 237–294, 585–644.

Geschwind, N. (1970). The organization of language and the brain. *Science, 170,* 940–944.

Geschwind, N. (1985). Mechanisms of change after brain lesions. *Annals of the New York Academy of Sciences, 457,* 1–11.

Ghent, L. (1956). Perception of overlapping and embedded figures by children of different ages. *American Journal of Psychology, 69,* 575–587.

Gil, R., Pluchon, C., Toullat, G., Michenau, D., Rogez, R., & Levevre, J. P. (1985). Disconnexion visuo-verbale (aphasie optique) pour les objets, les images, les couleurs et les visages avec alexie 'abstractive'. *Neuropsychologia, 23,* 333–349.

Gipson, P. (1986). The production of phonology and auditory priming. *British Journal of Psychology, 77,* 359–375.

Glanzer, M. (1972). Storage mechanisms in recall. In G. H. Bower (Ed.), *The psychology of learning and motivation* (Vol. 5). New York: Academic Press.

Glanzer, M. (1976). Intonation grouping and related words in free recall. *Journal of Verbal Learning and Verbal Behavior, 15,* 85–92.

Glanzer, M., & Cunitz, A. R. (1966). Two storage mechanisms in free recall. *Journal of Verbal Learning and Verbal Behavior, 5,* 351–360.

Glanzer, M., Dorfman, D., & Kaplan, B. (1981). Short-term storage in the processing of text. *Journal of Verbal Learning and Verbal Behavior, 20,* 656–670.

Glucksberg, S. (1984). The functional equivalence of common and multiple codes. *Journal of Verbal Learning and Verbal Behavior, 23,* 100–104.

Glushko, R. J. (1979). The organisation and activation of orthographic knowledge in reading aloud. *Journal of Experimental Psychology: Human Performance and Perception, 5,* 674–691.

Godwin-Austen, R. B. (1965). A case of visual disorientation. *Journal of Neurology, Neurosurgery and Psychiatry, 28,* 453–458.

Goldblum, M. C. (1980). Un equivalent de la dyslexie profonde dans la modalité auditive. *Grammatica*, 7, 157–177.

Goldblum, M. C. (1985). Word comprehension in surface dyslexia. In K. E. Patterson, M. Coltheart, & J. C. Marshall (Eds.), *Surface dyslexia*. London: Erlbaum.

Goldstein, K. (1944). Mental changes due to frontal lobe damage. *Journal of Psychology, 17*, 187–208.

Goldstein, K. (1948). *Language and language disturbance*. New York: Grune & Stratton.

Goodglass, H. (1968). Studies in the grammar of aphasics. In S. Rosenberg & J. Koplin (Eds.), *Developments in applied psycholinguistics*. New York: Macmillan.

Goodglass, H., & Baker, E. (1976). Semantic field, naming and auditory comprehension in aphasia. *Brain and Language, 3*, 359–374.

Goodglass, H., Blumstein, S. E., Gleason, J. B., Hyde, M. R., Green, E., & Statlender, S. (1979). The effect of syntactic coding on sentence comprehension in aphasia. *Brain and Language, 7*, 201–209.

Goodglass, H., Gleason, J. B., & Hyde, M. R. (1970). Some dimensions of auditory language comprehension in aphasia. *Journal of Speech and Hearing Research, 13*, 595–606.

Goodglass, H., & Kaplan, E. (1972). *The assessment of aphasia and related disorders*. Philadelphia: Lea and Febiger.

Goodglass, H., Kaplan, E., Weintraub, S., & Ackerman, N. (1976). The 'tip of the tongue' phenomenon in aphasia. *Cortex, 12*, 145–153.

Goodglass, H., Klein, B., Carey, P., & James, K. J. (1966). Specific semantic word categories in aphasia. *Cortex, 2*, 74–89.

Goodglass, H., Quadfasel, F. A., & Timberlake, W. H. (1964). Phrase length and the type and severity of aphasia. *Cortex, 1*, 133–153.

Goodman, R. A., & Caramazza, A. (1985). *Phonologically plausible errors: Implications for a model of the phoneme–grapheme conversion mechanism in the spelling process*. (Rep. No. 11). Baltimore: Johns Hopkins Cognitive Neuropsychology Laboratory.

Goodman, R. A., & Caramazza, A. (1986a). Aspects of the spelling process: Evidence from a case of acquired dysgraphia. *Language and Cognitive Processes, 1*, 263–296.

Goodman, R. A., & Caramazza, A. (1986b). Dissociation of spelling errors in written and oral spelling: The role of allographic conversion in writing. *Cognitive Neuropsychology, 3*, 179–206.

Gordon, B. (1982). Confrontation naming: Computational model and disconnection simulation. In M. A. Arbib, D. Caplan, & J. C. Marshall (Eds.), *Neural models of language processes*. New York: Academic Press.

Gordon, H. W. (1974). Olfaction and cerebral separation. In M. Kinsbourne & W. L. Smith (Eds.), *Hemisphere disconnection and cerebral function*. Springfield, Ill.: Thomas.

Graf, P., & Schacter, D. L. (1985). Implicit and explicit memory for new associations in normal and amnesic subjects. *Journal of Experimental Psychology: Learning, Memory and Cognition, 11*, 501–518.

Graf, P., Squire, L., & Mandler, G. (1984). The information that amnesic patients do not forget. *Journal of Experimental Psychology: Learning, Memory and Cognition, 10*, 164–178.

Grafman, J. (1985). *A frame of reference for describing preserved and impaired memory processes following frontal lobe lesions*. Unpublished manuscript.

Grafman, J., Passafiume, D., Faglioni, P., & Boller, F. (1982). Calculation disturbances in adults with focal hemispheric damage. *Cortex, 18*, 37–50.

Grant, D. A., & Berg, E. A. (1948). A behavioural analysis of degree of reinforcement and ease of shifting to new responses in a Weigl-type card-sorting problem. *Journal of Experimental Psychology, 38*, 404–411.

Green, D. W., & Shallice, T. (1976). Direct visual access in reading for meaning. *Memory and Cognition, 4*, 753–758.

Green, E. (1969). Psycholinguistic approaches to aphasia. *Linguistics, 53*, 30–50.

Green, E., & Howes, D. H. (1977). The nature of conduction aphasia: A study of anatomic and clinical features and of underlying mechanisms. In H. Whitaker & H. A. Whitaker (Eds.), *Studies in neurolinguistics* New York: Academic Press.

Greenblatt, S. H. (1973). Alexia without agraphia or hemianopsia: Anatomical analysis of an autopsied case. *Brain, 96*, 307–316.

Gregory, R. L. (1961). The brain as an engineering problem. In W. H. Thorpe & O. L. Zangwill (Eds.), *Current problems in animal behaviour*. Cambridge: Cambridge University Press.

Gregory, R. L., & Heard, P. (1981). Border locking and the Café Wall illusion. *Perception, 8*, 365–380.

Groeger, J. A. (1984). Evidence of unconscious semantic processing for a forced error situation. *British Journal of Psychology, 75*, 305–314.

Groeger, J. A. (1986). Predominant and non-predominant analysis: Effects of level of presentation. *British Journal of Psychology, 77*, 109–116.

Hanson, N. (1958). *Patterns of discovery*. Cambridge: Cambridge University Press.

Harlow, J. M. (1868). Recovery from the passage of an iron bar through the head. *Publications of the Massachusetts Medical Society, 2*, 327–346.

Hart, J., Berndt, R. S., & Caramazza, A. (1985). Category-specific naming deficit following cerebral infarction. *Nature, 316*, 439–440.

Hasher, L., & Zachs, R. T. (1979). Automatic and effortful processes in memory. *Journal of Experimental Psychology: General, 108*, 356–368.

Hatfield, F. M., & Patterson, K. E. (1983). Phonological spelling. *Quarterly Journal of Experimental Psychology, 35A*, 451–468.

Head, H. (1926). *Aphasia and kindred disorders of speech*. Cambridge: Cambridge University Press.

Healy, A. F. (1975). Coding of temporal-spatial patterns in short-term memory. *Journal of Verbal Learning and Verbal Behavior, 14*, 481–495.

Hebb, D. O. (1945). Man's frontal lobe: A critical review. *Archives of Neurology and Psychiatry, 54*, 10–24.

Hebb, D. O. (1949). *The organization of behavior*. New York: Wiley.

Hécaen, H. (1964). Mental symptoms associated with tumours of the frontal lobe. In J. M. Warren & K. Akert (Eds.), *The frontal granular cortex and behavior*. New York: McGraw-Hill.

Hécaen, H., & Ajuriaguerra, J. de (1956). Agnosie visuelle pour les objets inanimés par lésion unilatérale gauche. *Revue Neurologique, 94*, 222–233.

Hécaen, H., & Albert, M. L. (1978). *Human neuropsychology*. New York: Wiley.

Hécaen, H. & Angelergues, R. (1963). *La cécité psychique*. Paris: Masson & Cie.

Hécaen, H., Goldblum, M. C., Masure, M. C., & Ramier, A. M. (1974). Une nouvelle observation d'agnosie d'objet. Deficit de l'association ou de la categorisation, specifique de la modalité visuelle. *Neuropsychologia, 12*, 447–464.

Hécaen, H., & Kremin, H. (1976). Neurolinguistic research on reading disorders resulting from left hemisphere lesions: Aphasic and 'pure' alexia. In H. Whitaker & H. A. Whitaker (Eds.), *Studies in neurolinguistics* (Vol. 2). New York: Academic Press.

Heilman, K. M., & Scholes, R. J. (1976). The nature of comprehension errors in Broca's conduction and Wernicke's aphasics. *Cortex, 12*, 258–265.

Heilman, K. M., & Sypert, G. W. (1977). Korsakoff's syndrome arising from bilateral fornix lesions. *Neurology, 27*, 490–493.

Heilman, K. M., Tucker, D. M., & Valenstein, E. (1976). A case of mixed transcortical aphasia with intact naming. *Brain, 99*, 415–426.

Heilman, K. M., & Valenstein, E. (1979). Mechanisms underlying hemispatial neglect. *Annals of Neurology, 5*, 166–170.

Heilman, K. M., & Valenstein, E. (Eds.). (1985). *Clinical neuropsychology* (2nd ed.). New York: Oxford University Press.

Heilman, K. M., & Watson, R. T. (1977). Mechanisms underlying the unilateral neglect syndrome. In E. A. Weinstein & R. P. Friedland (Eds.), *Advances in neurology* (Vol. 18). New York: Raven Press.

Heilman, K. M., Watson, R. T., & Valenstein, E. (1985). Neglect and related disorders. In K. M. Heilman & E. Valenstein (Eds.), *Clinical neuropsychology* (2nd ed.). New York: Oxford University Press.

Heimburger, R. F., Demyer, W. C., & Reitan, R. M. (1964). Implications of Gerstmann's syndrome. *Journal of Neurology, Neurosurgery and Psychiatry, 27*, 52–57.

Helm-Estabrooks, N. A., Fitzpatrick, B. M., & Barresi, B. (1981). Response of an agrammatic patient to a syntax stimulation program for aphasia. *Journal for Speech and Hearing Disorders, 46*, 422–427.

Henderson, L. (1981). Information processing approaches to acquired dyslexia. *Quarterly Journal of Experimental Psychology, 35A*, 507–522.

Henderson, L. (1982). *Orthography and word recognition in reading*. London: Academic Press.

Henschen, S. E. (1919). Uber Sprach Musik- und Rechenmechanismen und ihre Lokalisation in Gehirn. *Zeitschrift für die Gesamte Neurologie und Psychiatry, 52*, 273–298.

Henschen, S. E. (1920). *Klinische und anatomische Beiträge zur Pathologie des Gehirns*. Stockholm: Almquist & Wiksell.

Herrmann, D. J., & Harwood, J. R. (1980). More evidence for the existence of separate semantic and episodic stores in long-term memory. *Journal of Experimental Psychology: Human Learning and Memory, 6*, 467–478.

Hier, D. B., & Mohr, J. P. (1977). Incongruous oral and written naming. *Brain and Language, 4*, 115–126.

Hillyard, S. A., & Picton, T. W. (1979). Event-related potentials and selective information processing in man. In J. Desmedt (Ed.), *Progress in clinical neurophysiology* (Vol. 6). Basle: Karger.

Hines, D. (1976). Recognition of verbs, abstract nouns and concrete nouns from the left and right visual half fields.*Neuropsychologia, 14*, 211–216.

Hinton, G. E. (1979). Some demonstrations of the effects of structural descriptions in mental imagery. *Cognitive Science, 3*, 231–250.

Hinton, G. E., & Anderson, J. A (Eds.). (1981). *Parallel models of associative memory*. Hillsdale, N.J.: Erlbaum.

Hinton, G. E., & Sejnowski, T. J. (1986). Learning and relearning in Boltzmann machines. In D. E. Rumelhart & J. L. McClelland (Eds.), *Parallel distributed processing: Explorations in the microstructure of cognition* (Vol. 1.). Cambridge, Mass.: MIT Press.

Hirst, W. (1982). The amnesic syndrome: Descriptions and explanations. *Psychological Bulletin, 91*, 435–460.

Hirst, W., Johnson, M. K., Kim, J. K., Phelps, E. A., Risse, C., & Volpe, B. T. (1986). Recognition and recall in amnesics. *Journal of Experimental Psychology: Learning Memory and Cognition, 12*, 445–451.

Hirst, W., & Volpe, B. T. (1984). Automatic and effortful encoding with amnesia. In M. S. Gazzaniga (Ed.), *Handbook of cognitive neuroscience*. New York: Plenum Press.

Hitch, G. J. (1978). The role of short-term working memory in mental arithmetic. *Cognitive Psychology, 10*, 302–323.

Hodder, I. (1982). *The present past*. London: Batsford.

Holender, D. (1986). Semantic activation without conscious identification in dichotic listening, parafoveal vision, and visual masking: A survey and appraisal. *Behavioral and Brain Sciences, 9*, 1–66.

Holmes, G. (1918). Disturbances of visual orientation. *British Journal of Ophthalmology, 2*, 449–468.

Holmes, J. M. (1973). *Dyslexia: A neurolinguistic study of traumatic and developmental disorders of reading*. Unpublished doctoral dissertation, University of Edinburgh.

Homa, D. Rhoads, D., & Chambliss, D. (1979). Evolution of conceptual structure. *Journal of Experimental Psychology: Human Learning and Memory, 5*, 11–23.

Hotopf, N. (1980). Slips of the pen. In U. Frith (Ed.), *Cognitive processes in spelling*. London: Academic Press.

Howard, D. (1985a). *The semantic organisation of the lexicon: Evidence from aphasia*. Unpublished doctoral dissertation, University of London.

Howard, D. (1985b). Agrammatism. In S. K. Newman & R. Epstein (Eds.), *Current perspectives in dysphasia*. Edinburgh: Churchill Livingstone.

Howard, D. (1987). Reading without letters? In M. Coltheart, G. Sartori, & R. Job (Eds.), *The cognitive neuropsychology of language*. London: Erlbaum.

Howard, D., & Orchard-Lisle, V. (1984). On the origin of semantic errors in naming: Evidence from the case of a global aphasic. *Cognitive Neuropsychology, 1,* 163–190.

Hull, C. L. (1920). Quantitative aspects of the evolution of concepts. *Psychological Monographs, 28* (123).

Humphreys, G. W., & Riddoch, M. J. (1984). Routes to object constancy: Implications from neurological impairments of object constancy. *Quarterly Journal of Experimental Psychology, 36A,* 385–415.

Humphreys, G. W., & Riddoch, M. J. (1985). Author's correction to 'Routes to object constancy' *Quarterly Journal of Experimental Psychology, 37A,* 493–495.

Humphreys, G. W., Riddoch, M. J., & Quinlan, P. T. (1985). Interactive processes in perceptual organisation: Evidence from visual agnosia. In M. I. Posner & O. S. M. Marin (Eds.), *Attention and performance* (Vol. 11). Hillsdale, N.J.: Erlbaum.

Humphreys, G. W., Riddoch, M. J., & Quinlan, P. T. (1988). Cascade processes in picture identification. *Cognitive Neuropsychology, 5,* 67–104.

Huppert, F. D., & Piercy, M. (1978). Dissociation between learning and remembering in organic amnesia. *Nature, 275,* 317–318.

Illis, L. S., & Gostling, J. V. T. (1972). *Herpes simplex encephalitis*. Bristol: Scientechnica.

Irigaray, L. (1973). *Le langage des déments*. The Hague: Mouton.

Isserlin, M. (1922). Uber Agrammatismus. *Zeitschrift für die Gesamte Neurologie und Psychiatrie, 75,* 332–416.

Jackson, J. H. (1874). On the nature of the duality of the brain. *Medical Press and Circular, 1,* 19, 41, 63. (Reprinted 1915 in *Brain, 38,* 80–103).

Jacoby, L. L. (1983a). Perceptual enhancement: Persistent effects of an experience. *Journal of Experimental Psychology: Learning, Memory, and Cognition, 9,* 21–38.

Jacoby, L. L. (1983b). Remembering the data: analyzing interactive processes in reading. *Journal of Verbal Learning and Verbal Behaviour, 22,* 485–508.

Jacoby, L. L., & Dallas, M. (1981). On the relationship between autobiographical memory and perceptual learning. *Journal of Experimental Psychology: General, 110,* 306–340.

Jacoby, L. L., & Witherspoon, D. (1982). Remembering without awareness. *Canadian Journal of Psychology, 32,* 300–324.

Jakobson, R. (1955). *Aphasia as a linguistic topic*. Clark University Monographs on Psychology and Related Disciplines, Worcester, Mass. (Reprinted 1971 in *Roman Jakobson, Selected Writings, Vol. 2*. The Hague: Mouton).

James, W. (1890). *The principles of psychology*. New York: Holt.

Jarvella, R. J. (1971). Syntactic processing of connected speech. *Journal of Verbal Learning and Verbal Behavior, 10,* 409–416.

Jarvella, R. J. (1979). Immediate memory and discourse processing. in G. H. Bower (Ed.), *The psychology of learning and motivation* (Vol. 13). New York: Academic Press.

Job, R., & Sartori, G. (1984). Morphological decomposition: Evidence from crossed phonological dyslexia. *Quarterly Journal of Experimental Psychology, 36A,* 435–458.

Johnson, M. K. (1983). A multiple-entry modular memory system. In G. H. Bower (Ed.), *The psychology of learning and motivation* (Vol. 17). New York: Academic Press.

Johnson, S. C. (1967). Hierarchical clustering schemes. *Psychometrika, 32,* 241–254.

Johnson-Laird, P. N. (1983). *Mental models*. Cambridge: Cambridge University Press.

Johnson-Laird, P. N., & Stevenson, R. (1970). Memory for syntax. *Nature, 227,* 412.

Jones, G. V. (1985). Deep dyslexia, imageability, and ease of predication. *Brain and Language, 24,* 1–19.

Jouandet, M., & Gazzaniga, M. S. (1979). The frontal lobes. In M. S. Gazzaniga (Ed.), *Handbook of behavioral neurobiology* (Vol. 2). New York: Plenum Press.

Kahn, D. (1980). Syllable-structure specification in phonological rules. In M. Aronoff & M.-L. Keen (Eds.), *On Juncture*. San Francisco: Amni Libri.

Kahne, S., Lefkowitz, I., & Rose, C. (1979). Automatic control by distributed intelligence. *Scientific American, 240*, 54–66.

Kahneman, D. (1973). *Attention and effort*. Englewood Cliffs, N.J.: Prentice-Hall.

Kapur, N., & Coughlan, A. K. (1980). Confabulation and frontal lobe dysfunction. *Journal of Neurology, Neurosurgery and Psychiatry, 43*, 461–463.

Kapur, N., & Lawton, F. E. (1983). Dysgraphia for letters: A form of motor memory deficit? *Journal of Neurology, Neurosurgery and Psychiatry, 46*, 573–575.

Katz, J. J., & Fodor, J. A. (1963). The structure of a semantic theory. *Language, 39*, 170–210.

Kay, J., & Lesser, R. (1985). The nature of phonological processing in oral reading: Evidence from surface dyslexia. *Quarterly Journal of Experimental Psychology, 37A*, 39–81.

Kay, J., & Marcel, A. J. (1981). One process not two in reading aloud: Lexical analogies do the work of non-lexical rules. *Quarterly Journal of Experimental Psychology, 33A*, 397–413.

Kay, J., & Patterson, K. E. (1985). Routes to meaning in surface dyslexia. In K. E. Patterson, M. Coltheart, & J. C. Marshall (Eds.), *Surface dyslexia*. London: Erlbaum.

Kean, M.-L. (1977). The linguistic interpretation of aphasic syndromes: Agrammatism, an example. *Cognition, 5*, 9–46.

Keil, F. C. (1981). Constraints on knowledge and cognitive development. *Psychological Review, 88*, 197–227.

Kempley, S. T., & Morton, J. (1982). The effects of priming with regularly and irregularly related words in auditory word recognition. *British Journal of Psychology, 73*, 441–454.

Kertesz, A., Lesk, D., & McCabe, P. (1977). Isotope localisation of infarcts in aphasia. *Archives of Neurology, 34*, 590–601.

Kertesz, A., & Phipps, J. B. (1977). Numerical taxonomy of aphasia. *Brain and Language, 4*, 1–10.

Kertesz, A., & Poole, E. (1974). The aphasia quotient: The taxonomic approach to measurement of aphasic disability. *Canadian Journal of Neurological Science, 1*, 7–16.

Kertesz, A., & Sheppard, A. (1981). The epidemiology of aphasic and cognitive impairment in stroke. *Brain, 104*, 117–128.

Kimura, D., & Archibald, Y. (1974). Motor function of the left hemisphere. *Brain, 97*, 337–350.

Kinsbourne, M. (1971). Cognitive deficit: Experimental analysis. In J. L. McGaugh (Ed.), *Psychobiology*. New York: Academic Press.

Kinsbourne, M. (1972). Behavioral analysis of the repetition deficit in conduction aphasia. *Neurology, 22*, 1126–1132.

Kinsbourne, M. (1974a). Cerebral control and mental evolution. In M. Kinsbourne & W. L. Smith (Eds.), *Hemisphere disconnection and cerebral function*. Springfield, Ill.: Thomas.

Kinsbourne, M. (1974b). Lateral interactions in the brain. In M. Kinsbourne & W. L. Smith (Eds.), *Hemisphere disconnection and cerebral function*. Springfield, Ill.: Thomas.

Kinsbourne, M., & Rosenfield, D. B. (1974). Agraphia selective for written spelling: An experimental case study. *Brain and Language, 1*, 215–225.

Kinsbourne, M., & Warrington, E. K. (1962a). A variety of reading disability associated with right hemisphere lesions. *Journal of Neurology, Neurosurgery and Psychiatry, 25*, 339–344.

Kinsbourne, M. & Warrington, E. K. (1962b). A disorder of simultaneous form perception. *Brain, 85*, 461–486.

Kinsbourne, M., & Warrington, E. K. (1965). A case showing selectively impaired oral spelling. *Journal of Neurology, Neurosurgery and Psychiatry, 28*, 563–567.

Kinsbourne, M., & Wood, F. (1975). Short-term memory processes and the amnesic syndrome. In D. Deutsch & J. A. Deutsch (Eds.), *Short-term memory*. New York: Academic Press.

Kleiman, G. M. (1975). Speech recoding in reading. *Journal of Verbal Learning and Verbal Behavior, 24*, 323–339.

Klein, B. von E. (1977). Inferring functional localisation from neurological evidence. In E. Walker (Ed.), *Explorations in the biology of language*. Montgomery, Vt.: Bradford Books.

Kleist, K. (1916). Uber Leitungsaphasie und grammatische Storungen. *Monatsschrift fur Psychiatrie und Neurologie, 40*, 118–199.

Kleist, K. (1934). *Gehirnpathologie*. Leipzig: Barth.

Klosowska, D. (1976). Relation between ability to program actions and location of brain damage. *Polish Psychological Bulletin, 7,* 245–255.

Knight, R. T. (1984). Decreased response to novel stimuli after prefrontal lesions in man. *Electroencephalography and Clinical Neurophysiology, 59,* 9–20.

Knight, R. T., Hillyard, S. A., Woods, D. L., & Neville, H. J. (1981). The effects of frontal cortical lesions on event-related potentials during auditory selective attention. *Electroencephalography and Clinical Neurophysiology, 52,* 571–582.

Kohler, W., & Van Restorff, H. (1935). Analyse von Vorgängen in Spurenfeld: II. Zur Theorie der Reproduktion. *Psychologische Forschung, 21,* 56–112.

Kolk, H. H. J. (1978). The linguistic interpretation of Broca's aphasia: A reply to M.-L. Kean. *Cognition, 6,* 353–361.

Kolk, H. H. J., & Van Grunsven, M. J. F. (1984). Metalinguistic judgements on sentence structure in agrammatism: A matter of task misinterpretation. *Neuropsychologia, 22,* 31–39.

Kolk, H. H. J., Van Grunsven, M. J. F., & Keyser, A. (1985). On parallelism between production and comprehension in agrammatism. In M.-L. Kean (Ed.), *Agrammatism.* New York: Academic Press.

Kolk, H. H. J., van Grunsven, M. J. F., & Kuper, A. (1982). *On parallelism in agrammatism: A case study.* Unpublished manuscript.

Kolodner, J. L. (1985). Memory for experience. In G. H. Bower (Ed.), *The psychology of learning and motivation* (Vol. 9). New York: Academic Press.

Konorski, J., & Lawicka, W. (1964). An analysis of errors in prefrontal animals on the delayed-response test. In J. M. Warren & K. Akert (Eds.), *The frontal granular cortex and behaviour.* New York: McGraw-Hill.

Kosslyn, S. M. (1980). *Image and mind.* Cambridge, Mass.: Harvard University Press.

Kremin, H. (1981). Deux stratégies de lecture dissociable par la pathologie: Description d'un cas de dyslexie profonde et d'un cas de dyslexie de surface. In C. L. Nespoulos (Ed.), *Études neurolinguistiques.* Toulouse: Le Mirail.

Kremin, H. (1982). Alexia: theory and research. In R. N. Malatesha & P. G. Aaron (Eds.), *Reading disorders: Varieties and treatments.* New York: Academic Press.

Kremin, H. (1984, June). *Spared naming without comprehension.* Paper presented at the International Neuropsychological Society European Conference, Aachen, West Germany.

Kremin, H. (1985). Routes and strategies in surface dyslexia. In K. E. Patterson, M. Coltheart, & J. C. Marshall (Eds.), *Surface dyslexia.* London: Erlbaum.

Kremin, H. (1987). Is there more than ah-oh-oh? Alternative strategies for writing and repeating lexically. In M. Coltheart, G. Sartori, & R. Job (Eds.), *The cognitive neuropsychology of language.* London: Erlbaum.

Kremin, H., & Goldblum, M. C. (1975). Étude de la compréhension syntaxique chez les aphasiques. *Linguistics, 154/5,* 31–46.

Kroll, N. E. A., Parks, T., Parkinson, S. R., Bieber, S. L., & Johnson, A. (1970). Short-term memory while shadowing: Recall of visually and of aurally presented letters. *Journal of Experimental Psychology, 85,* 220–224.

Kucera, H., & Francis, W. N. (1967). *Computational analysis of present-day American English.* Providence, R.I.: Brown University Press.

Kuhn, T. S. (1962). *The structure of scientific revolutions.* Chicago: University of Chicago Press.

Kussmaul, A. (1877). Die Störungen der Sprache. *Ziemssens Handbuch der Speciellen Pathologie und Therapie, 12,* 1–300.

Lakatos, I. (1963–64). Proofs and refutations. *British Journal for the Philosophy of Science, 14,* 1–25, 120–139, 221–243, 296–342.

Lakatos, I. (1970). Falsification and the methodology of scientific research programmes. In I. Lakatos & A. Musgrave (Eds.), *Criticism and the growth of knowledge.* Cambridge: Cambridge University Press.

Lakoff, G. (1980). What ever happened to deep structure? *Behavioral and Brain Sciences, 3,* 22–23.

Lambert, A. J. (1982). Right hemisphere language ability: Evidence from normal subjects. *Current Psychological Reviews, 22,* 139–152.

Lange, J. (1930). Fingeragnosie und Agraphie. *Monatschrift für Psychiatrie und Neurologie, 76,* 129–188.

Lapointe, S. G. (1985). A theory of verb form use in the speech of agrammatic aphasics. *Brain and Language, 24,* 100–155.

Lashley, K. S. (1929). *Brain mechanisms and intelligence.* Chicago: University of Chicago Press.

Lashley, K. S. (1950). In search of the engram. In *Symposia for the Society for Experimental Biology,* No. 4. Cambridge: Cambridge University Press.

Latour, B., & Woolgar, S. (1979). *Laboratory life.* Beverly Hills, Calif.: Sage.

Lecours, A. R., & Lhermitte, F. (1969). Phonemic paraphasias: Linguistic structures and tentative hypotheses. *Cortex, 5,* 193–228.

Lecours, A. R., & Lhermitte, F. (1976). The 'pure form' of the phonetic disintegration-syndrome (pure anarthria): Anatomo-clinical report of a historical case. *Brain and Language, 3,* 88–113.

Lecours, A. R., & Rouillon, F. (1976). Neurolinguistic analysis of jargonaphasia and jargonagraphia. In H. Whitaker & H. A. Whitaker (Eds.), *Studies in neurolinguistics* (Vol. 2). New York: Academic Press.

Le Doux, J. E., Wilson, D. H., & Gazzaniga, M. S. (1979). Beyond commissurotomy: Clues to consciousness. In M. S. Gazzaniga (Ed.), *Handbook of behavioral neurobiology.* (Vol. 2). New York: Plenum Press.

Lee, C. L., & Estes, W. K. (1977). Order and position in primary memory for letter strings. *Journal of Verbal Learning and Verbal Behavior, 16,* 395–418.

Lenneberg, E. H. (1973). The neurology of language. *Daedalus, 102,* 115–133.

Lesser, R. (1978). *Linguistic investigations of aphasia.* London: Arnold.

Levin, H. S., & Spiers, P. A. (1985). Acalculia. In K. M. Heilman & E. Valenstein (Eds.), *Clinical neuropsychology* (2nd ed.). New York: Oxford University Press.

Levine, D. N., & Calvanio, R. (1978). A study of the visual defect in verbal alexia-simultanagnosia. *Brain, 101,* 65–81.

Levine, D. N., Calvanio, R., & Popovics, A. (1982). Language in the absence of inner speech. *Neuropsychologia, 20,* 391–409.

Levy, B. A. (1971). Role of articulation in auditory and visual short-term memory. *Journal of Verbal Learning and Verbal Behavior, 10,* 123–132.

Levy, J., Trevarthen, C., & Sperry, R. W. (1972). Perception of bilateral chimeric figures following hemisphere disconnexion. *Brain, 95,* 61–78.

Lezak, M. R. (1976). *Neuropsychological assessment.* New York: Oxford University Press.

Lhermitte, F. (1983). 'Utilization behaviour' and its relation to lesions of the frontal lobes. *Brain, 106,* 237–255.

Lhermitte, F., & Beauvois, M.-F. (1973). A visual-speech disconnexion syndrome: Report of a case with optic-aphasia, agnosic alexia and colour agnosia. *Brain, 96,* 695–714.

Lhermitte, F., Chedru, F., & Chain, F. (1973). A propos d'un cas d'agnosie visuelle. *Revue Neurologique, 128,* 301–322.

Lhermitte, F., & Derouesné, J. (1974). Paraphasies et jargonaphasies dans le langage oral avec conservation du langage écrit. Genèse des neologismes. *Revue Neurologique, 130,* 21–38.

Lhermitte, F., Derouesné, J., & Signoret, J.-L. (1972). Analyse neuropsychologique du syndrome frontale. *Revue Neurologique, 127,* 415–440.

Lhermitte, F., & Signoret, J.-L. (1972). Analyse neuropsychologique et differenciation des syndromes amnesiques. *Revue Neurologique, 126,* 161–178.

Lhermitte, F., & Signoret, J.-L. (1982). L'aphasie de J. M. Charcot à Th. Alajouanine. *Revue Neurologique, 138,* 893–919.

Liberman, A. M. (1957). Some results of research on speech perception. *Journal of the Acoustical Society of America, 29,* 117–123.

Libet, B., Gleason, C. A., Wright, E. W., & Pearl, D. K. (1983). Time of conscious intention to act in relation to onset of cerebral activity (readiness-potential): The unconscious initiation of a freely voluntary act. *Brain, 106*, 623–642.

Libet, B., Wright, E. W., Feinstein, B., & Pearl, D. K. (1979). Subjective referral of the timing of a conscious sensory experience: A functional role for the somatosensory specific projection system. *Brain, 102*, 193–224.

Lichtheim, L. (1885). On aphasia. *Brain, 7*, 433–484.

Liepmann, H. (1900). Das Krankheitschild der Apraxie (motorischen Asymbolie). *Monatsschrift fur Psychiatrie und Neurologie, 8*, 15–44, 102–132, 182–197.

Linebarger, M. C., Schwartz, M. F., & Saffran, E. M. (1983). Sensitivity to grammatical structure in so-called agrammatic aphasics. *Cognition, 13*, 361–392.

Lissauer, H. (1890). Ein Fall von Seelenblindheit nebsteinen Betrag zur Theorie derselben. *Archiv fur Psychiatrie und Nervenkrankheiten, 21*, 222–270. (English translation by M. Jackson in *Cognitive Neuropsychology*, in press.)

Logue, V., Durward, M., Pratt, R. T. C., Piercy, M., & Nixon, W. L. B. (1968). The quality of survival after rupture of an anterior cerebral aneurysm. *British Journal of Psychiatry, 114*, 137–160.

Low, A. A. (1931). A case of agrammatism in the English language. *Archives of Neurology and Psychiatry, 25*, 556–597.

Luria, A. R. (1966). *Higher cortical functions in man*. London: Tavistock.

Luria, A. R. (1969). Frontal lobe syndromes. In P. J. Vinken & G. W. Bruyn (Eds.), *Handbook of clinical neurology* (Vol. 2). Amsterdam: North Holland.

Luria, A. R. (1970a). The functional organisation of the brain. *Scientific American, 222*, 66–78.

Luria, A. R. (1970b). *Traumatic aphasia*. The Hague: Mouton.

Luria, A. R. (1973). *The working brain*. London: Penguin.

Luria, A. R. (1976). *The neuropsychology of memory*. Washington, D.C.: Winston.

Luria, A. R., & Tsvetkova, L. S. (1964). The programming of constructive activity in local brain injuries. *Neuropsychologia, 2*, 95–107.

Lynch, G., McGaugh, J. L., & Weinberger, N. M. (1984). *The neurobiology of learning and memory*. New York: Guilford Press.

Lyon, D. R. (1977). Individual differences in immediate serial recall: A matter of mnemonics. *Cognitive Psychology, 9*, 403–411.

McCarthy, R. A., & Warrington, E. K. (1984). A two-route model of speech production: Evidence from aphasia. *Brain 107*, 463–485.

McCarthy, R. A., & Warrington, E. K. (1985). Category specificity in an agrammatic patient: The relative impairment of verb retrieval and comprehension. *Neuropsychologia, 23*, 709–727.

McCarthy, R. A., & Warrington, E. K. (1986a). Phonological reading: Phenomena and paradoxes. *Cortex, 22*, 359–380.

McCarthy, R. A., & Warrington, E. K. (1986b). Visual associative agnosia: A clinico-anatomical study of a single case. *Journal of Neurology, Neurosurgery and Psychiatry, 49*, 1233–1240.

McClelland, J. L. (1976). Preliminary letter identification in the perception of words and nonwords. *Journal of Experimental Psychology: Human Perception and Performance, 2*, 80–91.

McClelland, J. L. (1977). Letter and configuration information in word identification. *Journal of Verbal Learning and Verbal Behavior, 16*, 137–150.

McClelland, J. L. (1985). Putting knowledge in its place: A scheme for programming parallel structures on the fly. *Cognitive Science, 9*, 113–146.

McClelland, J. L., & Mozer, M. C. (1986). Perceptual interactions in two-word displays: Familiarity and similarity effects. *Journal of Experimental Psychology: Human Perception and Performance, 12*, 18–35.

McClelland, J. L., & Rumelhart, D. E. (1981). An interaction model of context effects in letter perception: Part 1. An account of basic findings. *Psychological Review, 88*, 375–407.

McClelland, J. L., & Rumelhart, D. E. (1985). Distributed memory and the representation of general and specific information. *Journal of Experimental Psychology: General, 114*, 159–188.

McCloskey, M., Caramazza, A., & Basili, A. (1985). Cognitive mechanisms in number processing and calculation. *Brain and Cognition, 4,* 171–196.

McCloskey, M., & Santee, J. (1981). Are semantic and episodic memory distinct systems? *Journal of Experimental Psychology: Human Learning and Memory, 7,* 66–71.

McDermott, D. (1978). Planning and acting. *Cognitive Science, 2,* 71–109.

McDermott, J., & Forgy, C. (1978). Production system conflict resolution strategies. In D. A. Waterman & F. Hayes-Roth (Eds.), *Pattern-directed inference systems.* New York: Academic Press.

McFarland, H. R., & Fortin, D. (1982). Amusia due to right tempero-parietal infarct. *Archives of Neurology, 39,* 725–727.

McFie, J. (1960). Psychological testing in clinical neurology. *Journal of Nervous and Mental Diseases, 131,* 383–393.

McFie, J. (1975). *Assessment of organic intellectual impairment.* London: Academic Press.

McFie, J., Piercy, M. F., & Zangwill, O. (1950). Visual-spatial agnosia associated with lesions of the right cerebral hemisphere. *Brain, 73,* 167–190.

McGlone, J. (1977). Sex differences in the cerebral organisation of verbal functions in patients with unilateral brain lesion. *Brain, 100,* 775–793.

McGlone, J. (1980). Sex differences in human brain asymmetry: A critical survey. *Behavioural and Brain Sciences, 3,* 215–263.

Mack, J. L., & Boller, F. (1978). Associative visual agnosia and its related deficits: The role of the minor hemisphere in asymmetry meaning to visual perception. *Neuropsychologia, 15,* 345–349.

MacKay, D. M. (1966a). Cerebral organisation and the conscious control of action. In J. C. Eccles (Ed.), *Brain and conscious experience.* Heidelberg: Springer Verlag.

MacKay, D. M. (1966b). Discussion of Dr. Sperry's paper. In J. C. Eccles (Ed.), *Brain and conscious experience.* Heidelberg: Springer Verlag.

McKenna, P., & Warrington, E. K. (1978). Category-specific naming preservation: A single case study. *Journal of Neurology, Neurosurgery and Psychiatry, 41,* 571–574.

McKoon, G., Ratliff, R., & Dell, G. S. (1986). A critical evaluation of the semantic-episodic distraction. *Journal of Experimental Psychology: Learning, Memory, and Cognition, 12,* 295–306.

McKoon, G., Ratliff, R., & Dell, G. S. (1986). A critical evaluation of the semantic-episodic distinction. *Journal of Experimental Psychology: Learning, Memory, and Cognition, 12,* 295–306.

McLeod, P. D. (1977). A dual task response modality effect: Support for multiprocessor models of attention. *Quarterly Journal of Experimental Psychology, 29,* 651–667.

McLeod, P. D., McLaughlin, C., & Nimmo-Smith, I. (1985). Information encapsulation and automaticity: Evidence from the visual control of finely tuned actions. In M. Posner & O. S. M. Marin (Eds.), *Attention and performance* (Vol. 11). Hillsdale, N.J.: Erlbaum.

Mair, W. G. P., Warrington, E. K., & Weiskrantz, L. (1979). Memory disorder in Korsakoff's psychosis. *Brain, 102,* 749–783.

Malmo, R. B. (1942). Interference factors in delayed response in monkeys after removal of frontal lobes. *Journal of Neurophysiology, 5,* 295–308.

Mandler, G. (1975). *Mind and emotion.* New York: Wiley.

Mandler, G. (1979). Organisation and repetition: Organisational principles with special reference to rote learning. In L.-G. Nilsson (Ed.), *Perspectives on memory research.* Hillsdale, N.J.: Erlbaum.

Mandler, G. (1980). Recognizing: the judgment of previous occurrence. *Psychological Review, 87,* 252–271.

Mandler, G. (1985). *Cognitive psychology: An essay in cognitive science.* Hillsdale, N.J.: Erlbaum.

Mandler, G. (in press). Memory: conscious and unconscious. In P. R. Solomon, G. R. Goethals, C. M. Kelley, & B. R. Stephens (Eds.), *Memory: An interdisciplinary approach,* New York: Springer.

Marcel, A. J. (1980). Surface dyslexia and beginning reading: A revised hypothesis of the pronunciation of print and its impairments. In M. Coltheart, K. E. Patterson, & J. C. Marshall (Eds.), *Deep dyslexia.* London: Routledge.

Marcel, A. J. (1983a). Conscious and unconscious perception: Experiments on visual masking and word recognition. *Cognitive Psychology, 15,* 197–237.

Marcel, A. J. (1983b). Conscious and unconscious perception: An approach to the relations between phenomenal experience and perceptual processes. *Cognitive Psychology, 15,* 238–300.

Marcel, A. J., & Bisiach, E. (Eds.). (in press). *Consciousness in contemporary science.* Oxford: Oxford University Press.

Marcel, A. J., & Patterson, K. E. (1978). Word recognition and production: Reciprocity in clinical and normal studies. In J. Requin (Ed.), *Attention and performance* (Vol. 7). Hillsdale, N.J.: Erlbaum.

Marcel, A. J., & Patterson, K. E. (1986, April). *Articulating non-lexical reading processes in phonological dyslexia.* Paper presented to the joint conference of the Experimental Psychology Society and Societa Italiana di Psicologia, Padua.

Marcie, P., & Hécaen, H. (1979). Agraphia: Writing disorders associated with unilateral cortical lesions. In K. M. Heilman & E. Valenstein (Eds.), *Clinical neuropsychology.* New York: Oxford University Press.

Margolin, D. I. (1984). The neuropsychology of writing and spelling: Semantic, phonological, motor and perceptual processes. *Quarterly Journal of Experimental Psychology, 36A,* 459–489.

Margolin, D. I., & Binder, L. (1984). Multiple component agraphia in a patient with atypical cerebral dominance: An error analysis. *Brain and Language, 22,* 26–40.

Margolin, D. I., Marcel, A. J., & Carlson, N. R. (1985). Common processes in dysnomia and post-semantic dyslexia: Processing deficits and selective attention. In K. E. Patterson, M. Coltheart, & J. C. Marshall (Eds.), *Surface dyslexia.* London: Erlbaum.

Margrain, S. A. (1967). Short-term memory as a function of input modality. *Quarterly Journal of Experimental Psychology, 19,* 109–114.

Marie, P. (1906a). Révision de la question de l'aphasie: La troisième convolution frontale gauche ne joue aucun role speciale dans la fonction du langage. *Semaine Medicale 21,* 241–247. (Reprinted in Cole, M. F., & Cole, M. [Eds.], [1971], *Pierre Marie's papers on speech disorders.* New York: Hafner).

Marie, P. (1906b). Révision de la question sur l'aphasie: Que faut-il penser des aphasies sous-corticales (aphasies pures)? *Semaine Medicale* (Paris), *26,* 493–500.

Marin, O. S. M., Saffran, E. M., & Schwartz, D. F. (1976). Dissociations of language in aphasia: Implications for normal functions. *Annals of the New York Academy of Sciences, 280,* 868–884.

Markowitsch, H. J. (1984). Can amnesia be caused by damage of a single brain structure? *Cortex, 20,* 27–45.

Marr, D. (1976). Early processing of visual information. *Philosophical Transactions of the Royal Society of London B, 275,* 483–524.

Marr, D. (1982). *Vision.* San Francisco: Freeman.

Marr, D., & Nishihara, H. K. (1978). Representation and recognition of the spatial organisation of three-dimensional shapes. *Proceedings of the Royal Society of London B, 200,* 269–294.

Marsden, C. D. (1982). The mysterious motor function of the basal ganglia. *Neurology, 32,* 514–539.

Marshall, J.C. (1976). Neuropsychological aspects of orthographic representation. In R. J. Wales & E. C. T. Walker (Eds.), *New approaches to the language mechanisms.* Amsterdam: North Holland.

Marshall, J.C. (1984a). Multiple perspectives on modularity. *Cognition, 17,* 209–242.

Marshall, J.C. (1984b). Towards a rational taxonomy of acquired dyslexias. In R. N. Malatesha & H. A. Whitaker (Eds.), *Dyslexia: a global issue.* The Hague: Martinus Nijhoff.

Marshall, J.C., & Morton, J. (1978). On the mechanics of Emma. In A. Sinclair, R. J. Jarvella, & W. J. M. Levelt (Eds.), *Child's conception of language.* Berlin: Springer.

Marshall, J.C., & Newcombe, F. (1966). Syntactic and semantic errors in paralexia. *Neuropsychologia, 4,* 169–176.

Marshall, J.C., & Newcombe, F. (1973). Patterns of paralexia: A psycholinguistic approach. *Journal of Psycholinguistic Research, 2,* 175–199.

Marshall, J.C., & Newcombe, F. (1977). Variability and constraint in acquired dyslexia. In H. Whitaker & H. A. Whitaker (Eds.), *Studies in neurolinguistics* (Vol. 3). New York: Academic Press.

Marshall, J.C., & Newcombe, F. (1980). The conceptual status of deep dyslexia: An historical perspective. In M. Coltheart, K. E. Patterson, & J. C. Marshall (Eds.), *Deep dyslexia*. London: Routledge.

Marshall, M., Newcombe, F., and Marshall, J. C. (1970). The microstructure of word-finding difficulties in a dysphasic patient. In G. B. Flores d'Arcais & W. J. M. Levelt (Eds.), *Advances in psycholinguistics*. Amsterdam: North Holland.

Marslen-Wilson, W. D., & Teuber, H.-L. (1975). Memory for remote events in anterograde amnesia: Recognition of public figures from news photographs. *Neuropsychologia, 13*, 347–352.

Marslen-Wilson, W. D., & Tyler, L. K. (1980). The temporal structure of spoken language understanding. *Cognition, 8*, 1–71.

Martin, A., & Fedio, P. (1983). Word production and comprehension in Alzheimer's disease: The breakdown of semantic knowledge. *Brain and Language, 19*, 121–141.

Martin, M., & Jones, G. V. (1979). Modality dependency of loss of recency in free recall. *Psychological Research, 40*, 273–289.

Martin, R., & Caramazza, A. (1982). Short-term memory performance in the absence of phonological coding. *Brain and Cognition, 1*, 50–70.

Mayes, A. R., & Meudell, P. R. (1981). How similar is immediate memory in amnesic patients to delayed memory in normal subjects? A replication, extension and reassessment of the amnesic coding effect. *Neuropsychologia, 19*, 647–654.

Mayes, A. R., Meudell, P. R., & Neary, D. (1978). Must amnesia be caused by either encoding or retrieval disorders? In M. M. Gruneberg, P. E. Morris, & R. N. Sykes (Eds.), *Practical aspects of memory*. London: Academic Press.

Mayes, A. R., Meudell, P. R., & Neary, D. (1980). Do amnesics adopt inefficient encoding strategies with faces and random shapes? *Neuropsychologia, 18*, 527–540.

Mayes, A. R., Meudell, P. R., & Pickering, A. (1985). Is organic amnesia caused by a selective deficit in remembering contextual information? *Cortex, 21*, 167–202.

Meadows, J. C. (1974). Disturbed perception of colors associated with localized cerebral lesions. *Brain, 97*, 615–632.

Messerli, P., Tissot, A., & Rodriguez, J. (1976). Recovery from aphasia: Some factors of prognosis. In Y. Lebrun & R. Hoops (Eds.), *Recovery in aphasics*. Amsterdam: Swets & Zeitlinger.

Mesulam, M. M. (1981). A cortical network for directed attention and unilateral neglect. *Annals of Neurology, 10*, 309–325.

Mettler, F. A. (1949). *Selective partial ablation of the frontal cortex: A correlative study of its effects on human psychotic subjects*. New York: Hoeber.

Mettler, F. A. (1952). *Psychosurgical problems*. New York: Blakiston.

Meudell, P., & Mayes, A. (1982). Normal and abnormal forgetting: Some comments on the human amnesic syndrome. In A. Ellis (Ed.), *Normality and pathology in cognitive functions*. London: Academic Press.

Meudell, P., Mayes, A., & Neary, D. (1980). Amnesia is not caused by cognitive slowness. *Cortex, 16*, 413–419.

Meyer, D. E., Schvaneveldt, R. W., & Ruddy, M. G. (1974). Functions of graphemic and phonemic codes in visual word recognition. *Memory and Cognition, 2*, 309–321.

Miceli, G., Caltagirone, C., Gainotti, G., Masullo, C., Silveri, M. C., & Villa, G. (1981). Influence of age, sex, literacy and pathologic lesion on incidence, severity and type of aphasia. *Acta Neurologica Scandinavia, 64*, 370–382.

Miceli, G., Mazzucchi, A., Menn, L., & Goodglass, H. (1983). Contrasting cases of Italian agrammatic aphasia without comprehension disorder. *Brain and Language, 19*, 65–97.

Miceli, G., Silveri, M. C., & Caramazza, A. (1987). The role of the phoneme–grapheme conversion system and of the graphemic output buffer in writing. In M. Coltheart, G. Sartori, & R. Job (Eds.), *The cognitive neuropsychology of language*. London: Erlbaum.

Miceli, G., Silveri, M. C., Villa, G., & Caramazza, A. (1984). On the basis of the agrammatic's difficulty in producing main verbs. *Cortex, 20*, 207–220.

Michel, F. (1979). Préservation du langage écrit malgré un déficit majeur du langage oral. *Lyon Medical, 241*, 141–149.

428   References

Michel, F., & Andreewsky, E. (1983). Deep dysphasia: An auditory analog of deep dyslexia in the auditory modality. *Brain and Language, 18,* 212–223.

Milberg, W., & Blumstein, S. E. (1981). Lexical decision and aphasia: Evidence for semantic processing. *Brain and Language, 14,* 371–385.

Miller, D., & Ellis, A. W. (1987). Speech and writing errors in neologistic jargonaphasia: A lexical activation hypothesis. In M. Coltheart, G. Sartori, & R. Job (Eds.), *The cognitive neuropsychology of language.* London: Erlbaum.

Miller, G. A., Galanter, E., & Pribram, K. H. (1960). *Plans and the structure of behavior.* New York: McGraw-Hill.

Miller, G. A., & Johnson-Laird, P. N. (1976). *Language and perception.* Cambridge, Mass.: Harvard University Press.

Milner, B. (1958). Psychological deficits produced by temporal-lobe excision. *Research Publications, Association for Research in Nervous and Mental Disease, 36,* 244–257.

Milner, B. (1962). Les troubles de mémoire accompagnant des lésions hippocampiques bilatérales. In *Physiologie de l'hippocampe* (CNRS Report No. 107).

Milner, B. (1963). Effects of different brain lesions on card-sorting. *Archives of Neurology, 9,* 90–100.

Milner, B. (1964). Some effects of frontal lobectomy in man. In J. M. Warren & K. Akert (Eds.), *The frontal granular cortex and behavior.* New York: McGraw-Hill.

Milner, B. (1965). Visually-guided maze learning in man: Effects of bilateral hippocampal, bilateral frontal and unilateral cerebral lesions. *Neuropsychologia, 3,* 317–338.

Milner, B. (1966). Amnesia following operations on the temporal lobes. In C. W. M. Whitty & O. L. Zangwill (Eds.), *Amnesia.* London: Butterworth.

Milner, B. (1968). Visual recognition and recall after right temporal-lobe excision in man. *Neuropsychologia, 6,* 191–209.

Milner, B. (1971). Interhemispheric differences in the localisation of psychological processes in man. *British Medical Bulletin, 27,* 272–277.

Milner, B. (1975). Psychological aspects of focal epilepsy and its neurosurgical management. In D. O. Purpura, J. K. Penry, & R. D. Walter (Eds.), *Advances in neurology* (Vol. 8). New York: Raven Press.

Milner, B. (1982). Some cognitive effects of frontal-lobe lesions in man. *Philosophical Transactions of the Royal Society of London B, 298,* 211–226.

Milner, B., Corkin, S., & Teuber, H.-L. (1968). Further analysis of the hippocampal amnesic syndrome: 14-year follow-up of H. M. *Neuropsychologia, 6,* 215–234.

Milner, B., Petrides, M., & Smith, M. L. (1985). Frontal lobes and the temporal organisation of memory. *Human Neurobiology, 4,* 137–142.

Minsky, M. L., & Papert, S. (1969). *Perceptrons.* Cambridge, Mass.: MIT Press.

Mishkin, M. (1964). Preservation of central sets after frontal lesions in monkeys. In J. M. Warren & K. Akert (Eds.), *The frontal granular cortex and behavior.* New York: McGraw-Hill.

Mishkin, M. (1982). A memory system in the monkey. *Philosophical Transactions of the Royal Society of London B, 298,* 85–95.

Mishkin, M., Malamut, B., & Bachevalier, J. (1984). Memories and habits: Two neural systems. In G. Lynch, J. L. McGaugh, & N. M. Weinberger (Eds.), *The neurobiology of learning and memory.* New York: Guilford Press.

Mitchell, D. C. (1972). Short-term visual memory and pattern masking. *Quarterly Journal of Experimental Psychology, 24,* 394–405.

Mohr, J. P. (1976). Broca's area and Broca's aphasia. In H. Whitaker & H. A. Whitaker (Eds.), *Studies in neurolinguistics* (Vol. 1). New York: Academic Press.

Mohr, J. P., Pessin, M. S., Finkelstein, S., Funkenstein, H. H., Duncan G. W., & Davis, K. R. (1978). Broca aphasia: Pathologic and clinical. *Neurology 28,* 311–324.

Mollon, J. D., Newcombe, F., Polden, P. G., & Ratcliff, G. (1980). On the presence of three cone mechanisms in a case of total achromatopsia. In G. Verriest (Ed.), *Colour vision deficiencies* (Vol. 5). Bristol: Hilger.

Monsell, S. (1985). Repetition and the lexicon. In A. N. Ellis (Ed.), *Progress in the psychology of language* (Vol. 2). London: Erlbaum.

Moran, J., & Desimone, R. (1985). Selective attention gates visual processing in the extrastriate cortex. *Science, 229,* 782–784.

Morton, J. (1969). The interaction of information in word recognition. *Psychological Review, 76,* 165–178.

Morton, J. (1970). A functional model of memory. In D. A. Norman (Ed.), *Models of human memory.* New York: Academic Press.

Morton, J. (1979a). Facilitation in word-recognition experiments causing changes in the logogen model. In P. A. Kolers, M. E. Wrolstad, & H. Bouma (Eds.), *Processing of visible language* (Vol. 1). New York: Plenum Press.

Morton, J. (1979b). Word recognition. In J. Morton & J. C. Marshall (Eds.), *Psycholinguistics* (Series 2). London: Elek.

Morton, J. (1980a). The logogen model and orthographic structure. In U. Frith (Ed.), *Cognitive approaches in spelling.* London: Academic Press.

Morton, J. (1980b). Two auditory parallels to deep dyslexia. In M. Coltheart, K. E. Patterson, & J. C. Marshall (Eds.), *Deep dyslexia.* London: Routledge.

Morton, J. (1981). The status of information processing models of language. *Philosophical Transactions of the Royal Society of London B, 295,* 387–396.

Morton, J. (1984). Brain-based and non-brain based models of language. In D. Caplan, A. R. Lecours, & A. Smith (Eds.), *Biological perspectives in language.* Cambridge, Mass.: MIT Press.

Morton, J., Hammersley, R. H., & Bekerian, D. A. (1985). Headed records: A model for memory and its failure. *Cognition, 20,* 1–23.

Morton, J., & Patterson, K. E. (1980). A new attempt at an interpretation, or, an attempt at a new interpretation. In M. Coltheart, K. E. Patterson, & J. C. Marshall (Eds.), *Deep dyslexia.* London: Routledge.

Moscovitch, M. (1973). Language and the cerebral hemispheres: Reaction-time studies and their implication for models of cerebral dominance. In P. Pliner (Ed.), *Communication and affect.* New York: Academic Press.

Moscovitch, M. (1982). Multiple dissociations of function in amnesia. In L. S. Cermak (Ed.), *Human memory and amnesia.* Hillsdale, N.J.: Erlbaum.

Mountcastle, V. B. (1978). Brain mechanisms of directed attention. *Journal of the Royal Society of Medicine, 71,* 14–27.

Mountcastle, V. B., Anderson, R. A., & Mutter, B. C. (1981). The influence of attentive fixation upon the excitability of the light sensitive neurons of the posterior parietal cortex. *Journal of Neuroscience, 1,* 1218–1245.

Moutier, F. (1908). *L'Aphasie de Broca.* Paris: Steinheil.

Mozer, M. C. (1983). Letter migration in word perception. *Journal of Experimental Psychology: Human Perception and Performance, 9,* 531–546.

Murdock, B. B., Jr. (1961). The retention of individual items. *Journal of Experimental Psychology, 62,* 618–625.

Murdock, B. B., Jr. (1962). The serial position effect of free recall. *Journal of Experimental Psychology, 64,* 482–488.

Murdock, B. B., Jr. (1967). Recent developments in short-term memory. *British Journal of Psychology, 58,* 421–433.

Murray, D. J. (1968). Articulation and acoustic confusability of short-term memory. *Journal of Experimental Psychology, 78,* 679–684.

Murrell, G. A., & Morton, J. (1974). Word recognition and morphemic structure. *Journal of Experimental Psychology, 102,* 963–968.

Nagel, T. (1971). Brain bisection and the unity of conscious experience. *Synthese, 22,* 396–413.

Navon, D. (1984). Resources – a theoretical soupstone. *Psychological Review, 91,* 216–234.

Navon, D., & Gopher, D. (1979). On the economy of the human processing system: A model of multiple capacity. *Psychological Review, 86,* 214–255.

Neisser, U. (1981). *Memory observed: Remembering in natural contexts.* San Francisco: Freeman.

Nelson, H. E. (1976). A modified card sorting task sensitive to frontal lobe defects. *Neuropsychologia, 12,* 313–324.

Nelson, H. E., & McKenna, P. (1975). The use of current reading ability in the assessment of dementia. *British Journal of Social and Clinical Psychology, 14,* 259–267.

Nelson, H. E., & O'Connell, A. (1978). Dementia: The estimation of premorbid intelligence levels using the new adult reading test. *Cortex, 14,* 234–244.

Nespoulous, J.-L., Dordain, M., Perron, C., Ska, B., Bub, D., Caplan, D., Mehler, J., & Lecours, A. R. (in press). Agrammatism in sentence production without comprehension deficits: Reduced availability of syntactic structures and/or of grammatical morphemes: A case study. *Brain and Language.*

Newcombe, F. (1969). *Missile wounds of the brain.* London: Oxford University Press.

Newcombe, F., & Marshall, J. C. (1980a). Transcoding and lexical stabilization in deep dyslexia. In M. Coltheart, K. E. Patterson, & J. C. Marshall (Eds.), *Deep dyslexia.* London: Routledge.

Newcombe, F., & Marshall, J. C. (1980b). Response monitoring and response blocking in deep dyslexia. In M. Coltheart, K. E. Patterson, & J. C. Marshall (Eds.), *Deep dyslexia.* London: Routledge.

Newcombe, F., & Marshall, J. C. (1984). Task- and modality-specific aphasias. In F. C. Rose (Ed.), *Advances in neurology 42: Progress in aphasiology.* New York: Raven Press.

Newcombe, F., & Ratcliff, G. (1974). Agnosia: A disorder of object recognition. In F. Michel & B. Schott (Eds.), *Les syndromes de disconnexion.* Lyon: Colloque International de Lyon.

Newcombe, F., & Ratcliff, G. (1979). Long-term psychological consequences of cerebral lesions. In M. S. Gazzaniga (Ed.), *Handbook of behavioral neurobiology* (Vol. 2). New York: Plenum Press.

Newell, A. (1973). You can't play 20 questions with nature and win. In W. G. Chase (Ed.), *Visual information processing.* New York: Academic Press.

Newell, A., & Simon, H. (1972). *Human problem solving.* Englewood Cliffs, N.J.: Prentice-Hall.

Nielson, J. M. (1946). *Agnosia, apraxia, aphasia: Their value in cerebral localization* (2nd ed.). New York: Hoeber.

Nolan, K. A., & Caramazza, A. (1982). Modality-independent impairments in word processing in a deep dyslexic patient. *Brain and Language, 16,* 237–264.

Nolan, K. A., & Caramazza, A. (1983). An analysis of writing in a case of deep dyslexia. *Brain and Language, 20,* 305–328.

Norman, D. A. (1968). Toward a theory of memory and attention. *Psychological Review, 75,* 522–536.

Norman, D. A. (1981). Categorisation of action slips. *Psychological Review, 88,* 1–15.

Norman, D. A. (1986). Reflections on cognition and parallel distributed processing. In J. L. McClelland & D. E. Rumelhart (Eds.), *Parallel distributed processing: Explorations in the microstructure of cognition* (Vol. 2). Cambridge, Mass.: MIT Press.

Norman, D. A., & Bobrow, D. G. (1975). On data-limited and resource-limited processes. *Cognitive Psychology, 7,* 44–64.

Norman, D. A., & Bobrow, D. G. (1979). Descriptions: An intermediate stage in memory retrieval. *Cognitive Psychology, 11,* 107–123.

Norman, D. A., & Rumelhart, D. E. (1975). *Explorations in cognition.* San Francisco: Freeman.

Norman, D. A., & Shallice, T. (1980). *Attention to action: Willed and automatic control of behavior.* Center for Human Information Processing (Technical Report No. 99). (Reprinted in revised form in R. J. Davidson, G. E. Schwartz, & D. Shapiro [Eds.] [1986] *Consciousness and self-regulation* [Vol. 4]. New York: Plenum Press.)

Obler, L. K., Albert, M. L., Goodglass, H., & Benson, D. F. (1978). Aphasia type and aging. *Brain and Language, 6,* 318–322.

Ogden, J. A. (1985a). Autotopagnosia: Occurrence in a patient without nominal aphasia and with an intact ability to point to parts of animals and objects. *Brain, 108,* 1009–1022.

Ogden, J. A. (1985b). Contralesional neglect of constructed visual images in right- and left-handed brain-damaged patients. *Neuropsychologia, 23,* 273–277.

Ojemann, G. A. (1978). Organization of short-term verbal memory in language areas of human cortex: Evidence from electrical stimulation. *Brain and Language, 5,* 331–340.

O'Keefe, J. (1985). Is consciousness the gateway to the hippocampal cognitive map: A speculative essay on the neural basis of mind. In D. Oakley (Ed.), *Brain and mind*. London: Methuen.

O'Keefe, J., & Nadel, L. (1978). *The hippocampus as a cognitive map*. London: Oxford University Press.

Oscar-Berman, M. (1973). Hypothesis testing and focusing behavior during concept formation by amnesic Korsakoff patients. *Neuropsychologia, 11*, 191–198.

Paillard, J. (1982). Apraxia and the neurophysiology of motor control. *Philosophical Transactions of the Royal Society of London B, 298*, 111–134.

Paivio, A. (1971). *Imagery and verbal processes*. London: Holt, Rinehart and Winston.

Parisi, D. (1987). Grammatical disturbances of speech production. In M. Coltheart, G. Sartori, & R. Job (Eds.), *The cognitive neuropsychology of language*. London: Erlbaum.

Parisi, D., & Pizzamiglio, L. (1970). Syntactic comprehension in aphasia. *Cortex, 6*, 204–215.

Parkin, A. J. (1982). Phonological recoding in lexical decision: Effects of spelling-to-sound regularity depend on how regularity is defined. *Memory and Cognition, 10*, 43–53.

Parkin, A. J. (1984). Amnesic syndrome: A lesion-specific disorder? *Cortex, 20*, 479–508.

Parkin, A. J., & Underwood, G. (1983). Orthographic versus phonological irregularity in lexical decisions. *Memory and Cognition, 11*, 351–355.

Pasik, P., & Pasik, T. (1982). Visual functions in monkeys after total removal of visual cerebral cortex. In W. D. Neff (Ed.), *Contributions to sensory physiology* (Vol. 7). New York: Academic Press.

Patterson, K. E. (1978). Phonemic dyslexia: Errors of meaning and meaning of errors. *Quarterly Journal of Experimental Psychology, 30*, 587–601.

Patterson, K. E. (1979). What is right with 'deep' dyslexic patients? *Brain and Language, 8*, 111–129.

Patterson, K. E. (1980). Derivational errors. In M. Coltheart, K. E. Patterson, & J. C. Marshall (Eds.), *Deep dyslexia*. London: Routledge.

Patterson, K. E. (1981). Neuropsychological approaches to the study of reading. *British Journal of Psychology, 72*, 151–174.

Patterson, K. E. (1982). The relation between reading and psychological coding: Further neuropsychological observations. In A. W. Ellis (Ed.), *Normality and pathology in cognitive functions*. London: Academic Press.

Patterson, K. E. (1986). Lexical but nonsemantic spelling? *Cognitive Neuropsychology, 3*, 341–367.

Patterson, K. E., & Besner, D. (1984). Is the right hemisphere literate? *Cognitive Neuropsychology, 1*, 315–342.

Patterson, K. E., Coltheart, M., & Marshall, J. C. (Eds.). (1985). *Surface dyslexia*. London: Erlbaum.

Patterson, K. E., & Kay, J. (1982). Letter-by-letter reading: Psychological descriptions of a neurological syndrome. *Quarterly Journal of Experimental Psychology, 34A*, 411–441.

Patterson, K. E., & Marcel, A. J. (1977). Aphasia, dyslexia and the phonological coding of written words. *Quarterly Journal of Experimental Psychology, 29*, 307–318.

Patterson, K. E., & Morton, J. (1980). 'Little words – no!' In M. Coltheart, K. E. Patterson, & J. C. Marshall, (Eds.), *Deep dyslexia*. London: Routledge.

Patterson, K. E., & Morton, J. (1985). From orthography to phonology: An attempt at an old interpretation. In K. E. Patterson, M. Coltheart, & J. C. Marshall (Eds.), *Surface dyslexia*. London: Erlbaum.

Patterson, K. E., & Shewell, C. (1987). Speak and spell: Dissociations and word-class effects. In M. Coltheart, G. Sartori, & R. Job (Eds.), *The cognitive neuropsychology of language*. London: Erlbaum.

Perenin, M. T., & Jeannerod, M. (1978). Visual function within the hemianopic field following early cerebral hemidecortication in man: I. Spatial localisation. *Neuropsychologia, 16*, 1–13.

Peretz, I., & Morais, J. (1980). Modes of processing melodies and ear asymmetry in non-musicians. *Neuropsychologia, 18*, 477–489.

Peretz, I., & Morais, J. (1983). Task determinants of ear differences in melody processing. *Brain and Cognition, 2*, 313–330.

Perret, E. (1974). The left frontal lobe in man and suppression of habitual responses in verbal categorical behavior. *Neuropsychologia, 12*, 323–330.

Petrides, M., & Milner, B. (1982). Deficits on subject-ordered tasks after frontal- and temporal-lobe lesions in man. *Neuropsychologia, 20,* 249–262.

Pfeifer, B. (1910). Les troubles psychiques dans les tumeurs cerebrales. *Archives de Psychologie, 47,* 558–591.

Philipchalk, R., & Rowe, E. J. (1971). Sequential and nonsequential memory for verbal and non-verbal auditory stimuli. *Journal of Experimental Psychology, 91,* 341–343.

Phillips, W. A., & Christie, D. F. M. (1977). Components of visual memory. *Quarterly Journal of Experimental Psychology, 29,* 117–133.

Piaget, J. (1936). *La naissance de l'intelligence chez l'enfant.* Neuchatel: Delachaux et Niestlé.

Pick, A. (1973). *Aphasia* (J. W. Brown, Trans.). Springfield, Ill.: Thomas. (Original work published 1931)

Piercy, M., Hécaen, H., & Ajuriguerra, J. de (1960). Constructional apraxia associated with unilateral lesions – left and right sided cases compared. *Brain, 83,* 225–242.

Pillon, B., Signoret, J.-L., & Lhermitte, F. (1981). Agnosie visuelle associative. Rôle de l'hemisphere gauche dans la perception visuelle. *Revue Neurologique, 137,* 831–842.

Poeck, K. (1983). What do we mean by 'aphasic syndromes'?: A neurologist's view. *Brain and Language, 20,* 79–89.

Poeck, K. (1984). Neuropsychological demonstration of splenial interhemispheric disconnection in a case of 'optic anomia'. *Neuropsychologia, 22,* 707–713.

Poeck, K., De Bleser, R., & Von Kayserlingk, D. G. (1984a). Computed tomography localisation of standard aphasic syndromes. In F. C. Rose (Ed.), *Advances in neurology 42: Progress in aphasiology.* New York: Raven Press.

Poeck, K., De Bleser, R., & Von Kayserlingk, D. G. (1984b). Neurolinguistic status and localisation of lesion in aphasic patients with exclusively consonant–vowel recurring utterances. *Brain, 107,* 199–217.

Poeck, K., & Orgass, B. (1966). Gerstmann's syndrome and aphasia. *Cortex, 2,* 421–427.

Pöppel, E., Held, R., & Frost, D. (1973). Residual visual function after brain wounds involving the central visual pathways in man. *Nature, 243,* 295–296.

Poppelreuter, W. (1923). Zur Psychologie und Pathologie des Optischen Wohrnehmung. *Zeitschrift für die Gesamte Neurologie und Psychiatrie, 83,* 26–152.

Porteus, S. D., & Kepner, R. D. (1944). Mental changes after bilateral prefrontal lobotomy. *Genetic Psychology Monographs, 29,* 3–115.

Posner, M. I. (1978). *Chronometric explorations of mind.* Hillsdale, N.J.: Erlbaum.

Posner, M. I. (1980). Orienting of attention. *Quarterly Journal of Experimental Psychology, 32,* 3–25.

Posner, M. I., Boies, S. J., Eichelman, W. H., & Taylor, R. L. (1969). Retention of visual and name codes of single letters. *Journal of Experimental Psychology: Monographs, 79,* Vol. 1, pt. 2.

Posner, M. I., Cohen, Y., & Rafal, R. D. (1982). Neural systems control of spatial orienting. *Philosophical Transactions of the Royal Society of London B, 298,* 187–198.

Posner, M. I., Inhof, A. W., Friedrich, F. J., & Cohen, A. (1987). Isolating attentional systems: A cognitive-anatomical analysis. *Psychobiology, 15,* 107–12.

Posner, M. I., & Klein, R. M. (1973). On the functions of consciousness. In S. Kornblum (Ed.), *Attention and performance* (Vol. 4). New York: Academic Press.

Posner, M. I., Walker, J. A., Friedrich, F. J., & Rafal, R. D. (1984). Effects of parietal injury on covert orienting of visual attention. *Journal of Neuroscience, 4,* 1863–1874.

Postman, L. (1975). Verbal learning and memory. *Annual Review of Psychology, 26,* 291–335.

Potter, M. C. (1979). Mundane symbolism: The relations among names, objects and ideas. In N. Smith & M. B. Franklin (Eds.), *Symbolic functioning in childhood.* Hillsdale, N.J.: Erlbaum.

Potter, M. C., & Faulconer, B. A. (1975). Time to understand pictures and words. *Nature, 253,* 437–438.

Puccetti, R. (1973). Brain bisection and personal identity. *British Journal for the Philosophy of Science, 24,* 339–355.

Puccetti, R. (1981). The case for mental duality: Evidence from split-brain data and other considerations. *Behavioral and Brain Sciences, 4,* 93–123.

Puccetti, R., & Dykes, R. W. (1978). Sensory cortex and the mind–brain problem. *Behavioral and Brain Sciences, 3,* 337–375.

Putnam, H. (1960). Minds and machines. In S. Hook (Ed.), *Dimensions of mind.* New York: New York University Press.

Putnam, H. (1984). Models and modules. *Cognition, 17,* 253–264.

Pylyshyn, Z. W. (1980). Computation and cognition: Issues in the foundation of cognitive science. *Behavioral and Brain Sciences, 3,* 111–169.

Radford, A. (1981). *Transformational syntax.* Cambridge: Cambridge University Press.

Ratcliff, G., & Davies-Jones, A. B. (1972). Defective visual localisation in focal brain wounds. *Brain, 95,* 49–60.

Ratcliff, G., & Newcombe, F. (1982). Object recognition: Some deductions from the clinical evidence. In A. W. Ellis (Ed.), *Normality and pathology in cognitive function.* London: Academic Press.

Ratliff, R., & McKoon, G. (1986). More on the distinction between episodic and semantic memories. *Journal of Experimental Psychology: Learning, Memory, and Cognition, 12,* 312–313.

Reason, J. T. (1979). Actions not as planned. In G. Underwood & R. Stevens (Eds.), *Aspects of consciousness* (Vol. 1). London: Academic Press.

Reason, J. T. (1984). Lapses of attention. In R. Parasuraman, R. Davies, & J. Beatty (Eds.), *Varieties of attention.* Orlando, Fla.: Academic Press.

Reiff, R., & Scheerer, M. (1959). *Memory and hypnotic age regression.* New York: International Universities Press.

Rey, A. (1941). L'examen psychologique dans les cas d'encephalopathie traumatique. *Archives de Psychologie, 28,* 286–340.

Ribot, T. (1882). *Diseases of memory.* New York: Appleton.

Richardson, J. T. E. (1975). The effect of word imageability in acquired dyslexia. *Neuropsychologia, 13,* 281–288.

Riddoch, G. (1917). Dissociation of visual perception due to occipital injuries with especial reference to appreciation of movement. *Brain, 40,* 15–57.

Riddoch, M. J., Humphreys, G. W., Coltheart, M., & Funnell, E. (1988). Semantic systems or system? Neuropsychological evidence re-examined. *Cognitive Neuropsychology, 5,* 3–25.

Rieger, C. (1978). Grind-1: First report on the Magic Grinder story comprehension project. *Discourse Processes, 1,* 267–303.

Rieger, C., & Small, S. (1979). *Word expert parsing.* University of Maryland Computer Science Technical Report No. 734.

Rizzolatti, G., Gentilucci, M., & Matelli, M. (1985). Selective spatial attention: One center, one circuit or many circuits. In M. I. Posner & O. S. M. Marin (Eds.), *Attention and performance* (Vol. 11). Hillsdale, N.J.: Erlbaum.

Robbins, T. W., & Sahakian, B. (1983). Behavioral effects of psychomotor drugs: Clinical and neuropsychological implications. In I. Creese (Ed.). *Stimulants: neurochemical, behavioral and clinical perspectives.* New York: Raven Press.

Robinson, J. A. (1976). Sampling autobiographical memory. *Cognitive Psychology, 8,* 578–595.

Rochford, G. (1974). Are jargon aphasics dysphasic? *British Journal of Disorders of Communication, 9,* 35–44.

Roeltgen, D. P., & Heilman, K. M. (1983). Apractic agraphia in a patient with normal praxis. *Brain and Language, 18,* 35–46.

Roeltgen, D. P., & Heilman, K. M. (1984). Lexical agraphia, further support for the two-strategy hypothesis of linguistic agraphia. *Brain, 107,* 811–827.

Roeltgen, D. P., Gonzalez-Rothi, L., & Heilman, K. M. (1986). Linguistic semantic agraphia: A dissociation of the lexical spelling system from semantics. *Brain and Language, 27,* 257–280.

Roeltgen, D. P., Sevush, S., & Heilman, K. M. (1983). Phonological agraphia: Writing by the lexical-semantic route. *Neurology, 33,* 755–765.

Rollins, H., & Hendricks, R. (1980). Processing of words presented simultaneously to eye and ear. *Journal of Experimental Psychology: Human Perception and Performance, 6,* 99–109.

Rondot, P., de Recondo, J., & Ribadeau Dumas, J. L. C. (1977). Visuomotor ataxia. *Brain, 100,* 355–376.

Rosati, G., & De Bastiani, P. (1979). Pure agraphia: A discrete form of aphasia. *Journal of Neurology, Neurosurgery and Psychiatry, 42,* 266–269.

Rosch, E., Mervis, C., Gray, W., Johnson, D., & Boyes-Braem, P. (1976). Basic objects in natural categories. *Cognitive Psychology, 8,* 382–439.

Rosenthal, V. (1984). *Modularity of scientific reason: a methodological perspective.* Paper presented at the Second Cognitive Neuropsychology Workshop, Bressanone, Italy.

Ross Russell, R. W., & Bharucha, N. (1984). Visual localization in patients with occipital infarction. *Journal of Neurology, Neurosurgery and Psychiatry, 47,* 153–158.

Rosvold, H. E., & Mishkin, M. (1961). Non-sensory effects of frontal lesions on discrimination learning and performance. In J. F. Delafrasnaye (Ed.), *Brain mechanisms and learning.* Springfield, Ill.: Thomas.

Routh, D. A. (1976). An 'across-the-board' modality effect in immediate serial recall. *Quarterly Journal of Experimental Psychology, 28,* 285–304.

Rowe, E. J. (1974). Ordered recall of sounds and words in short-term memory. *Bulletin of the Psychonomic Society, 4,* 559–561.

Rozin, P. (1976). The evolution of intelligence and access to the cognitive unconscious. In J. M. Sprague & A. N. Epstein (Eds.), *Progress in physiological psychology* (Vol. 6). New York: Academic Press.

Rubens, A. B. (1979). Agnosia. In K. M. Heilman & E. Valenstein (Eds.), *Clinical neuropsychology.* New York: Oxford University Press.

Rubinstein, H., Lewis, S. S., & Rubinstein, M. A. (1971). Evidence for phonemic recoding in visual word recognition. *Journal of Verbal Learning and Verbal Behavior, 10,* 645–657.

Rumelhart, D. E., Hinton, G. E., & Williams, R. J. (1986). Learning internal representations by error propagation. In J. L. McClelland & D. E. Rumelhart (Eds.), *Parallel distributed processing: Explorations in the microstructure of cognition* (Vol. 1). Cambridge, Mass.: MIT Press.

Rumelhart, D. E., & McClelland, J. L. (1982). An interactive activation model of context effects in letter perception: Part 2. The contextual enhancement effect and some tests and extensions of the model. *Psychological Review, 89,* 60–94.

Rumelhart, D. E., & Ortony, A. (1977). The representation of knowledge in memory. In R. C. Anderson, R. J. Spiro, & W. E. Montague (Eds.), *Schooling and the acquisition of knowledge.* Hillsdale, N.J.: Erlbaum.

Rumelhart, D. E., Smolensky, P., McClelland, J. L., & Hinton, G. E. (1986). Schemata and sequential thought processes in PDP models. In J. L. McClelland and D. E. Rumelhart (Eds.), *Parallel distributed processing: explorations in the microstructure of cognition* (Vol. 2). Cambridge, Mass.: MIT Press.

Rumelhart, D. E., & Zipser, D. (1985). Feature discovery by competitive learning. *Cognitive Science, 9,* 75–112.

Ryan, J. (1969). Grouping and short-term memory: Different means and patterns of grouping. *Quarterly Journal of Experimental Psychology, 21,* 137–147.

Rylander, G. (1939). Personality changes after operations on the frontal lobes. *Acta Psychiatrica et Neurologica Scandanavia,* Supplement No. 20.

Sachs, J. S. (1967). Recognition memory for syntactic and semantic aspects of connected discourse. *Perception and Psychophysics, 2,* 437–442.

Saffran, E. M. (1980). Reading in deep dyslexia is not ideographic. *Neuropsychologia, 18,* 219–223.

Saffran, E. M. (1982). Neuropsychological approaches to the study of language. *British Journal of Psychology, 73,* 317–337.

Saffran, E. M. (1984). Acquired dyslexia: Implications for models of reading. In G. E. Mackinnon & T. G. Waller (Eds.), *Reading research: Advances in theory and practice* (Vol. 4). New York: Academic Press.

Saffran, E. M. (1985a, March). *Short-term memory impairment and language comprehension: Specify-*

ing the nature of the interaction. Paper presented at the Second Venice Conference on Cognitive Neuropsychology, Venice.

Saffran, E. M. (1985b). Lexicalisation and reading performance in surface dyslexia. In K. E. Patterson, M. Coltheart, & J. C. Marshall (Eds.), *Surface dyslexia*. London: Erlbaum.

Saffran, E. M. (in press). Short-term memory impairment and language processing. In A. Caramazza (Ed.), *Advances in cognitive neuropsychology and neurolinguistics*. Hillsdale, N.J.: Erlbaum.

Saffran, E. M., Bogyo, L. C., Schwartz, M. F., & Marin, O. S. M. (1980). Does deep dyslexia reflect right-hemisphere reading? In M. Coltheart, K. E. Patterson, J. C. Marshall (Eds.), *Deep dyslexia*. London: Routledge.

Saffran, E. M., & Marin, O. S. M. (1975). Immediate memory for word lists and sentences in a patient with a deficient auditory short-term memory. *Brain and Language, 2,* 420–433.

Saffran, E. M., & Marin, O. S. M. (1977). Reading without phonology. *Quarterly Journal of Experimental Psychology, 29,* 515–525.

Saffran, E. M., Schwartz, M. F., & Marin, O. S. M. (1976). Semantic mechanisms in paralexia. *Brain and Language, 3,* 255–265.

Saffran, E. M., Schwartz, M. F., & Marin, O. S. M. (1979, February). *Neuropsychological evidence for mechanisms of reading: I. Deep dyslexia*. Paper presented to the Seventh International Neuropsychology Society Meeting, New York.

Saffran, E. M., Schwartz, M. F., & Marin, O. S. M. (1980a). The word order problem in agrammatism: II. Production. *Brain and Language, 10,* 249–262.

Saffran, E. M., Schwartz, M. F., & Marin, O. S. M. (1980b). Evidence from aphasia: Isolating the components of a production model. In B. Butterworth (Ed.), *Language production* (Vol. 1). London: Academic Press.

Salamé, P., & Baddeley, A. D. (1982). Disruption of short-term memory by unattended speech: Implications for the structure of working memory. *Journal of Verbal Learning and Verbal Behaviour, 21,* 150–164.

Salmaso, D., & Denes, G. (1982). Role of the frontal lobes on an attention task: A signal detection analysis. *Perception and Motor Skills, 54,* 1147–1150.

Sanders, H. I., & Warrington, E. K. (1971). Memory for remote events in amnesic patients. *Brain, 94,* 661–668.

Sandson, J., & Albert, M. L. (1984). Varieties of perseveration. *Neuropsychologia, 22,* 715–732.

Sartori, G. (1988). From neuropsychological data to theory and vice-versa. In G. Denes, P. Bisiacchi, C. Semenza, E. Andreewsky (Eds.), *Perspectives in cognitive neuropsychology*. London: Erlbaum.

Sartori, G., Barry, C., & Job, R. (1984). Phonological dyslexia: A review. In R. N. Malatesha & H. A. Whitaker (Eds.), *Dyslexia: A global issue*. The Hague: Martinus Nijhoff.

Sartori, G., & Job, R. (1988). The oyster with four legs: A neuropsychological study on the interaction of visual and semantic information. *Cognitive Neuropsychology, 5,* 105–132.

Sasanuma, S. (1980). Acquired dyslexia in Japanese: Clinical features and underlying mechanisms. In M. Coltheart, K. E. Patterson, & J. C. Marshall (Eds.), *Deep dyslexia*. London: Routledge.

Sasanuma, S. (1985). Surface dyslexia and dysgraphia: How are they manifested in Japanese? In K. E. Patterson, M. Coltheart, & J. C. Marshall (Eds.), *Surface dyslexia*. London: Erlbaum.

Scarborough, D. L., Cortese, C., & Scarborough, H. S. (1977). Frequency and repetition effects in lexical memory. *Journal of Experimental Psychology: Human Perception and Performance, 3,* 1–17.

Schacter, D. L., & Graf, P. (1986). Preserved learning in amnesic patients: Perspectives from research on direct priming. *Journal of Clinical and Experimental Neuropsychology, 8,* 727–743.

Schacter, D. L., & Tulving, E. (1982). Memory, amnesia and the episodic/semantic distinction. In P. L. Isaacson & N. E. Spear (Eds.), *Expression of knowledge*. New York: Plenum Press.

Schank, R. C. (1982). *Dynamic memory*. Cambridge: Cambridge University Press.

Schank, R. C., & Abelson, R. (1977). *Scripts, plans, goals, and understanding*. Hillsdale, N.J.: Erlbaum.

Schmidt, R. A. (1975). A schema theory of discrete motor skill learning. *Psychological Review, 82,* 225–260.

Schuell, H. (1950). Paraphasia and paralexia. *Journal of Speech and Hearing Disorders, 15*, 291–306.

Schuell, H., & Jenkins, J. J. (1959). The nature of language deficit in aphasia. *Psychological Review, 66*, 45–67.

Schuell, H., Jenkins, J. J., & Carroll, J. M. (1962). Factor analysis of the Minnesota Test for differential diagnosis of aphasia. *Journal of Speech and Hearing Research, 5*, 349–369.

Schwartz, M. F. (1984). What the classical aphasia categories don't do for us and why. *Brain and Language, 21*, 3–8.

Schwartz, M. F., Linebarger, M. C., & Saffran, E. M. (1985). The status of the syntactic theory of agrammatism. In M.-L. Kean (Ed.), *Agrammatism*. New York: Academic Press.

Schwartz, M. F., Marin, O. S. M., & Saffran, E. M. (1979). Dissociation of language function in dementia: A case study. *Brain and Language, 7*, 277–306.

Schwartz, M. F., Saffran, E. M., & Marin, O. S. M. (1977, February). *An analysis of agrammatic reading in aphasia*. Paper presented at the meeting of the International Neuropsychological Society, Santa Fe, N. Mex.

Schwartz, M. F., Saffran, E. M., & Marin, O. S. M. (1980a). Fractionating the reading process in dementia: Evidence for word-specific print-to-sound associations. In M. Coltheart, K. E. Patterson, & J. C. Marshall (Eds.), *Deep dyslexia*. London: Routledge.

Schwartz, M. F., Saffran, E. M., & Marin, O. S. M. (1980b). The word order problem in agrammatism: 1. Comprehension. *Brain and Language, 10*, 249–262.

Schwartz, M. F., & Schwartz, B. (1984). In defence of organology. *Cognitive Neuropsychology, 1*, 25–42.

Scoville, W. B., & Milner, B. (1957). Loss of recent memory after bilateral hippocampal lesions. *Journal of Neurology, Neurosurgery and Psychiatry, 20*, 11–21.

Searle, J. (1980). Minds, brains and programs. *Behavioral and Brain Sciences*, 417–457.

Seidenberg, M. S. (1985). The time course of phonological code activation in two writing systems. *Cognition, 19*, 1–30.

Seidenberg, M. S., Waters, G. S., Barnes, M. A., & Tanenhaus, M. K. (1984). When does irregular spelling or pronunciation influence word recognition? *Journal of Verbal Learning and Verbal Behavior, 23*, 383–404.

Sejnowski, T. J., & Rosenberg, C. R. (1986). *NETtalk: A parallel network that learns to read aloud.* Johns Hopkins University Electrical Engineering and Computer Science Technical Report JHU/EECS-86/01.

Semenza, C., & Zettin, M. (in press). Generating proper names: A case of selective inability. *Cognitive Neuropsychology*.

Semmes, J., Weinstein, S., Ghent, L., & Teuber, H.-L. (1963). Correlates of impaired orientation in personal and extrapersonal space. *Brain, 86*, 747–772.

Seymour, P. H. K. (1973). A model for reading, naming and comparison. *British Journal of Psychology, 64*, 35–49.

Seymour, P. H. K. (1979). *Human visual cognition*. London: Collier Macmillan.

Seymour, P. H. K., & MacGregor, C. J. (1984). Developmental dyslexia: A cognitive experimental analysis of phonological, morphemic and visual impairments. *Cognitive Neuropsychology, 1*, 43–82.

Shallice, T. (1972). Dual functions of consciousness. *Psychological Review, 79*, 383–393.

Shallice, T. (1975). On the contents of primary memory. In P. M. A. Rabbitt & S. Dornic (Eds.), *Attention and performance* (Vol. 5). London: Academic Press.

Shallice, T. (1978). The dominant action system: An information-processing approach to consciousness. In K. S. Pope & J. L. Singer (Eds.), *The stream of consciousness: Scientific investigations into the flow of human experience*. New York: Plenum Press.

Shallice, T. (1979a). Neuropsychological research and the fractionation of memory systems. In L.-G. Nilsson (Ed.), *Perspectives on memory research*. Hillsdale, N.J.: Erlbaum.

Shallice, T. (1979b). Case-study approach in neuropsychological research. *Journal of Clinical Neuropsychology, 1*, 183–211.

Shallice, T. (1981a). Phonological agraphia and the lexical route in writing. *Brain, 104,* 413–429.

Shallice, T. (1981b). Neurological impairment of cognitive processes. *British Medical Bulletin, 37,* 187–192.

Shallice, T. (1982). Specific impairments of planning. *Philosophical Transactions of the Royal Society of London B, 298,* 199–209.

Shallice, T. (1984). More functionally isolable subsystems but fewer 'modules'? *Cognition, 17,* 243–252.

Shallice, T. (1987). Impairments of semantic processing: Multiple dissociations. In M. Coltheart, G. Sartori, & R. Job (Eds.), *The cognitive neuropsychology of language.* London: Erlbaum.

Shallice, T. (in press). Information-processing models of consciousness: Possibilities and problems. In A. J. Marcel & E. Bisiach (Eds.), *Consciousness in contemporary science.* Oxford: Oxford University Press.

Shallice, T., & Butterworth, B. (1977). Short-term memory impairment and spontaneous speech. *Neuropsychologia, 15,* 729–735.

Shallice, T., & Coughlan, A. K. (1980). Modality specific word comprehension deficits in deep dyslexia. *Journal of Neurology, Neurosurgery and Psychiatry, 43,* 866–872.

Shallice, T., & Evans, M. E. (1978). The involvement of the frontal lobes in cognitive estimation. *Cortex, 14,* 294–303.

Shallice, T., & McCarthy, R. (1985). Phonological reading: From patterns of impairment to possible procedures. In K. E. Patterson, M. Coltheart, & J. C. Marshall (Eds.), *Surface dyslexia.* London: Erlbaum.

Shallice, T., & McGill, J. (1978). The origins of mixed errors. In J. Requin (Ed.), *Attention and performance* (Vol. 7). Hillsdale, N.J.: Erlbaum.

Shallice, T., McLeod, P., & Lewis, K. (1985). Isolating cognitive modules with the dual-task paradigm: Are speech perception and production separate processes? *Quarterly Journal of Experimental Psychology, 37A,* 507–532.

Shallice, T., & Saffran, E. M. (1986). Lexical processing in the absence of explicit word identification: Evidence from a letter-by-letter reader. *Cognitive Neuropsychology, 3,* 429–458.

Shallice, T., & Warrington, E. K. (1970). Independent functioning of the verbal memory stores: A neuropsychological study. *Quarterly Journal of Experimental Psychology, 22,* 261–273.

Shallice, T., & Warrington, E. K. (1974). The dissociation between short-term retention of meaningful sounds and verbal material. *Neuropsychologia, 12,* 553–555.

Shallice, T., & Warrington, E. K. (1975). Word recognition in a phonemic dyslexic patient. *Quarterly Journal of Experimental Psychology, 27,* 187–199.

Shallice, T., & Warrington, E. K. (1977a). Auditory–verbal short-term memory impairment and spontaneous speech. *Brain and Language, 4,* 479–491.

Shallice, T., & Warrington, E. K. (1977b). The possible role of selective attention in acquired dyslexia. *Neuropsychologia, 15,* 31–41.

Shallice, T., & Warrington, E. K. (1980). Single and multiple component central dyslexic syndromes. In M. Coltheart, K. E. Patterson, & J. C. Marshall (Eds.), *Deep dyslexia.* London: Routledge.

Shallice, T., & Warrington, E. K., & McCarthy, R. (1983). Reading without semantics. *Quarterly Journal of Experimental Psychology, 35A,* 111–138.

Shepard, R. N., & Metzler, J. (1971). Mental rotation of three-dimensional objects. *Science, 171,* 701–703.

Shiffrin, R. M., & Schneider, W. (1977). Controlled and automatic human information processing: II. Perceptual learning, automatic attending, and a general theory. *Psychological Review, 84,* 127–190.

Shimamura, A. P. (1986). Priming effects in amnesia: Evidence for a dissociable memory function. *Quarterly Journal of Experimental Psychology, 38A,* 619–644.

Shulman, H. G. (1970). Encoding and retention of semantic and phonemic information in short-term memory. *Journal of Verbal Learning and Verbal Behavior, 9,* 499–508.

Signoret, J.-L., Castaigne, P., Lhermitte, F., Abelanet, R., & Lavorel, P. (1984). Rediscovery of Leborgne's brain: Anatomical description with CT scan. *Brain and Language, 22,* 303–319.

Signoret, J.-L., & Lhermitte, F. (1976). The amnesic syndrome and the encoding process. In M. R. Rosenzweig & E. L. Bennett (Eds.), *Neural mechanisms of learning and memory*. Cambridge, Mass.: MIT Press.

Silveri, M. C., & Gainotti, G. B. (1987). *Interaction between vision and language in category specific semantic impairment for living things*. Unpublished manuscript.

Simon, H. A. (1969). *The sciences of the artificial*. Cambridge, Mass.:MIT Press.

Smith, A. (1966). Intellectual functions in patients with lateralized frontal tumours. *Journal of Neurology, Neurosurgery and Psychiatry, 29*, 52–59.

Smith, E. E., Shoben, E. J., & Rips, L. J. (1974). Structure and process in semantic memory: A featural model for semantic decision. *Psychological Review, 81*, 214–241.

Smith, E. E., & Spoehr, K. T. (1974). The perception of printed English: A theoretical perspective. In B. H. Kantowitz (Ed.), *Human information processing: Tutorials in performance and cognition*. Potomac, Md.: Erlbaum.

Smith, K. U., & Akelaitis, A. J. (1942). Studies on the corpus callosum I. *Archives of Neurology and Psychiatry, 47*, 519–543.

Smith, M. L., & Milner, B. (1984). Differential effects of frontal-lobe lesions on cognitive estimation and spatial memory. *Neuropsychologia, 22*, 697–705.

Snodgrass, J. G. (1984). Concepts and their surface representations. *Journal of Verbal Learning and Verbal Behavior, 23*, 3–22.

Speedie, L. J., Rothi, L. J., & Heilman, K. M. (1982). Spelling dyslexia: A form of cross-cuing. *Brain and Language, 15*, 340–352.

Spelke, E., Hirst, W., & Neisser, U. (1976). Skills of divided attention. *Cognition, 4*, 205–230.

Sperling, G. (1967). Successive approximations to a model for short-term memory. *Acta Psychologia, 27*, 285–292.

Sperling, G., & Melcher, M. J. (1978). Visual search, visual attention and the attention operating characteristic. In J. Requin (Ed.), *Attention and performance* (Vol. 7). Hillsdale, N.J.: Erlbaum.

Sperling, G., & Speelman, R. G. (1970). Acoustic similarity and auditory short-term memory: Experiments and a model. In D. A. Norman (Ed.), *Models of human memory*. New York: Academic Press.

Sperry, R. W. (1968). Mental unity following surgical disconnection of the cerebral hemispheres. *The Harvey Lectures Series, 62*, 293–323.

Sperry, R. W. (1984). Consciousness, personal identity and the divided brain. *Neuropsychologia, 22*, 661–673.

Spreen, O., Benton, A. L., & Van Allen, M. W. (1966). Dissociation of visual and tactile naming in amnesic aphasia. *Neurology, 16*, 807–814.

Squire, L. R. (1981). Two forms of human amnesia: An analysis of forgetting. *Journal of Neuroscience, 1*, 635–640.

Squire, L. R., & Cohen, N. J. (1982). Remote memory, retrograde amnesia and the neuropsychology of memory. In L. S. Cermak (Ed.), *Human memory and amnesia*. Hillsdale, N.J.: Erlbaum.

Squire, L. R., & Shimamura, A. P. (1986). Characterizing amnesic patients for neurobehavioral study. *Behavioral Neuroscience, 100*, 866–877.

Squire, L. R., & Slater, P. C. (1978). Anterograde and retrograde memory impairment in chronic amnesia. *Neuropsychologia, 16*, 313–322.

Staller, J., Buchanan, D., Singer, M., Lappin, J., & Webb, W. (1978). Alexia without agraphia: An experimental case study. *Brain and Language, 5*, 378–387.

Stemberger, J. P. (1984). Structural errors in normal and agrammatic speech. *Cognitive Neuropsychology, 1*, 281–313.

Stemberger, J. P. (1985). An interactive activation model of language production. In A. W. Ellis (Ed.), *Progress in the psychology of language* (Vol. 1). London: Erlbaum.

Stengel, E., & Lodge Patch, I. C. (1955). 'Central' aphasia associated with parietal symptoms. *Brain, 78*, 401–416.

Sternberg, S. (1969). The discovery of processing stages: Extensions of Donders' method. *Acta Psychologia, 30*, 276–315.

Strawson, P. F. (1959). *Individuals*. London: Methuen.

Strub, R. L., & Gardner, H. (1974). The repetition deficit in conduction aphasia: Mnestic or linguistic? *Brain and Language, 1*, 241–255.

Stuss, D. T., Alexander, M. P., Lieberman, A., & Levine, H. (1978). An extraordinary form of confabulation. *Neurology, 28*, 1166–1172.

Stuss, D. T., & Benson, D. F. (1984). Neuropsychological studies of the frontal lobes. *Psychological Bulletin, 95*, 3–28.

Stuss, D. T., & Benson, D. F. (1986). *The frontal lobes*. New York: Raven Press.

Stuss, D. T., Benson, D. F., Kaplan, E. F., Weir, W. S., Naeser, M. A., Lieberman, I., & Ferrill, D. (1983). The involvement of orbitofrontal cerebrum in cognitive tasks. *Neuropsychologia, 21*, 235–248.

Stuss, D. T., Kaplan, E. F., Benson, D. F., Weir, W. S., Naeser, M. A., & Levine, H. L. (1981). Long-term effects of prefrontal leucotomy: An overview of neuropsychologic residuals. *Journal of Clinical Neuropsychology, 3*, 13–32.

Sunderland, A. (1984). *Cognitive factors in unilateral neglect*. Unpublished doctoral dissertation, Brunel University.

Sussman, G. J. (1975). *A computational model of skill acquisition*. New York: American Elsevier.

Sutherland, N. S. (1968). Outline of a theory of visual pattern recognition in animals and man. *Proceedings of the Royal Society of London B, 171*, 297–317.

Sutherland, N. S. (1973). Object recognition. In E. C. Carterette & M. P. Friedmann (Eds.), *Handbook of perception* (Vol. 3). New York: Academic Press.

Talland, G. A. (1965). *Deranged memory*. New York: Academic Press.

Taylor, A. M., & Warrington, E. K. (1971). Visual agnosia: A single case report, *Cortex, 7*, 152–161.

Taylor, A. M., & Warrington, E. K. (1973). Visual discrimination in patients with localised cerebral lesions. *Cortex, 9*, 82–93.

Te Linde, J. (1982). Picture–word differences in decision latency: A test of common coding assumptions. *Journal of Experimental Psychology: Learning Memory and Cognition, 8*, 584–598.

Temple, C. M. (1985). Surface dyslexia: Variations within a syndrome. In K. E. Patterson, M. Coltheart, & J. C. Marshall (Eds.), *Surface dyslexia*. London: Erlbaum.

Teuber, H. L. (1955). Physiological psychology. *Annual Review of Psychology, 9*, 267–296.

Teuber, H. L., Battersby, W. S., & Bender, M. B. (1951). Performance of complex visual tasks after cerebral lesions. *Journal of Nervous and Mental Diseases, 114*, 413–429.

Teuber, H. L., Battersby, W. S., & Bender, M. B. (1960). *Visual field defects after penetrating missile wounds of the brain*. Cambridge, Mass.: Harvard University Press.

Teuber, H. L., & Milner, B. (1968). Alteration of perception and memory in man: Reflections on methods. In L. Weiskrantz (Ed.), *Analysis of behavioral change*. New York: Harper & Row.

Tissot, R., Mounin, G., & Lhermitte, F. (1973). *L'Agrammatisme*. Paris: Dessart.

Tranel, E., & Damasio, A. R. (1985). Knowledge without awareness: An autonomic index of facial recognition by prosopagnosics. *Science, 228*, 1453–1454.

Treisman, A. (1960). Contextual cues in selective listening. *Quarterly Journal of Experimental Psychology, 12*, 242–248.

Treisman, A. (1986). Properties, parts and objects. In K. R. Boff, L. Kaufman, & J. P. Thomas (Eds.), *Handbook of perception and human performance* (Vol. 2). New York: Wiley.

Treisman, A., & Davies, A. (1973). Divided attention to ear and eye. In S. Kornblum (Ed.), *Attention and performance* (Vol. 4). London: Academic Press.

Treisman, A., & Gelade, G. (1980). A feature integration theory of attention. *Cognitive Psychology, 12*, 97–136.

Treisman, A., & Souther, J. (1985). Illusory words: The roles of attention and of top-down constraints in conjoining letters to form words. *Journal of Experimental Psychology: Human Performance and Perception, 12*, 3–17.

Trevarthen, C. B. (1965). Functional interactions between the cerebral hemispheres of the split-brain monkey. In E. G. Ettlinger (Ed.), *Functions of the Corpus Callosum*. London: Churchill.

Trevarthen, C. B. (1968). Two mechanisms of vision in primates. *Psychologische Forschung, 31,* 299–337.

Tulving, E. (1972). Episodic and semantic memory. In E. Tulving & W. Donaldson (Eds.), *Organization of memory.* New York: Academic Press.

Tulving, E. (1976). Ecphoric processes in recall and recognition. In J. Brown (Ed.), *Recall and recognition.* London: Wiley.

Tulving, E. (1983). *Elements of episodic memory.* Oxford: Oxford University Press.

Tulving, E. (1986). What kind of a hypothesis is the distinction between episodic and semantic memory? *Journal of Experimental Psychology: Learning, Memory and Cognition, 12,* 307–311.

Tulving, E., et al. (1984). Multiple book review of *Elements of episodic memory. Behavioral and Brain Sciences, 7,* 223–268.

Tulving, E., & Madigan, S. A. (1970). Memory and verbal learning. *Annual Review of Psychology, 21,* 437–484.

Tulving, E., & Patterson, R. D. (1968). Functional units and retrieval processes in free recall. *Journal of Experimental Psychology, 77,* 239–248.

Tulving, E., & Pearlstone, Z. (1966). Availability versus accessibility of information in memory for words. *Journal of Verbal Learning and Verbal Behavior, 5,* 381–391.

Tulving, E., Schacter, D. L., & Stark, H. A. (1982). Priming effects in word-fragment completion are independent of recognition memory. *Journal of Experimental Psychology: Learning, Memory and Cognition, 8,* 336–342.

Tzortzis, C., & Albert, M. L. (1974). Impairment of memory for sequences in conduction aphasia. *Neuropsychologia, 12,* 355–366.

Valenstein, E. S. (1973). *Brain control: A critical examination of brain stimulation and psychosurgery.* New York: Wiley.

Vallar, G., & Baddeley, A. D. (1984a). Fractionation of working memory: Neuropsychological evidence for a phonological short-term store. *Journal of Verbal Learning and Verbal Behavior, 23,* 151–161.

Vallar, G., & Baddeley, A. D. (1984b). Phonological short-term store, phonological processing and sentence comprehension: A neuropsychological case study. *Cognitive Neuropsychology, 1,* 121–141.

Vallar, G., & Papagno, C. (1986). Phonological short-term store and the nature of the recency effect: Evidence from neuropsychology. *Brain and Cognition, 5,* 428–442.

Van Essen, D. C. (1979). Visual areas of mammalian cerebral cortex. *Annual Review of Neuroscience, 2,* 227–263.

Venezky, R. L. (1970). *The structure of English orthography.* The Hague: Mouton.

Victor, M., Adams, R. D., & Collins, G. H. (1971). *The Wernicke-Korsakoff syndrome.* Oxford: Blackwell.

Vincent, F., Sadowsky, C., Saunders, R., & Reeves, A. (1977). Alexia without agraphia, hemianopia or color-naming defect: A disconnection syndrome. *Neurology, 27,* 689–691.

Von Cramon, D. Y., Hebel, N., & Schuri, U. (1985). A contribution to the anatomical basis of thalamic amnesia. *Brain, 108,* 993–1008.

Von Monakow, C. (1910). *Uber Lokalisation der Hirnfunktionen.* Wiesbaden: Von Bergmann.

Von Stockert, T. R. (1972). Recognition of syntactic structure in aphasic patients. *Cortex, 8,* 323–354.

Von Stockert, T. R., & Bader, L. (1976). Some relations of grammar and lexicon in aphasia. *Cortex, 12,* 49–60.

Wada, J., & Rasmussen, T. (1960). Intracarotid injection of sodium amytal for the lateralisation of cerebral speech dominance. *Journal of Neurosurgery, 17,* 266–282.

Walsh, K. W. (1978). *Neuropsychology: A clinical approach.* Edinburgh: Churchill Livingstone.

Wanner, E., & Maratsos, M. (1978). An ATN approach to comprehension. In M. Halle, J. Bresnan, & G. A. Miller (Eds.), *Linguistic theory and psychological reality.* Cambridge, Mass.: MIT Press.

Warrington, E. K. (1969). Constructional apraxia. In P. J. Vinken & G. W. Bruyn (Eds.), *Handbook of clinical neurology* (Vol. 4). Amsterdam: North Holland.

Warrington, E. K. (1974). Deficient recognition memory in organic amnesia. *Cortex, 10,* 289–291.

Warrington, E. K. (1975). The selective impairment of semantic memory. *Quarterly Journal of Experimental Psychology, 27*, 635–657.

Warrington, E. K. (1981). Concrete word dyslexia. *British Journal of Psychology, 72*, 175–196.

Warrington, E. K. (1982a). The double dissociation of short- and long-term memory deficits. In L. S. Cermak (Ed.), *Human memory and amnesia*. Hillsdale, N.J.: Erlbaum.

Warrington, E. K. (1982b). Neuropsychological studies of object recognition. *Philosophical Transactions of the Royal Society of London B, 298*, 15–33.

Warrington, E. K. (1982c). The fractionation of arithmetical skills: A single case study. *Quarterly Journal of Experimental Psychology, 34A*, 31–51.

Warrington, E. K. (1984). *Recognition Memory Test*. Windsor: NFER Nelson.

Warrington, E. K. (1985). Agnosia: The impairment of object recognition. In P. J. Vinken, G. W. Bruyn, & H. L. Klawans (Eds.), *Handbook of Clinical Neurology, 45*, Amsterdam: Elsevier.

Warrington, E. K. (1986). Visual deficits associated with occipital lobe lesions in man. *Experimental Brain Research Supplementum, 11*, 247–261.

Warrington, E. K., & James, M. (1967). Disorders of visual perception in patients with localised cerebral lesions. *Neuropsychologia, 5*, 253–266.

Warrington, E. K., & James, M. (1986). Visual object recognition in patients with right hemisphere lesions: Axes or features. *Perception, 15*, 355–366.

Warrington, E. K., James, M., & Maciejewski, C. (1986). The WAIS as a lateralising and localising diagnostic instrument: A study of 656 patients with unilateral cerebral lesions. *Neuropsychologia, 24*, 223–239.

Warrington, E. K., Logue, V., & Pratt, R. T. C. (1971). The anatomical localisation of selective impairment of auditory verbal short-term memory. *Neuropsychologia, 9*, 377–387.

Warrington, E. K., & McCarthy, R. (1983). Category specific access dysphasia. *Brain, 106*, 859–878.

Warrington, E. K., & McCarthy, R. (1987). Categories of knowledge: Further fractionation and an attempted integration. *Brain, 110*, 1273–1296.

Warrington, E. K., & Rabin, P. (1971). Visual span of apprehension in patients with unilateral cerebral lesions. *Quarterly Journal of Experimental Psychology, 23*, 423–431.

Warrington, E. K., & Sanders, H. I. (1971). The fate of old memories. *Quarterly Journal of Experimental Psychology, 23*, 432–442.

Warrington, E. K., & Shallice, T. (1969). The selective impairment of auditory verbal short-term memory. *Brain, 92*, 885–896.

Warrington, E. K., & Shallice, T. (1972). Neuropsychological evidence of visual storage in short-term memory tasks. *Quarterly Journal of Experimental Psychology, 24*, 30–40.

Warrington, E. K., & Shallice, T. (1979). Semantic access dyslexia. *Brain, 102*, 43–63.

Warrington, E. K., & Shallice, T. (1980). Word-form dyslexia. *Brain, 103*, 99–112.

Warrington, E. K., & Shallice, T. (1984). Category specific semantic impairments. *Brain, 107*, 829–853.

Warrington, E. K., & Taylor, A. M. (1973). The contribution of the right parietal lobe to object recognition. *Cortex, 9*, 152–164.

Warrington, E. K., & Taylor, A. M. (1978). Two categorical stages of object recognition. *Perception, 7*, 695–705.

Warrington, E. K., & Weiskrantz, L. (1968). New method of testing long-term retention with special reference to amnesic patients. *Nature, 217*, 972–974.

Warrington, E. K., & Weiskrantz, L. (1970). Amnesic syndrome: Consolidation or retrieval? *Nature, 228*, 628–630.

Warrington, E. K., & Weiskrantz, L. (1978). Further analysis of the prior learning effect in amnesic patients. *Neuropsychologia, 16*, 169–177.

Warrington, E. K., & Weiskrantz, L. (1982). Amnesia: A disconnection syndrome. *Neuropsychologia, 20*, 233–249.

Warrington, E. K., & Zangwill, O. L. (1957). A study of dyslexia. *Journal of Neurology, Neurosurgery and Psychiatry, 20*, 208–215.

Watkins, O. C., & Watkins, M. J. (1977). Serial recall and the modality effect. *Journal of Experimental Psychology: Human Learning and Memory, 3,* 712–718.

Watt, R. (1987). An outline of the primal sketch in human vision. *Pattern Recognition Letters, 5,* 139–150.

Waugh, N. C., & Norman, D. A. (1965). Primary memory. *Psychological Review, 72,* 89–104.

Wechsler, D. (1917). A study of retention in Korsakoff psychosis. *Psychiatric Bulletin of New York State Hospitals, 2,* 403–451.

Wechsler, D. (1958). *The measurement and appraisal of adult intelligence.* New York: Williams & Wilkins.

Weigl, E. (1961). The phenomenon of temporary deblocking in aphasia. *Zeitschrift für Phonetische Sprachewissenschaft und Kommunikationsforschung, 14,* 337–361.

Weigl, E. (1964). Some critical remarks concerning the problem of so-called simultanagnosia. *Neuropsychologia, 2,* 189–207.

Weigl, E., & Bierwisch, M. (1970). Neuropsychology and linguistics: Topics of common research. *Foundations of Language, 6,* 1–18.

Weisenburg, T., & McBride, K. E. (1935). *Aphasia.* New York: Commonwealth Fund.

Weiskrantz, L. (1968). Some traps and pontifications. In L. Weiskrantz (Ed.), *Analysis of behavioral change.* New York: Harper & Row.

Weiskrantz, L. (1980). Varieties of residual experience. *Quarterly Journal of Experimental Psychology, 32,* 365–386.

Weiskrantz, L. (1982). Comparative aspects of studies of amnesia. *Philosophical Transactions of the Royal Society of London B, 298,* 97–109.

Weiskrantz, L. (1985). On issues and theories of the human amnesic syndrome. In N. Weinberger, J. L. McGaugh, & G. Lynch (Eds.), *Memory systems of the brain.* New York: Guilford Press.

Weiskrantz, L. (1986). *Blindsight.* Oxford: Clarendon Press.

Weiskrantz, L., (in press). Residual vision in a scotoma: A follow-up study of 'form' discrimination. *Brain.*

Weiskrantz, L., Warrington, E. K., Sanders, M. D., & Marshall, J. (1974). Visual capacity of the hemianopic field following a restricted occipital ablation. *Brain, 97,* 709–728.

Wernicke, C. (1874). *Der Aphasische Symptomenkomplex.* Breslau: Cohn & Weigart. (Translated in *Boston Studies in Philosophy of Science, 4,* 34–97)

Wetzel, C. D., & Squire, L. R. (1982). Cued recall in anterograde amnesia. *Brain and Language, 15,* 70–81.

Wickelgren, W. A. (1965). Acoustic similarity and retroactive interference in short-term memory. *Journal of Verbal Learning and Verbal Behavior, 4,* 53–61.

Wickelgren, W. A. (1968). The sparing of short-term memory in an amnesic patient: Implications for strength theory of memory. *Neuropsychologia, 6,* 235–244.

Wickelgren, W. A. (1979). Chunking and consolidation: A theoretical synthesis. *Psychological Review, 86,* 44–60.

Wilkins, A. J., & Moscovitch, M. (1978). Selective impairment of semantic memory after temporal lobectomy. *Neuropsychologia, 16,* 73–79.

Wilkins, A. J., Shallice, T., & McCarthy, R. (1987). Frontal lesions and sustained attention. *Neuropsychologia, 25,* 359–365.

Williams, M. D., & Hollan, J. D. (1981). The process of retrieval from very long-term memory. *Cognitive Science, 5,* 87–119.

Wilson, H. R., & Bergen, J. R. (1979). A four mechanism model for spatial vision. *Vision Research, 19,* 19–32.

Wing, A. M., & Baddeley, A. D. (1980). Spelling errors in handwriting: A corpus and a distributional analysis. In U. Frith (Ed.), *Cognitive processes in spelling.* London: Academic Press.

Winnick, W. A., & Daniel, S. A. (1970). Two kinds of response priming in tachistoscopic recognition. *Journal of Experimental Psychology, 84,* 74–81.

Winocur, G., Kinsbourne, M., & Moscovitch, M. (1981). The effect of cueing on release from proactive interference in Korsakoff amnesic patients. *Journal of Experimental Psychology: Human Learning and Memory, 7,* 56–65.

Winocur, G., Oxbury, S., Roberts, R., Agnetti, V., & Davis, C. (1985). Amnesia in a patient with bilateral lesions to the thalamus. *Neuropsychologia, 22,* 123–143.

Wolpert, I. (1924). Die Simultanagnosie – Storung der Gesamtauffassung. *Zeitschrift für die gesamte Neurologie und Pscyhiatrie, 93,* 397–415.

Wood, C. C. (1978). Variations on a theme of Lashley: Lesion experiments on the neural model of Anderson, Silverstein, Ritz & Jones. *Psychological Review, 85,* 582–591.

Wood, C. C. (1982). Implications of simulated lesion experiments for the interpretation of lesions in real nervous systems: In M. A. Arbib, D. Caplan, & J. C Marshall (Eds.), *Neural models of language processes.* New York: Academic Press.

Wood, F., Ebert, V., & Kinsbourne, M. (1982). The episodic–semantic memory distinction and amnesia: Clinical and experimental observations. In L. S. Cermak (Ed.), *Human memory and amnesia.* Hillsdale, N.J.: Erlbaum.

Woods, R. T., & Piercy, M. (1974). A similarity between amnesic memory and normal forgetting. *Neuropsychologia, 12,* 437–445.

Wurtz, R. H., Goldberg, M. E., & Robinson, D. L. (1982). Brain mechanisms of visual attention. *Scientific American, 246,* 124–135.

Yamadori, A., & Albert, M. L. (1973). Word category aphasia. *Cortex, 9,* 112–125.

Young, R. M. (1970). *Mind, brain and adaptation in the nineteenth century.* Oxford: Clarendon Press.

Young, R., and O'Shea, T. (1981). Errors in children's subtraction. *Cognitive Science, 5,* 153–177.

Zaidel, E. (1975). A technique for presenting lateralised visual input with prolonged exposure. *Visual Research, 15,* 283–289.

Zaidel, E. (1976). Auditory vocabulary in the right hemisphere following brain bisection and hemidecortication. *Cortex, 12,* 191–211.

Zaidel, E. (1978). Lexical organisation in the right hemisphere. In P. Buser & A. Rougeul-Buser (Eds.), *Cerebral correlates of conscious experience.* Amsterdam: Elsevier.

Zaidel, E. (1982). Reading by the disconnected right hemisphere: An aphasiological perspective. In Y. Zotterman (Ed.), *Dyslexia: Neuronal, cognitive and linguistic aspects.* Oxford: Pergamon Press.

Zaidel, E. (1983a). Disconnection syndrome as a model for laterality effects in the normal brain. In J. B. Hellige (Ed.), *Cerebral hemisphere asymmetry: Method, theory and applications.* New York: Praeger.

Zaidel, E. (1983b). A response to Gazzaniga: Language in the right hemisphere, convergent perspectives. *American Psychologist, 38,* 542–546.

Zaidel, E., & Peters, A. M. (1981). Phonological encoding and ideographic reading by the disconnected right hemisphere: Two case studies. *Brain and Language, 14,* 205–234.

Zaidel, E., & Schweiger, A. (1984). On wrong hypotheses about the right hemisphere: Commentary on K. Patterson and D. Besner 'Is the right hemisphere literate?' *Cognitive Neuropsychology, 1,* 351–364.

Zaidel, E., Zaidel, D. W., & Sperry, R. W. (1981). Left and right intelligence: Case studies of Raven's Progressive Matrices following brain bisection and hemi-decortication. *Cortex, 17,* 167–186.

Zangwill, O. L. (1946). Some qualitative observations on verbal memory in cases of cerebral lesion. *British Journal of Psychology, 37,* 8–19.

Zangwill, O. L. (1960). *Cerebral dominance and its relation to psychological function.* Springfield, Ill.: Thomas.

Zangwill, O. L. (1966). The amnesic syndrome. In C. W. M. Whitty & O. L. Zangwill (Eds.), *Amnesia.* London: Butterworth.

Zeki, S. M. (1978). Functional specialisation in the visual cortex of the rhesus monkey. *Nature, 274,* 423–428.

Zeki, S. M. (1980). The representation of colours in the cerebral cortex. *Nature, 284,* 412–418.

Zihl, J. (1980). 'Blindsight': Improvement of visually guided eye movements by systematic practice in patients with cerebral blindness. *Neuropsychologia, 18,* 71–77.

Zihl, J., Von Cramon, D., & Mai, N. (1983). Selective disturbance of movement vision after bilateral brain damage. *Brain, 106,* 313–340.

Zola-Morgan, S., Cohen, N. J., & Squire, L. R. (1983). Recall of remote episodic memory in amnesia. *Neuropsychologia, 21,* 487–500.

Zurif, E. B., & Caramazza, A. (1976). Psycholinguistic structures in aphasia: Studies in syntax and semantics. In H. Whitaker & H. A. Whitaker (Eds.), *Studies in neurolinguistics* (Vol. 1). New York: Academic Press.

Zurif, E. B., Caramazza, A., & Myerson, R. (1972). Grammatical judgements of agrammatic aphasics. *Neuropsychologia, 10,* 405–417.

Zurif, E. B., Caramazza, A., Myerson, R., & Galvin, J. (1974). Semantic feature representations for normal and aphasic language. *Brain and Language, 1,* 167–187.

Subject Index

Author Index

454

Index of Patients Cited

461